Manual of Nephrology

Sixth Edition

Edited by
Robert W. Schrier, M.D.
Professor of Medicine
University of Colorado
Health Sciences Center
Denver, Colorado

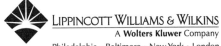
LIPPINCOTT WILLIAMS & WILKINS
A **Wolters Kluwer** Company

Philadelphia • Baltimore • New York • London
Buenos Aires • Hong Kong • Sydney • Tokyo

Acquisitions Editor: Lisa McAllister
Developmental Editor: Erin McMullan
Project Manager: Nicole Walz
Senior Manufacturing Manager: Benjamin Rivera
Production Editor: Barbara Stabb, TechBooks
Cover Designer: Vasilia Kiethas
Design Coordinator: Risa Clow
Compositor: TechBooks
Printer: RR Donnelley, Crawfordsville

Sixth Edition
© 2005 by LIPPINCOTT WILLIAMS & WILKINS
530 Walnut Street
Philadelphia, PA 19106-3780 USA
LWW.com

Library of Congress Cataloging-in-Publication Data
Manual of nephrology / edited by Robert W. Schrier.—6th ed.
    p. ;   cm.
    Includes bibliographical references and index.
    ISBN 0-7817-5020-2 (alk. paper)
        1. Kidneys—Diseases—Handbooks, manuals, etc.   I. Schrier, Robert W.
    [DNLM: 1. Kidney Diseases—diagnosis–Handbooks.   2. Kidney
Diseases—therapy—Handbooks.   3. Metabolic Diseases—diagnosis—Handbooks.
4. Metabolic Diseases—therapy—Handbooks. WJ 39 M294 2005]
    RC903.M194 2005
    616.6′1—dc22

                                                              2004016510

10 9 8 7 6 5 4 3 2 1

Contents

Preface

The sixth edition of the *Manual of Nephrology* continues to focus on the practical clinical aspects of the diagnosis and management of patients with electrolyte and acid-base disorders, urinary tract infections, kidney stones, glomerulonephritis and vasculitis, acute or chronic renal failure, hypertension, kidney disease and hypertension in pregnancy, and drug dosing with renal impairment. Because of the growing number of patients with end stage renal disease (ESRD), separate chapters are now included on treatment by chronic renal replacement therapy with dialysis and kidney transplantation. The *Manual of Nephrology* should continue to be of excellent clinical value for those caregivers encountering patients with the above disorders. This would include house officers, medical students, primary care physicians, nephrology fellows, nurse practitioners, and busy subspecialists outside of nephrology.

I am very appreciative of the outstanding contributions by the authors who have made every effort to update each chapter with recent advances in the diagnosis and management of the spectrum of hypertensive and kidney disorders. This includes adding several new authors who are outstanding clinician-educators. The *Manual of Nephrology* is again dedicated to Professor Hugh de Wardener who has made enormous contributions to the fields of hypertension and nephrology as a clinician, scientist, and educator for over 60 years.

Robert W. Schrier

Contributing Authors

Sharon G. Adler, MD	Professor of Medicine, Division of Nephrology and Hypertension, University of California, Los Angeles, UCLA School of Medicine
George R. Aronoff, MD	Professor of Medicine and Pharmacology, Chief Division of Nephrology, University of Louisville School of Medicine, Louisville, Kentucky
Phyllis August, MD	Professor of Medicine and Obstetrics and Gynecology, Weill Medical College of Cornell University, New York, New York
Tomas Berl, MD	Professor and Head, Division of Renal Diseases and Hypertension, University of Colorado Health Sciences Center, Denver, Colorado
Michael Conchol, MD	Assistant Professor of Medicine, Division of Renal Diseases and Hypertension, University of Colorado Health Sciences Center, Denver, Colorado
Robert E. Cronin, MD	Professor of Medicine, VA Medical Center, Dallas, Texas
Charles L. Edelstein, MD	Associate Professor of Medicine, Division of Renal Diseases and Hypertension, University of Colorado Health Sciences Center, Denver, Colorado
David H. Ellison, MD	Professor of Medicine, Head, Division of Nephrology and Hypertension, Oregon Health and Science University, Portland, Oregon
Kenneth Fairley, MD	Professorial Associate, Department of Medicine, University of Melbourne Hospital, Melbourne, Australia
Sarah Faubel, MD	Assistant Professor of Medicine, Division of Renal Diseases and Hypertension, University of Colorado Health Sciences Center, Denver, Colorado

Eric Gibney, MD	Fellow, Division of Renal Diseases and Hypertension, University of Colorado Health Sciences Center, Denver, Colorado
Alkesh Jani, MD	Assistant Professor of Medicine, Division of Renal Diseases and Hypertension, University of Colorado Health Sciences Center, Denver, Colorado
William D. Kaehny, MD	Professor of Medicine/Program Director, Medicine Residency Training Program School of Medicine, University of Colorado Health Sciences Center, Denver, Colorado
Catherine L. Kelleher, MD	Assistant Professor of Medicine, Division of Renal Diseases and Hypertension, University of Colorado Health Sciences Center, Denver, Colorado
Marilyn E. Levi, MD	Associate Professor of Medicine, Division of Infectious Diseases, University of Colorado Health Sciences Center, Denver, Colorado
Stuart L. Linas, MD	Professor of Medicine, Division of Renal Diseases and Hypertension, University of Colorado Health Sciences Center, Denver, Colorado
Marshall D. Lindheimer, MD	Professor Emeritus, Departments of Medicine and Obstetrics, and Gynecology, University of Chicago, Chicago, Illinois
Charles R. Nolan, MD	Professor of Medicine, University of Texas Health Sciences Center at San Antonio, San Antonio, Texas
Chirag Parikh, MD	Assistant Professor of Medicine, Division of Renal Diseases and Hypertension, University of Colorado Health Sciences Center, Denver, Colorado
Jay Redington, MD	Associate Professor of Medicine, Denver Veterans Administration Medical Center, Division of Infectious Disease and Ambulatory Care Denver, Colorado
Robert F. Reilly, MD	Associate Professor of Medicine, Division of Nephrology, Yale University Medical School, New Haven, Connecticut

L. Barth Reller, MD

Professor of Medicine and Pathology, Departments of Medicine and Pathology, Duke University Medical Center, Durham, North Carolina

Robert W. Schrier, MD

Professor of Medicine, Division of Renal Diseases and Hypertension, University of Colorado Health Sciences Center, Denver, Colorado

David M. Spiegel, MD

Associate Professor of Medicine, Division of Renal Diseases and Hypertension, University of Colorado Health Sciences Center, Denver, Colorado

Alexander Wiseman, MD

Associate Professor of Medicine, Division of Renal Diseases and Hypertension, University of Colorado Health Sciences Center, Denver, Colorado

The Edematous Patient: Cardiac Failure, Cirrhosis, and Nephrotic Syndrome

David H. Ellison and Robert W. Schrier

I. **Body fluid distribution.** Of the total fluids in the human body two-thirds reside inside the cell (i.e., intracellular fluid) and one-third resides outside cells (i.e., extracellular fluid [ECF]). The patient with generalized edema has an excess of ECF. The ECF resides in two locations: in the vascular compartment (plasma fluid) and between the cells of the body, but outside of the vascular compartment (interstitial fluid). In the vascular compartment, approximately 85% of the fluid resides on the venous side of the circulation and 15% on the arterial side (Table 1-1). An excess of interstitial fluid constitutes edema. On applying digital pressure, the interstitial fluid can generally be moved from the area of pressure, leaving and an indentation; this is described as *pitting*. This demonstrates that the excess interstitial fluid can move freely within its space between the body's cells. If digital pressure does not cause pitting in the edematous patient, then interstitial fluid cannot move freely. Such nonpitting edema can occur with lymphatic obstruction (i.e., lymphedema) or regional fibrosis of subcutaneous tissue, which may occur with chronic venous stasis.

Although generalized edema always signifies an excess of ECF, specifically in the interstitial compartment, the intravascular volume may be decreased, normal, or increased. Because two-thirds of ECF resides in the interstitial space and only one-third in the intravascular compartment, a rise in total ECF volume may occur as a consequence of excess interstitial fluid (i.e., generalized edema) even though intravascular volume is decreased.

A. **Starling's Law** states that the rate of fluid movement across a capillary wall is proportional to the hydraulic permeability of the capillary, the transcapillary hydrostatic pressure difference, and the transcapillary oncotic pressure difference. As shown in Figure 1-1, under normal conditions, fluid leaves the capillary at the arterial end because the transcapillary hydrostatic pressure difference favoring transudation exceeds the transcapillary oncotic pressure difference, which favors fluid resorption. In contrast, fluid returns to the capillary at the venous end because the transcapillary oncotic pressure difference exceeds the hydrostatic pressure difference. Because serum albumin is the major determinant of capillary oncotic pressure, which acts to maintain fluid in the capillary, hypoalbuminemia can lead to excess transudation of fluid from the vascular to interstitial compartment. Although hypoalbuminemia might be expected to lead commonly to edema, several factors act to buffer the effects of hypoalbuminemia on fluid transudation. First, an increase in transudation tends to dilute interstitial fluid, thus reducing the interstitial protein concentration. Second, increases in interstitial fluid volume increase interstitial fluid hydrostatic pressure. Third, the lymphatic flow into the jugular veins, which returns transudated fluid to the circulation, increases. In fact, in cirrhosis, where hepatic fibrosis causes high capillary hydrostatic pressures in association with hypoalbuminemia, the lymphatic flow can increase 20-fold to 20 L per day, attenuating the tendency to accumulate interstitial fluid. When these safety factors are overwhelmed, interstitial fluid accumulation can lead to edema. Another factor that must be borne in mind as a cause of edema is an increase in the fluid permeability of the capillary wall (an increase in hydraulic conductivity). This increase is the cause of edema associated with

1

Table 1-1. Body fluid distribution

Compartment	Amount	Volume (L) in 70 kg man
Total body fluid	60% of body weight	42
Intracellular fluid (ICF)	40% of body weight	28
Extracellular fluid (ECF)	20% of body weight	14
Interstitial fluid	Two-thirds of ECF	9.4
Plasma fluid	One-third of ECF	4.6
Venous fluid	85% of plasma fluid	3.9
Arterial fluid	15% of plasma fluid	0.7

hypersensitivity reactions and angioneurotic edema, and it may be a factor in edema associated with diabetes mellitus and idiopathic cyclic edema.

B. These comments refer to **generalized edema** (i.e., an increase in total body interstitial fluid), but it should be noted that such edema may have a **predilection for specific areas** of the body for various reasons. The formation of ascites because of portal hypertension has already been mentioned. With the normal hours of upright posture, an accumulation of the edema fluid in the dependent parts of the body should be expected, whereas excessive hours at bed rest in the supine position predispose to edema accumulation in the sacral and periorbital areas of the body. The physician must also be aware of the potential presence of localized edema, which must be differentiated from generalized edema.

C. Although generalized edema may have a predilection for certain body sites, it is nevertheless a **total-body phenomenon** of excessive interstitial fluid. Localized edema, on the other hand, is caused by local factors and therefore is not a total-body phenomenon. Venous obstruction, as can occur with thrombophlebitis, may cause localized edema of one lower extremity. Lymphatic obstruction (e.g., from malignancy) can also cause an excessive accumulation of interstitial fluid and, thus, edema. The physical

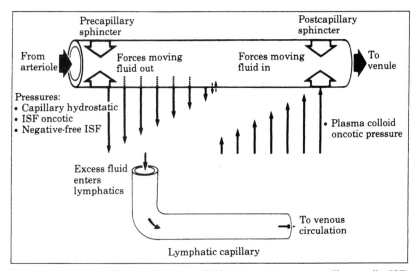

Figure 1-1. Effect of Starling forces on fluid movement across capillary wall. (ISF, interstitial fluid.)

examination of a patient with ankle edema should, therefore, include a search for venous incompetence (e.g., varicose veins) and for evidence of lymphatic disease. It should be recognized, however, that deep venous disease may not be detectable on physical examination and therefore may necessitate other diagnostic approaches (e.g., noninvasive). Thus, if the venous disease is bilateral, the physician may mistakenly search for causes of generalized edema (e.g., cardiac failure and cirrhosis), when indeed the bilateral ankle edema is due to local factors. Pelvic lymphatic obstruction (e.g., malignancy) can also cause bilateral lower-extremity edema and thereby mimic generalized edema. Trauma, burns, inflammation, and cellulitis are other causes of localized edema.

II. **Body fluid volume regulation.** The edematous patient has long presented a challenge in the understanding of body fluid volume regulation. In the normal subject, if ECF is expanded by the administration of isotonic saline, the kidney will excrete the excessive amount of sodium and water, thus returning ECF volume to normal. Such an important role of the kidney in volume regulation has been recognized for many years. What has not been understood, however, is why the kidneys continue to retain sodium and water in the edematous patient. It is understandable that when kidney disease is present and renal function is markedly impaired (i.e., acute or chronic renal failure), the kidney continues to retain sodium and water even to a degree causing hypertension and pulmonary edema. Much more perplexing are those circumstances in which the kidneys are known to be normal and yet continue to retain sodium and water in spite of the expansion of ECF and edema formation (e.g., cirrhosis, congestive heart failure). For example, if the kidneys from a cirrhotic patient are transplanted to a patient without liver disease, excessive renal sodium and water retention no longer occur. The conclusion has emerged, therefore, that neither total ECF nor its interstitial component, both of which are expanded in the patient with generalized edema, is the modulator of renal sodium and water excretion. Rather, as Peters suggested in the 1950s, some body fluid compartment other than total ECF or interstitial fluid volume must be the regulator of renal sodium and water excretion.

   A. The term **effective blood volume** was coined to describe this undefined, enigmatic body fluid compartment that signals the kidney, through unknown pathways, to retain sodium and water in spite of an expansion of total ECF. That the kidney must be responding to cardiac output was suggested, providing an explanation for sodium and water retention in low-output cardiac failure. This idea, however, did not provide a universal explanation for generalized edema because many patients with decompensated cirrhosis, who were avidly retaining sodium and water, were found to have normal or elevated cardiac outputs.

   B. **Total plasma or blood volume** was then considered as a possible candidate for the effective blood volume modulating renal sodium and water excretion. However, it was soon apparent that expanded plasma and blood volumes were frequently present in the renal sodium and water-retaining states, such as congestive heart failure and cirrhosis. The venous component of the plasma in the circulation has also been proposed as the modulator of renal sodium and water excretion and thus of volume regulation, because a rise in the left atrial pressure is known to cause a water diuresis and natriuresis, mediated in part by a suppression of vasopressin and a decrease in neurally mediated renal vascular resistance. A rise in right and left atrial pressure also has been found to cause a rise in atrial natriuretic peptide. However, despite these effects on the low-pressure venous side of the circulation, renal sodium and water retention are hallmarks of congestive heart failure, a situation in which pressures in the atria and venous component of the circulation are routinely increased.

   C. The **arterial portion of body fluids** (Table 1-1) is the remaining component that may be pivotal in the regulation of renal sodium and water excretion. More recently, the relationship between cardiac output and peripheral

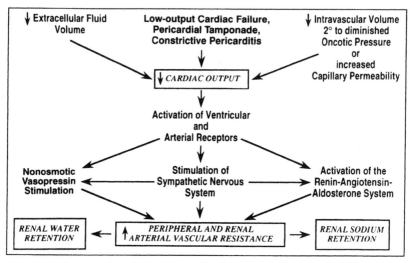

Figure 1-2. Decreased cardiac output as the initiator of arterial underfilling. (From Schrier RW. A unifying hypothesis of body fluid volume regulation. *J R Coll Physicians Lond* 1992;26:296. Reprinted with permission.)

arterial resistance [the effective arterial blood volume (EABV)] has been proposed as a regulator of renal sodium and water reabsorption. This relationship establishes the "fullness" of the arterial vascular tree. In this context, a primary decrease in cardiac output or peripheral arterial vasodilation, or a combination thereof, may cause arterial underfilling and thereby initiate and sustain a sodium and water-retaining state, which leads to edema. The sodium- and water-retaining states that are initiated by a decline in cardiac output are shown in Figure 1-2 and include (a) ECF volume depletion (e.g., diarrhea, vomiting, hemorrhage); (b) low-output cardiac failure, pericardial tamponade, and constrictive pericarditis; and (c) intravascular volume depletion secondary to protein loss and hypoalbuminemia (e.g., nephrotic syndrome, burns or other protein-losing dermopathies, protein-losing enteropathy); and (d) increased capillary permeability (capillary leak syndrome). The causes of increased renal sodium and water retention leading to edema that are initiated by primary peripheral arterial vasodilation are equally numerous and are shown in Figure 1-3. Severe anemia, beri-beri, Paget's disease, and thyrotoxicosis are causes of high-output cardiac failure that may lead to sodium and water retention. A wide-open arteriovenous fistula, hepatic cirrhosis, sepsis, pregnancy, and vasodilating drugs (e.g., minoxidil or hydralazine) are other causes of peripheral arterial vasodilation that decrease renal sodium and water excretion.

D. Two major **compensatory processes** protect against arterial underfilling, as defined by the interrelationship of cardiac output and peripheral arterial vascular resistance. One compensatory process is very rapid and consists of a neurohumoral and systemic hemodynamic response. The other is slower and involves renal sodium and water retention. In the edematous patient, these compensatory responses have occurred to varying degrees depending on the point when the patient is seen during the clinical course. Because of the occurrence of these compensatory processes, mean arterial pressure is a poor index of the integrity of the arterial circulation. Whether a primary fall in cardiac output or peripheral arterial vasodilation is the initiator of

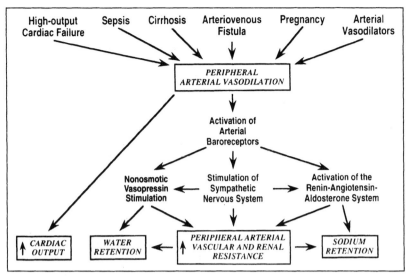

Figure 1-3. Peripheral arterial vasodilation as the initiator of arterial underfilling. (From Schrier RW. A unifying hypothesis of body fluid volume regulation. *J R Coll Physicians Lond* 1992;26:296. Reprinted with permission.)

arterial underfilling, the compensatory responses are quite similar. As depicted in Figures 1-2 and 1-3, the common neurohumoral response to a decreased EABV involves the stimulation of three vasoconstrictor pathways, namely the sympathetic nervous system, angiotensin, and vasopressin. In addition to direct effects, the sympathetic nervous system also increases angiotensin and vasopressin because increases in central sympathetic hypothalamic input and beta-adrenergic stimulation via the renal nerves are important components of the increased nonosmotic vasopressin release and stimulation of renin secretion, respectively. With a primary fall in cardiac output or primary peripheral arterial vasodilation, secondary increases in peripheral arterial vascular resistance or cardiac output occur, respectively, to acutely maintain arterial pressure. This rapid compensation allows time for the slower renal sodium and water retention to occur and further restore arterial circulatory integrity. With a decrease in ECF volume, such as occurs with acute gastrointestinal losses, sufficient sodium and water retention can occur to restore cardiac output to normal and thus terminate renal sodium and water retention before edema forms. Such may not be the case with low-output cardiac failure, because even these compensatory responses may not restore cardiac output to normal.

1. Thus, the **neurohumoral** and **renal sodium- and water-retaining mechanisms** persist as important compensatory processes in maintaining EABV. Specifically, neither the acute nor the chronic compensatory mechanisms are successful in restoring cardiac contractility, or reversing cardiac tamponade or constrictive pericardial tamponade. Compensatory renal sodium and water retention occurs with an expansion of the venous side of the circulation as arterial vascular filling improves but does not return to normal. The resultant rise in venous pressure enhances capillary hydrostatic pressure and thus transudation of fluid into the interstitial fluid, with resultant edema formation. In hypoalbuminemia and the capillary leak syndrome, excessive transudation of

fluid occurs across the capillary bed and also prevents the restoration of cardiac output; thus continuous renal sodium and water retention occurs and causes edema formation.

2. **Peripheral arterial vasodilation,** the other major initiator of arterial underfilling, also generally cannot be totally reversed by the compensatory mechanisms and thus may lead to edema formation. Peripheral arterial vasodilation results in dilatation of precapillary arteriolar sphincters, thus increasing capillary hydrostatic pressure and probably capillary surface area. A larger proportion of retained sodium and water thus is transudated across the capillary bed into the interstitium in these edematous disorders (see Fig. 1-3).

E. Another reason why low cardiac output or peripheral arterial vasodilation may lead to edema formation is the inability of patients with these disorders, as compared with normal subjects, to escape from the **sodium-retaining effect of aldosterone** (Fig. 1-4). In the normal subject receiving large exogenous doses of aldosterone or another mineralocorticoid hormone, a rise in the glomerular filtration rate and a decrease in proximal tubular sodium and water reabsorption lead to an increase in sodium and water delivery to the distal nephron site of aldosterone action. This increase in distal sodium delivery is the major mediator of escape from the sodium-retaining effect of mineralocorticoids in normal subjects, thus avoiding edema formation. In contrast, the renal vasoconstriction that accompanies the

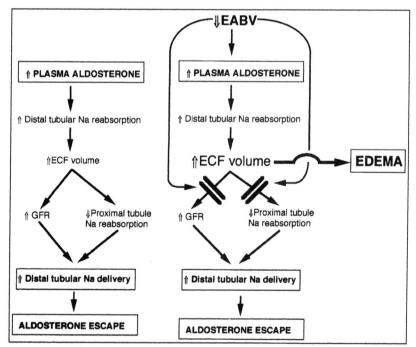

Figure 1-4. Aldosterone escape in a normal subject (left side) and failure of aldosterone escape in patients with arterial underfilling (right side). (EABS, effective arterial blood volume; ECF, extracellular fluid; GFR, glomerular filtration rate.) (From Schrier RW. Body fluid regulation in health and disease: a unifying hypothesis. *Ann Intern Med* 1990;113:155–59. Adapted with permission.)

compensatory neurohumoral response to arterial underfilling is associated with a decrease in distal sodium and water delivery to the distal nephron site of aldosterone action. This diminution in distal delivery, which occurs primarily because of a fall in the glomerular filtration rate and an increase in proximal tubular sodium reabsorption, results in a failure to escape from aldosterone and, therefore, causes edema formation. The importance of renal hemodynamics, particularly the glomerular filtration rate, in the aldosterone escape phenomena is emphasized by the observation that in pregnancy, a state of primary arterial vasodilation, aldosterone escape occurs despite arterial under-filling because of an associated 30% to 50% increase in the glomerular filtration rate. It still remains to be determined why pregnancy is associated with this large increase in the glomerular filtration rate, which occurs within 2 to 4 weeks of conception. The increase in the filtration rate cannot be due to plasma volume expansion, because this does not occur until several weeks after conception. The higher filtered load of sodium, and thus distal sodium load in pregnancy, no doubt allows the escape from the sodium-retaining effect of aldosterone. The occurrence of aldosterone escape in pregnancy attenuates edema formation when compared to other edematous disorders.

III. **Dietary and diuretic treatment of edema: general principles.** The daily sodium intake in this country is typically 4 to 6 g (1 g of sodium contains 43 mEq; 1 g of sodium chloride [NaCl] contains 17 mEq of sodium). By not using added salt at meals, the daily sodium intake can be reduced to 4 g (172 mEq), whereas a typical "low-salt" diet contains 2 g (86 mEq). Diets that are lower in NaCl content can be prescribed, but many individuals find them unpalatable. If salt substitutes are used, it is important to remember that these contain potassium chloride; therefore potassium-sparing diuretics (i.e., spironolactone, eplerenone, triamterene, amiloride) should not be used with salt substitutes. Other drugs that increase serum potassium concentration must also be used with caution in the presence of salt substitute intake [e.g., converting enzyme inhibitors, beta blockers, and nonsteroidal anti-inflammatory drugs (NSAIDs)]. When prescribing dietary therapy for an edematous patient, it is important to emphasize that sodium chloride restriction is required, even if diuretic drugs are employed. The therapeutic potency of diuretic drugs varies inversely with dietary salt intake.

All commonly used **diuretic drugs** act by increasing urinary sodium excretion. They can be divided into five classes, based on their predominant site of action along the nephron (Table 1-2). Osmotic diuretics (e.g., mannitol) and proximal diuretics (e.g., acetazolamide) are not employed as primary agents to treat edematous disorders. Loop diuretics (e.g., furosemide), distal convoluted tubule diuretics (DCT; e.g., hydrochlorothiazide), and collecting duct diuretics (e.g., spironolactone), however, all play important but distinct roles in treating edematous patients. The goal of the diuretic treatment of edema is to reduce extracellular fluid volume and to maintain the extracellular fluid volume at the reduced level. This requires an initial natriuresis, but, at steady-state, urinary sodium chloride excretion returns close to baseline despite continued diuretic administration. Importantly, an increase in sodium and water excretion does *not* prove therapeutic efficacy if extracellular fluid volume does not decline. Conversely, a return to "basal" levels of urinary sodium chloride excretion does not indicate diuretic resistance. The continued efficacy of a diuretic is documented by the rapid return to ECF volume expansion that occurs if the diuretic is discontinued.

A. When starting a loop diuretic as treatment for edema, it is important to establish a therapeutic goal, usually a target weight. If a low dose does not lead to natriuresis, it can be doubled repeatedly until the maximum recommended dose is reached (Table 1-3). When a **diuretic drug is administered by mouth,** the magnitude of the natriuretic response is determined by the intrinsic potency of the drug, the dose, the bioavailability, the amount delivered to the kidney, the amount that enters the tubule fluid (most diuretics

Table 1-2. Physiologic classification of diuretic drugs

Osmotic diuretics
Proximal diuretics
  Carbonic anhydrase inhibitors
    Acetazolamide
Loop diuretics (maximal FE_{Na} = 30%)
  Na-K-2Cl inhibitors
    Furosemide
    Bumetanide
    Torsemide
    Ethacrynic Acid
DCT diuretics (maximal FE_{Na} = 9%)
  Na-Cl inhibitors
    Chlorothiazide
    Hydrochlorothiazide
    Metolazone
    Chlorthalidone
    Indapamide[†]
    Many others
Collecting-duct diuretics (maximal FE_{Na} = 3%)
  Na channel blockers
    Amiloride
    Triameterene
  Aldosterone antagonists
    Spironolactone
    Eplerenone

[†]Indapamide may have other actions as well. DCT, Distal Convoluted Tubule; CD, Collecting Duct.

act from the luminal side), and the physiologic state of the individual. Except for proximal diuretics, the maximal natriuretic potency of a diuretic can be predicted from its site of action. Table 1-2 shows that loop diuretics can increase fractional sodium (Na) excretion to 30%, distal convoluted tubule (DCT) diuretics can increase it to 9%, and sodium channel blockers can increase it to 3% of the filtered load. The intrinsic diuretic potency of a diuretic is defined by its dose response curve, which is generally sigmoid. The steep sigmoid relation is the reason that loop diuretic drugs are often described as "threshold drugs." When starting loop diuretic treatment,

Table 1-3. Ceiling doses of loop diuretics

	Furosemide (mg)		Bumetanide (mg)		Torsemide (mg)	
	IV	PO	IV	PO	IV	PO
Renal insufficiency						
GFR 20–50 mL/min	80	80–160	2–3	2–3	50	50
GFR < 20 mL/min	200	240	8–10	8–10	100	100
Severe acute renal failure	500	NA	12	NA		
Nephrotic syndrome	120	240	3	3	50	50
Cirrhosis	40–80	80–160	1	1–2	10–20	10–20
Congestive heart failure	40–80	160–240	2–3	2–3	20–50	50

GFR, glomerular filtration rate.
Note: Ceiling dose indicates the dose that produces the maximal increase in fractional sodium excretion. Larger doses may increase net daily natriuresis by increasing the *duration* of natriuresis without increasing the maximal rate.

ensuring that each dose reaches the steep part of the dose-response curve before the dose frequency is adjusted is important. Because loop diuretics are rapid-acting, many patients note an increase in urine output within several hours of taking the drug; this can be helpful in establishing that an adequate dose has been reached. Because loop diuretics are short-acting, any increase in urine output more than 6 hours after a dose is unrelated to drug effects. Therefore, most loop diuretic drugs should be administered at least twice daily, when given by mouth.

B. The **bioavailability of diuretic drugs** varies widely among classes of drugs, among different drugs of the same class, and even within the same drug. The bioavailability of loop diuretics ranges from 10% to 100% (mean, 50% for furosemide; 80% to 100% for bumetanide and torsemide). Limited bioavailability can usually be overcome by appropriate dosing, but some drugs, such as furosemide, are variably absorbed by the same patient on different days, making precise titration difficult. Doubling the furosemide dose when changing from intravenous to oral therapy is customary, but the relation between intravenous and oral dose may vary. For example, the amount of sodium excreted during 24 hours is similar whether furosemide is administered to a normal individual by mouth or by vein, despite its 50% bioavailability. This paradox results from the fact that oral furosemide absorption is slower than its clearance, leading to "absorption-limited" kinetics. Thus, effective serum furosemide concentrations persist longer when the drug is given by mouth, because a reservoir in the gastrointestinal tract continues to supply furosemide to the body. This relation holds for a normal individual. Predicting the precise relation between oral and intravenous doses, therefore, is difficult.

IV. Diuretic resistance. Patients are considered to be **diuretic resistant** when an inadequate reduction in ECF volume is observed despite near maximal doses of loop diuretics. Several causes of resistance can be determined by considering factors that affect diuretic efficacy, as discussed above.

A. Causes of diuretic resistance

1. **Excessive dietary NaCl intake is one cause of diuretic resistance.** When NaCl intake is high, renal NaCl retention can occur between natriuretic periods, thus maintaining the ECF volume expansion. Measuring the sodium excreted during 24 hours can be useful in diagnosing excessive intake. If the patient is at steady state (the weight is stable), then the urinary sodium excreted during 24 hours is equal to dietary NaCl intake. If sodium excretion exceeds 100 to 120 mM (approximately 2–3 g sodium per day), then dietary NaCl consumption is too high and dietary counseling should be undertaken.

2. **Impaired diuretic delivery to its active site** in the kidney tubule is another cause of diuretic resistance. Most diuretics, including the loop diuretics, DCT diuretics, and amiloride, act from the luminal surface. Although diuretics are small molecules, most circulate while tightly bound to protein and reach tubule fluid primarily by tubular secretion. Loop and DCT diuretics are organic anions that circulate bound to albumin and reach tubule fluid primarily via the organic anion secretory pathway in the proximal tubule. Although experimental data suggest that diuretic resistance results when serum albumin concentrations are very low, because the volume of diuretic distribution increases, most studies suggest that this effect is only marginally significant clinically and is observed only when serum albumin concentration declines below 2 g/L. A variety of endogenous and exogenous substances that compete with diuretics for secretion into tubule fluid are more probable causes of diuretic resistance. Uremic anions, NSAIDS, probenecid, and penicillins all inhibit loop and DCT diuretic secretion into tubule fluid. Under some conditions, this may predispose to diuretic resistance, because the concentration of drug achieved in tubule fluid does not exceed the diuretic threshold. For example, chronic renal failure shifts the loop diuretic

dose-response curve to the right, therefore requiring a higher dose to achieve maximal effect.

3. **Diuretic binding to protein in tubule fluid** is another factor that may influence diuretic effectiveness. Diuretic drugs are normally bound to proteins in the plasma, but not once they are secreted into tubule fluid. This reflects the normally low protein concentrations in tubule fluid. In contrast, when serum proteins, such as albumin, are filtered in appreciable quantities, as in nephrotic syndrome, diuretic drugs interact with them and lose effectiveness. Despite experimental support, recent clinical studies have indicated that this phenomenon does not contribute significantly to diuretic resistance in nephrotic syndrome.

B. **Treatment of diuretic resistance.** Several strategies are available to achieve the effective control of ECF volume in patients who do not respond to full doses of effective loop diuretics.

1. A diuretic of another class may be added to a regimen that includes a loop diuretic (**Combination Diuretic Therapy** Table 1-4). This strategy produces true synergy; the combination of agents is more effective than the *sum* of the responses to each agent alone. DCT diuretics are most commonly combined with loop diuretics. DCT diuretics inhibit the adaptive changes in the distal nephron that increase the reabsorptive capacity of the tubule and limit the potency of loop diuretics. Because, DCT diuretics have longer half-lives than loop diuretics, they prevent or attenuate NaCl retention during the periods between doses of loop diuretics, thereby increasing their net effect. When two diuretics are combined, the DCT diuretic is generally administered some time before the loop diuretic (1 hour is reasonable) to ensure that NaCl transport in the distal nephron is blocked when it is flooded with solute. When intravenous therapy is indicated, chlorothiazide (500–1000 mg) may be employed. Metolazone is the DCT diuretic most frequently combined with loop diuretics, because its half-life is relatively long (as formulated in Zaroxylin) and because it has been reported to be effective even when renal failure is present. Other thiazide and thiazide-like diuretics, however, appear to be equally effective, even in severe renal failure. The dramatic effectiveness of combination diuretic therapy is accompanied by complications in a significant number of patients. Massive fluid and electrolyte losses have led to circulatory collapse during combination therapy, and patients must be followed carefully. The lowest effective dose of DCT diuretic should be added to the loop diuretic regimen; patients can frequently be treated with combination therapy for only a few days and then must be placed back on a single drug regimen. When continuous combination therapy is needed, low doses of DCT diuretic (2.5 mg metolazone or 25 mg hydrochlorothiazide) administered only 2 or 3 times per week may be sufficient.

Table 1-4. Combination diuretic therapy (to add to a ceiling dose of a loop diuretic)

Distal convoluted tubule diuretics:
   Metolazone 2.5–10 mg P.O. daily*
   Hydrochlorothiazide (or equivalent) 25–100 mg P.O. daily
   Chlorothiazide 500–1,000 mg intravenously
Proximal tubule diuretics:
   Acetazolamide 250–375 mg daily or up to 500 mg intravenously
Collecting-duct diuretics:
   Spironolactone 100–200 mg daily
   Amiloride 5–10 mg daily

*Metolazone is generally best given for a limited period (3–5 days) or should be reduced in frequency to 3 times per week once extracellular fluid volume has declined to the target level. Only in patients who remain volume expanded should full doses be continued indefinitely, based on the target weight.

Table 1-5. Continuous infusion of loop diuretics

Diuretic	Starting bolus mg	Infusion rate, mg/hr		
		GFR <25 mL/min	GFR 25–75 mL/min	GFR >75 mL/min
Furosemide	40	20 then 40	10 then 20	10
Bumetanide	1	1 then 2	0.5 then 1	05
Torsemide	20	10 then 20	5 then 10	

2. For hospitalized patients who are resistant to diuretic therapy, the continuous infusion of loop diuretics is an alternative approach. **Continuous diuretic infusions** (Table 1-5) have several advantages over bolus diuretic administration. First, because they avoid peaks and troughs of diuretic concentration, continuous infusions prevent periods of positive NaCl balance (post-diuretic NaCl retention) from occurring. Second, continuous infusions are more efficient than bolus therapy (the amount of NaCl excreted per mg of drug administered is greater). Third, some patients who are resistant to large doses of diuretics given by bolus respond to continuous infusion. Fourth, diuretic response can be titrated; in the intensive care unit, where obligate fluid administration must be balanced by fluid excretion, excellent control of NaCl and water excretion can be obtained. Finally, complications associated with high doses of loop diuretics, such as ototoxicity, appear to be less common when large doses are administered as a continuous infusion. Total daily furosemide doses exceeding 1 g have been tolerated well when administered over 24 hours. One approach is to administer a loading dose of 20 mg furosemide followed by a continuous infusion at 4 to 60 mg per hr. In patients with preserved renal function, therapy at the lower dosage range should be sufficient. When renal failure is present, higher doses may be used, but patients should be monitored carefully for side effects, such as ECF volume depletion and ototoxicity.

3. When therapy with diuretic drugs fails, **ultrafiltration** using hemodialysis equipment or a specialized ultrafiltration apparatus has been used. Although this approach is not recommended for routine use, in one controlled study, the response to volume removal via ultrafiltration was better sustained than after an equivalent volume removal via diuretics. In that study, loop diuretics induced a large rise in renin and angiotensin secretion, probably by stimulating the macula densa mechanism directly. This may explain the unique beneficial results sometimes observed following nonpharmacologic volume removal.

V. **Congestive heart failure**

A. Early **clinical symptoms** of cardiac failure occur before overt physical findings of pedal edema and pulmonary congestion. These symptoms relate to the compensatory renal sodium and water retention that accompanies arterial underfilling. The patient may present with a history of weight gain, weakness, dyspnea on exertion, decreased exercise tolerance, paroxysmal nocturnal dyspnea, and orthopnea. Nocturia may occur because cardiac output, and therefore renal perfusion, may be enhanced by the supine position. Patients with congestive heart failure may lose considerable weight during the first few days of hospitalization, even without the administration of diuretics because of this nocturia. Although overt edema is not detectable early in the course of congestive heart failure, the patient may complain of swollen eyes on awakening and tight rings and shoes, particularly at the end of the day. With incipient edema, as much as 3 to 4 L of fluid can be retained prior to the occurrence of overt edema.

The period of incipient edema is then followed by more overt symptoms and physical findings: basilar pulmonary rales, ankle edema, distended neck veins at 30 degrees, tachycardia, and a gallop rhythm with a third heart sound. Although the chest x-ray may only show cephalization of pulmonary markings early in cardiac failure, increased hilar markings, Kerley's B lines, and pleural effusions occur later, generally accompanied by an enlarged heart size.

B. Etiology. Two mechanisms that reduce cardiac output are recognized to cause congestive heart failure: systolic dysfunction and diastolic dysfunction. Because specific, life-saving therapy is available for systolic dysfunction, it is essential to determine whether systolic dysfunction is present when a patient presents with the symptoms and signs of heart failure. Although physical examination, chest x-ray, and electrocardiogram are useful in this regard, additional diagnostic tests are usually indicated. An echocardiogram provides information about systolic (the ejection fraction) and diastolic function, and about valvular disease, which may require surgery. Occult hypo- or hyperthyroidism and alcoholic cardiomyopathy may present as congestive heart failure; these are treatable. Uncontrolled hypertension may contribute to congestive heart failure, but disease of the coronary arteries is the most common cause. In one study, severe coronary artery disease was found in 9 of 38 patients undergoing cardiac transplantation for presumed idiopathic dilated cardiomyopathy, and in 3 of 4 patients with presumed alcoholic cardiomyopathy. These data suggest that cardiac catheterization may be indicated in virtually all patients who present with new-onset congestive heart failure. In patients with preexisting cardiac disease, a cardiac arrhythmia, pulmonary embolus, cessation of medicines, severe anemia or fever, dietary sodium indiscretion, and worsening of chronic obstructive lung disease with infection and resultant hypoxia are examples of potentially treatable precipitants of worsening of congestive heart failure. Drugs with a negative inotropic effect, such as verapamil, may worsen heart failure by decreasing cardiac output. A trial cessation of these drugs is the best means of determining their possible role in worsening congestive heart failure.

C. Treatment. When none of these specific primary or precipitating causes of congestive heart failure are detectable, then general principles of treatment must be considered.

Every patient with symptomatic systolic dysfunction or, if asymptomatic, an ejection fraction of less than 40% should be started on an **angiotensin converting enzyme (ACE) inhibitor,** unless a specific contraindication exists. ACE inhibitors (and angiotensin receptor inhibitors) are unique agents that reduce blood pressure (reduce afterload), shift the renal function curve to the left (promote continued sodium losses), and block maladaptive neuroregulatory hormones (Fig. 1-5). These agents should be started at low doses (enalapril 2.5 mg b.i.d. or captopril 6.25 mg t.i.d.), but increased if tolerated to 10 b.i.d. of enalapril or 50 t.i.d. of captopril, unless side effects occur. If cough or angioedema limits ACE inhibitor use, then an AT1 angiotensin receptor blocker should be used (although angioedema may develop with AT1 receptor blockers, the incidence is lower with this class of drugs). If neither class of drug can be employed safely, then therapy with hydralazine and isosorbide dihydrate or monohydrase should be used.

Beta blockers have been shown to improve symptoms and mortality in patients with systolic dysfunction. Both selective beta blockers (metoprolol) and nonselective beta blockers with alpha blocking properties (carvedilol) are approved by the Food and Drug Administration (FDA) for the treatment of congestive heart failure. Because beta blockers can lead to symptomatic exacerbations of heart failure, these drugs are initiated only when patients are clinically stable and without expansion of the ECF volume.

The role of **digitalis glycosides** has been clarified by recent controlled studies. Digoxin significantly improves symptoms and reduces the

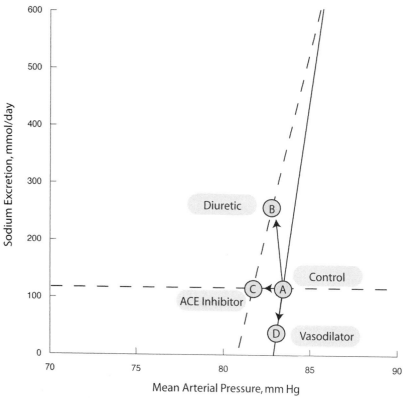

Figure 1-5. Relationship between cardiac output and left ventricular filling pressure under normal circumstances (upper curve) and low-output congestive heart failure (lower curve). Reduction of afterload (e.g., angiotensin-converting enzyme inhibitor or a vasodilator) or improved contractility (inotropic agents) may shift the lower curve to the middle curve. Diuretic-induced preload reduction or other causes of volume depletion may decrease cardiac output (e.g., shift from point A to point B on the lower curve). (From Schrier RW, ed. *Renal and Electrolyte Disorders,* 4th ed. Boston: Little, Brown, 1990. Reprinted with permission.)

incidence of hospitalization in patients with impaired left ventricular function, but it does not appear to prolong life. Thus, the drug is indicated for symptomatic treatment when combined with ACE inhibitors and diuretics. In certain clinical states of heart failure, however, cardiac glycosides have been shown to be of little therapeutic value, for example in association with thyrotoxicosis, chronic obstructive pulmonary disease, and cor pulmonale. Cardiac glycosides may actually worsen symptoms in patients with hypertrophic obstructive cardiomyopathy and subaortic stenosis, pericardial tamponade, and constrictive pericarditis. It should also be remembered that digoxin is excreted by the kidneys; therefore, the dosage interval should be increased in the patient with chronic renal disease (see Chapter 16). Also, the elderly patient should receive a decreased dose (e.g., 0.125 mg q.o.d.), even if the serum creatinine level is not increased. Because renal function deteriorates with age, serum creatinine levels may not rise because of a concomitant loss of muscle mass. Although potentially useful acute therapy, phosphodiesterase inhibitors, such as milrinone, which also increase

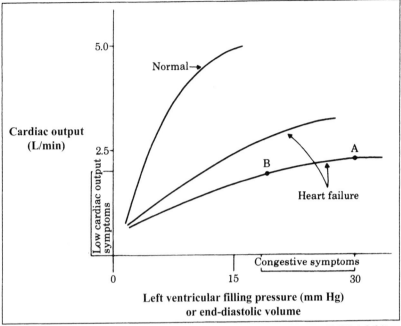

Figure 1-6. Comparison of diuretic, angiotensin converting enzyme (ACE) inhibitor, and vasodilator effects on mean arterial pressure and natriuresis. The normal renal function curve is shown (solid line). Adding a vasodilator reduces mean arterial pressure but also reduces natriuresis because blood pressure declines. A diuretic moves the individual to a new renal function curve (dashed line), thereby increasing natriuresis, but has little effect on blood pressure. An ACE inhibitor moves the individual to a new renal function curve, maintaining natriuresis at a lower blood pressure.

cardiac output, have been shown to increase mortality when used chronically; these drugs should be avoided.

If symptomatic pulmonary congestion or periperal edema is present, **diuretic therapy** is indicated (Fig. 1-5). A loop diuretic is usually employed as first-line therapy, although some patients may be managed using a thiazide. In patients with congestive heart failure, diuretic therapy must be instituted with full knowledge of the Starling-Frank curve of myocardial contractility (Fig. 1-6). The patient with congestive heart failure who responds to a diuretic will exhibit improved symptomatology as end-diastolic volume and pulmonary congestion decrease. However, because the Starling-Frank curve is usually either flat or up-sloping even in failing hearts, an improvement in cardiac output may not occur. If, during the diuretic treatment of a patient with congestive heart failure, the serum creatinine and blood urea nitrogen levels begin to rise, it is likely that cardiac output has fallen. This situation is especially pronounced in patients who receive ACE inhibitor therapy. ACE inhibitors impair renal autoregulation and make patients prone to prerenal azotemia. When mild azotemia develops in a patient treated with diuretics and an ACE inhibitor, it is usually advisable to reduce the diuretic dose or liberalize dietary salt intake, provided that pulmonary congestion is not present simultaneously. This approach has been shown to permit the continued administration of ACE inhibitors in many patients. Some pedal edema may be preferable to a diuretic-induced decline in cardiac output as estimated by the occurrence or worsening of prerenal azotemia. Patients with congestive heart failure are especially sensitive to renal functional deterioration if NSAIDs are used together with diuretics and ACE inhibitors. Thus, NSAIDS should be diligently avoided in this patient population.

Both congestive heart failure itself and treatment with loop diuretics stimulate the renin-angiotensin-aldosterone axis. Two large studies have provided evidence that **blocking mineralocorticoid (aldosterone) receptors** can improve mortality of such patients. In one trial, adding spironolactone (25 to 50 mg per day) to a regimen that included an ACE inhibitor and a diuretic (with or without digoxin) reduced all cause mortality by 30% and reduced hospitalization for heart failure by 35%. Gynecomastia, which is a relatively common side effect of spironolactone owing to its estrogenic side effects, does not appear to occur with eplerenone, a newer more selective drug.

Hyperkalemia is of concern when aldosterone blockade is instituted. It is currently recommended that serum potassium be monitored 1 week after initiating therapy with an aldosterone blocker, after 1 month, and every 3 months thereafter. An increase in serum potassium greater than 5.5 mEq per L should prompt an evaluation for medications such as potassium supplements or NSAIDs that might be contributing to the hyperkalemia. If such factors are not detected, the dose of aldosterone blocker should be reduced 25 mg every other day. It is prudent to avoid the use of aldosterone blockers in patients with a creatinine clearance of less than 30 mL per min and to be cautious in those with a creatinine clearance of between 30 and 50 mL per min. These patients must be followed very closely.

Complications of diuretic therapy are shown in Table 1-6. Although hyponatremia may be a complication of diuretic treatment, furosemide, when combined with ACE inhibitors, may ameliorate hyponatremia in some patients with congestive heart failure, possibly by improving cardiac output. Hypokalemia and hypomagnesemia are frequent complications of diuretic treatment in heart failure patients because of secondary hyperaldosteronism, which increases sodium delivery to the distal sites at which aldosterone stimulates potassium and hydrogen ion secretion. Severe renal magnesium wasting may also occur in the setting of secondary hyperaldosteronism and loop diuretic administration. Because both magnesium and potassium depletion cause similar deleterious effects on the heart, and potassium repletion is very difficult in the presence of magnesium depletion, supplemental replacement of both these cations is frequently necessary in patients with cardiac failure.

Table 1-6. Complications of diuretics

Contraction of the vascular volume
Orthostatic hypotension (from volume depletion)
Hypokalemia (loop and DCT diuretics)
Hyperkalemia (spironolactone, eplerenone, triamterene, and amiloride)
Gynecomastia (spironolactone)
Hyperuricemia
Hypercalcemia (thiazides)
Hypercholesterolemia
Hyponatremia (especially with DCT diuretics)
Metabolic alkalosis
Gastrointestinal upset
Hyperglycemia
Pancreatitis (DCT diuretics)
Allergic interstitial nephritis

The treatment of patients with congestive heart failure and preserved systolic function, is less clearly defined. Hypertension control is clearly paramount in these patients, because hypertension is a frequent cause of cardiac hypertrophy. Diuretics are usually necessary to improve symptoms of dyspnea and orthopnea. Beta blockers, ACE inhibitors, angiotensin receptor blockers, or non-dihydropyridine calcium antagonists may be beneficial in some patients with diastolic dysfunction.

VI. **Hepatic cirrhosis.** The pathogenesis of renal sodium and water retention is similar in all varieties of cirrhosis, including alcoholic, viral, and biliary cirrhosis. Studies in both humans and animals indicate that renal sodium and water retention precedes the formation of ascites in cirrhosis. Thus, the classic "underfill theory," which attributed the renal sodium and water retention of cirrhosis to ascites formation with resultant hypovolemia, seems untenable as a primary mechanism. Because plasma volume expansion secondary to renal sodium and water excretion occurs prior to ascites formation, the "overflow theory" of ascites formation was proposed. This postulated that an undefined process, triggered by the diseased liver (e.g., increased intrahepatic pressure), causes renal sodium and water retention that then overflows into the abdomen because of portal hypertension. This overflow theory, however, predicts that renal salt retention and ascites formation would be associated with decreased levels of vasopressin, renin, aldosterone, and norepinephrine. Because these hormones rise progressively as cirrhosis advances from the states of compensation (no ascites) to decompensation (ascites) to hepatorenal syndrome, the overflow hypothesis also does not seem to explain the renal sodium and water retention associated with advanced cirrhosis. More recently, the peripheral arterial vasodilation theory has been proposed. This theory, summarized in Figure 1-7, is compatible with virtually all known observations in

	Compensated cirrhosis (no ascites)	Decompensated cirrhosis (ascites)	Hepatorenal syndrome
Peripheral arterial vasodilation	↑	↑↑	↑↑↑
Plasma hormones (AVP, renin, aldosterone, NE)	Normal*	↑	↑↑
Plasma volume**	↑	↑↑	↑↑↑

Figure 1-7. Peripheral arterial vasodilation hypothesis. Stages of progression of cirrhosis. (AVP, arginine vasopressin; NE, norepinephrine.)
*Given the positive sodium and water balance that has occurred, these plasma hormones would be suppressed in normal subjects without liver disease.
**The progressive renal sodium and water retention increases extracellular fluid, interstitial fluid, and plasma volume. However, the concomitant occurrence of hypoalbuminemia in decompensated cirrhosis and hepatorenal syndrome may attenuate the degree of volume expansion.

patients during the various stages of cirrhosis. According to this theory, cirrhosis causes arterial vasodilation and a decline in blood pressure; hypotension stimulates renal NaCl retention. The cause of the primary arterial vasodilation in cirrhosis is not clear, but is known to occur early in the course of the disease before ascites formation, primarily in the splanchnic circulation. Although several mediators, including substance P, vasoactive intestinal peptide, endotoxin, and glucagon have been proposed to play a role in arterial vasodilation, recent information indicates that nitric oxide may be a crucial participant. The opening of existing splanchnic arteriovenous shunts may account for some early arterial vasodilation. Later, anatomically new portosystemic and arteriovenous shunting secondary to the portal hypertension may also occur.

A. Options for treating cirrhotic ascites and edema include dietary NaCl restriction, diuretic drugs, large-volume paracentesis, peritoneovenous shunting, portosystemic shunting [usually transjugular intrahepatic portosystemic shunting (TIPS)], and liver transplantation. Each of these approaches has a role in the treatment of cirrhotic ascites, but most patients can be treated successfully with dietary restriction, diuretics, and occasionally large-volume paracentesis.

The **initial therapy of cirrhotic ascites** is supportive, including dietary sodium restriction and cessation of alcohol. When these measures prove inadequate, diuretic treatment should begin with spironolactone. Spironolactone has several advantages. First, a controlled trial showed that spironolactone is more effective than furosemide alone in reducing ascites in cirrhotic patients. Second, spironolactone is a long-acting diuretic that can be given once per day in doses ranging from 25 mg to 400 mg per day. Third, unlike most other diuretics, hypokalemia does not occur when spironolactone is administered. Hypokalemia increases renal ammonia production and can precipitate encephalopathy. The most common side effect of spironolactone is painful gynecomastia. (Gynecomastia appears to be much less common with eplerenone, a newer, more selective antagonist, which may be substituted.) Although amiloride, another K-sparing diuretic, can be used as an alternative, spironolactone is more effective than amiloride in reducing ascites. In patients who do not respond to a low dose of spironolactone, spironolactone can be combined with furosemide, starting at 100 mg spironolactone and 40 mg furosemide (to a maximum of 400 mg spironolactone and 160 mg furosemide). This regimen has the advantages of once per day dosing and minimal hypokalemia.

B. The appropriate **rate of diuresis** depends on the presence or absence of peripheral edema. Because mobilizing ascitic fluid into the vascular compartment is slow (approximately 500 mL per day), the rate of daily diuresis should be limited to 0.5 kg per day if peripheral edema is absent. In the presence of peripheral edema, most patients can tolerate up to 1.0 kg per day of fluid removal. Because ascites in the decompensated cirrhotic patient is associated with substantial complications including (a) spontaneous bacterial peritonitis (50% to 80% mortality), which does not occur in the absence of ascites; (b) impaired ambulation, decreased appetite, and back and abdominal pain; (c) an elevated diaphragm with decreased ventilation predisposing to hypoventilation, atelectasis, and pulmonary infections; and (d) negative cosmetic and psychologic effects, the treatment of ascites with diuretics and sodium restriction is appropriate. This approach is successful in approximately 90% of patients, and complications are rare. Earlier studies of diuretic therapy complications often utilized more aggressive diuretic regimens.

An alternate approach to diuretics is **large-volume paracentesis.** Total paracentesis, occurring in increments over 3 days or, more commonly, at one setting has been shown to have few complications; in some studies paracentesis appears to have a lower incidence of complications than does diuretic treatment. When peripheral edema is absent, albumin (6 g for each L of ascitic fluid removed) may be infused to reduce hemodynamic compromise and the elaboration of vasoregulatory hormones. The use of albumin remains controversial in patients with concomitant peripheral edema. Patients often favor paracentesis because of the rapid improvement in symptoms; diuretics and salt restriction, however, continue to be the primary approach and are required between paracentesis, even in those patients who cannot be maintained on diuretics alone.

Portosystemic shunting is usually performed as TIPS. In two uncontrolled trials, TIPS led to an increase in urine output, a marked reduction in ascites, and a reduction in diuretic usage. Renal function also improved. Yet in a controlled trial, mortality increased in patients who received a TIPS as compared with controls, and TIPS can precipitate hepatic encephalopathy, especially in Child-Pugh Class C patients. A recent review of the literature confirmed that TIPS can effectively reduce or eliminate ascites, but carries a substantial complication rate. Therefore, it remains best reserved for truly refractory patients who will not receive a liver transplant. Similar considerations apply to peritoneovenous (LeVeen) shunting. In controlled trials, peritoneovenous shunting was shown to reduce ascites more effectively than paracentesis or diuretics, but this was associated with a high rate of complications (e.g., shunt clotting); the shunt carries no survival advantage. Despite reports that the high complication rate can be reduced, most centers reserve this therapy for patients who are truly refractory to more conventional approaches and who are not candidates for liver transplantation.

The development of ascites in a previously compensated cirrhotic patient is an indication for liver transplantation. In view of the morbidity and mortality associated with diuretic-resistant decompensated cirrhosis, liver transplantation is an important treatment for the ECF volume expansion that accompanies cirrhotic ascites. Worsening of ascites in a previously stable individual is most often caused by progressive liver disease, but should also compel the search for hepatocellular carcinoma and portal vein thrombosis.

C. **Treatment aimed at the peripheral arterial vasodilation** of cirrhosis has only been used in the acute setting of the patient with portal hypertension and bleeding esophageal varices. Nitric oxide may play an important role in cirrhosis-associated vasodilation. In a rat model of cirrhosis, the blockade of nitric oxide synthesis corrected many of the hemodynamic and neurohumoral perturbations and dramatically improved sodium and water retention. In a short-term human trial, however, blocking nitric oxide synthesis increased blood pressure but did not lead to natriuresis. Definitive evidence for this approach awaits longer-term studies. Portal venous hypertension is caused not only by the intrahepatic capillary fibrosis that causes resistance to flow but also by increased splanchnic flow. Therefore, the administration of vasopressin, which selectively constricts the splanchnic vasculature, has been shown to decrease portal venous pressure and thereby diminish esophageal variceal bleeding. A chronic oral vasopressin analogue that has selective V_1 (vascular) agonist activity but not V_2 (antidiuretic) activity and a reasonably long duration of action (hours) could be of value in the chronic treatment of portal hypertension and the prevention of esophageal variceal bleeding. Such a compound, however, remains to be developed. Because there are fewer V_1 receptors on the renal than the splanchnic vascular bed, such an approach could also increase renal perfusion pressure without causing further renal vasoconstriction.

VII. **Nephrotic syndrome.** Another major cause of edema is nephrotic syndrome, the clinical hallmarks of which include proteinuria (>3.5 gm per day), hypoalbuminemia, hypercholesterolemia, and edema. The degree of the edema may range from pedal edema to total body anasarca, including ascites and pleural effusions. The lower the plasma albumin concentration, the more likely the occurrence of anasarca; the degree of sodium intake is, however, also a determinant of the degree of edema. Nephrotic syndrome has many causes (see

Chapter 8). Systemic causes include diabetes mellitus, lupus erythematosus, drugs (e.g., phenytoin, heavy metals, NSAIDs), carcinomas, and Hodgkin's disease, and primary renal diseases such as minimal change nephropathy, membranous nephropathy, focal glomerulosclerosis, and membranoproliferative glomerulonephritis.

A. The **pathogenesis** of ECF volume expansion in nephrotic syndrome appears to be more variable than the pathogenesis of edema in congestive heart failure or cirrhotic ascites. Traditionally, ECF volume expansion in nephrotic syndrome was believed to depend on hypoalbuminemia and underfilling of the arterial circulation. Several observations have raised questions about this hypothesis. First, the interstitial oncotic pressure in normal individuals is higher than previously appreciated. Transudation of fluid during ECF volume expansion reduces the interstitial oncotic pressure, thus minimizing the change in transcapillary oncotic pressure. Second, patients recovering from minimal-change nephropathy frequently begin to excrete sodium before their serum albumin concentration rises. Third, the circulating concentrations of volume-regulatory hormones are not as high in nephrotic patients as in patients with severe cirrhosis or congestive heart failure. These and other observations have **suggested a role for primary renal NaCl retention** in the pathogenesis of nephrotic edema.

B. Whereas "primary" renal NaCl retention may contribute to nephrotic edema in many patients, it is not often the only mechanism; some component of **"underfill"** often plays a role as well. Evidence for its role includes the observation that "primary" renal NaCl retention alone does not lead to edema. Chronic aldosterone infusion, for example, leads to hypertension and escape from sodium retention in the absence of edema formation. Furthermore, levels of vasoactive hormones, although below the levels commonly seen in cirrhosis and congestive heart failure, are often higher than would be expected based on the level of ECF expansion. It appears, therefore, that nephrotic syndrome reflects a combination of primary renal NaCl retention and relative arterial underfilling. A preponderance of one or the other mechanism may be observed in nephrosis from different causes. In general, a normal or near-normal glomerular filtration rate is associated with hypovolemic, vasoconstrictor nephrotic syndrome, whereas a diminution in glomerular filtration rate, primary renal sodium retention, and evidence of volume expansion (e.g., decreased plasma renin activity) are characteristic of hypervolemic nephrotic syndrome.

C. Treatment. The initial focus of therapy must be aimed at those treatable, systemic causes of nephrotic syndrome such as systemic lupus erythematosus or drugs (e.g., phenytoin, NSAID). The treatment of the primary renal causes of nephrotic syndrome is described in Chapter 8.

The treatment of edema in nephrotic patients involves **dietary sodium restriction and diuretics.** Because these patients may not be as underfilled as patients with cirrhosis or congestive heart failure, diuretic treatments are often tolerated well. In general, loop diuretics are used as initial therapy. For several reasons, however, nephrotic patients are relatively resistant to these drugs. Although low serum albumin concentrations may increase the volume of diuretic distribution, and filtered albumin may bind to diuretics in the tubule lumen, these factors do not appear to be the predominant causes of diuretic resistance. Rather, diuretic resistance likely reflects a combination of reduced glomerular filtration rate and intense renal NaCl retention. When the glomerular filtration rate is reduced, endogenous organic anions impair diuretic secretion into the tubule lumen, where these drugs act to inhibit NaCl transport. Thus, higher doses of loop diuretics are often required to achieve natriuresis.

The administration of albumin to patients with nephrotic syndrome can be costly and may cause pulmonary edema. One report, however, suggested that mixing albumin with a loop diuretic (6.25 g albumin per 40 mg furosemide) may induce diuresis in severely hypoalbuminemic patients.

Recently, a double-blind, controlled study of nine nephrotic patients compared the effects of (a) 60 mg intravenous furosemide, (b) 60 mg intravenous furosemide plus 200 mL of a 20% solution of albumin, or (c) a sham infusion plus 200 mL of albumin. Co-administration of furosemide and albumin was significantly more effective than either albumin or furosemide alone. The authors noted that although adding albumin did increase natriuresis, the benefit was relatively small.

Suggested readings

Abraham W, Cadnapaphornchai M, and Schrier RW. Cardiac failure, liver disease and the nephrotic syndrome. In: Schrier RW, ed. *Diseases of the kidney and urinary tract*. 7th ed. Philadelphia: Lippincott Williams & Wilkins, 2004:2465–2510.

Brater DC. Diuretic therapy. *N Engl J Med* 1998;339:387–395.

Ellison DH. *Intensive diuretic therapy*. In: Seldin D, Giebisch G, eds. *Clinical physiology and use of diuretic agents*. San Diego: Academic Press, 1997:281–300.

Ellison DH. *Adaptation to diuretic drugs*. In: Seldin D, Giebisch G, eds. *Clinical physiology and use of diuretic agents*. San Diego: Academic Press, 1997;209–231.

Ellison DH. Diuretic therapy and resistance in congestive heart failure. *Cardiology* 2001;96:132–143.

Fliser D, Zurbruggen I, Mutschler E, et al. Coadministration of albumin and furosemide in patients with the nephrotic syndrome. *Kidney Int* 1999;55:629–634.

Schrier RW. Pathogenesis of sodium and water retention in high and low output cardiac failure, cirrhosis, nephrotic syndrome, and pregnancy. *N Engl J Med* 1988;319:16,1065–1072;319:17,1127–1134.

Schrier RW. A unifying hypothesis of body fluid volume regulation. *J R Coll Physicians Lond* 1992;26:297.

Schrier RW, Abraham WT. Hormones and hemodynamics in heart failure. *N Engl J Med* 1999;341:8:577–585.

Schrier RW, Arroyo V, Bernardi M, et al. Peripheral arterial vasodilation hypothesis: a proposal for the initiation of renal sodium and water retention in cirrhosis. *Hepatology* 1998;8:1151.

Schrier RW, Fassett RG. A critique of the overfill hypothesis of sodium and water retention in the nephrotic syndrome. *Kidney Int* 1998;53:1111–1117.

Schrier RW, Gurevitch AK, Abraham WT. Renal sodium excretion, edematous disorders, and diuretic use. In: Schrier RW, ed. *Renal and electrolyte disorders* 6th ed. Philadelphia: Lippincott Williams & Wilkins, 2002:64–114.

The Patient with Hyponatremia or Hypernatremia

Tomas Berl and Robert W. Schrier

Control of serum sodium and osmolality. Under physiologic conditions, the concentration of sodium in plasma is kept in a very narrow range, between 138 and 142 mEq per L, despite great variations in water intake. Because sodium is the predominant cation in extracellular fluid (ECF), this reflects the equally narrow range in which the tonicity (osmolality) of body fluids is regulated, between 280 and 290 mOsm per kg. Thus, calculated plasma osmolality can be expressed as follows:

$$P_{OSM} = 2[Na^+] + \frac{\text{blood urea nitrogen (mg/dL)}}{2.8} + \frac{\text{glucose (mg/dL)}}{18}$$

Serum sodium (concentration) and plasma osmolality are maintained in these normal ranges by the function of arginine vasopressin, a very sensitive osmoreceptor that controls the secretion of the antidiuretic hormone. This hormone, in turn, is critical in determining water excretion by allowing urinary dilution in its absence and urinary concentration in its presence. Hyponatremic disorders supervene when water intake exceeds the patient's renal diluting capacity. Conversely, hypernatremia supervenes in settings associated with renal concentrating defects accompanied by inadequate water intake.

Hyponatremia. *Hyponatremia,* defined as a plasma sodium concentration of less than 135 mEq per L, is a frequent occurrence in the hospitalized patient. It has been suggested that approximately 10% to 15% of patients in hospitals have a low plasma sodium concentration at some time during their stay. Hyponatremia in the ambulatory outpatient is a much less frequent occurrence and is usually associated with a chronic disease state.

I. **Interpretation of the serum sodium.** Under most clinical circumstances, a decrement in serum sodium reflects a hypo-osmolar state. However, recognizing the settings in which a normal or even low sodium level does not reflect a normal osmotic or a hypo-osmotic state is important. The addition to the ECF of osmotically active solutes that do not readily penetrate into cells, such as glucose, mannitol, or glycine, causes water to move from cells to ECF, thereby leading to cellular dehydration and a decrement in serum sodium concentration. This *translocational hyponatremia* does not reflect changes in total body water, but rather the movement of water from the intracellular to the extracellular compartment.

In hyperglycemia, for each 100 mg per dL rise in blood glucose, a 1.6 mEq per L fall in plasma sodium concentration occurs as water moves out of cells into the ECF. For example, in an untreated diabetic patient, as blood glucose rises from 200 to 1,200 mg per dL, the plasma sodium concentration is expected to fall from 140 to 124 mEq per L (1.6 mEq/L × 10 = 16 mEq) without a change in total body water and electrolytes. Conversely, treatment with insulin and lowering of the blood sugar from 1,200 to 200 mg per dL in this diabetic patient results in a comparable osmotic water movement from the ECF into cells and a return of plasma sodium concentration to 140 mEq per L without any change in total body water or electrolytes.

Hyponatremia can occur without a change in plasma osmolality, this is termed pseudohyponatremia. Pseudohyponatremia occurs when the solid phase of plasma, primarily lipids and proteins (usually 6% to 8%), is greatly increased, as in severe hypertriglyceridemia and paraproteinemic disorders.

This falsely low reading is a consequence of the flame photometry methods that measure the concentration of Na^+ in whole plasma and not only in the liquid phase. It is estimated that a rise in plasma lipids by 4.6 g per L or in plasma proteins of 10 g per dL lowers serum sodium concentration by 1 mEq per L. This is not a problem when undiluted serum is analyzed with an ion-specific electrode that measures the concentration of sodium in serum water.

II. **Approach to the hypo-osmolar hyponatremic patient.** In the absence of pseudohyponatremia or an excess of osmotically active solute in the ECF, the most important initial step in the diagnosis of hyponatremia is an assessment of the ECF volume status.

Sodium is the primary cation in the ECF compartment. Therefore, sodium, with its accompanying anions, dictates ECF osmolality and fluid volume. Thus, ECF volume provides the best index of total body exchangeable sodium. A careful physical examination focused on the evaluation of ECF volume status therefore allows for the classification of the hyponatremic patient into one of three categories: (a) hyponatremia in the presence of an excess of total body sodium, (b) hyponatremia in the presence of a deficit of total body sodium, and (c) hyponatremia with a near normal total body sodium. For example, the edematous patient is classified as having hyponatremia with an excess of total body sodium. The volume-depleted patient with flat neck veins, decreased skin turgor, dry mucous membranes, and orthostatic hypotension and tachycardia is classified as having hyponatremia with a deficit of total body sodium. The patient with neither edema nor evidence of ECF volume depletion is classified as having hyponatremia with near-normal total body sodium (Fig. 2-1).

A. In the **hypervolemic (edematous) hyponatremic patient,** both total body sodium and total body water are increased, water more so than sodium. These patients have cardiac failure, cirrhosis, nephrotic syndrome, or renal failure. When hyponatremia is secondary to cardiac and hepatic disease, the disease is advanced and readily evident on clinical examination. In the absence of the use of diuretics, the urinary sodium concentration in the hyponatremic edematous patient should be quite low (less than 10 mEq per L) because of avid tubular sodium reabsorption. The exception occurs in the presence of acute or chronic renal failure, in which, because of tubular dysfunction, the urinary sodium concentration is higher (greater than 20 mEq per L).

B. The diagnostic possibilities in the **hypovolemic hyponatremic patient** are entirely different. Again, a spot urinary sodium concentration is of value. If the volume-depleted hyponatremic patient has a low (less than 10 mEq per L) sodium concentration, the kidney is functioning normally by conserving sodium in response to ECF volume depletion. Conversely, if the urinary sodium concentration is greater than 20 mEq per L in a hypovolemic hyponatremic patient, the kidney is not responding appropriately to the ECF volume depletion, and renal losses of sodium and water must be considered as the likely cause of the hyponatremia.

1. In a hypovolemic hyponatremic patient with a **urinary sodium concentration of less than 10 mEq per L,** a gastrointestinal (or "third space") source of sodium and water losses must be sought. The source may be readily apparent if the patient presents with a history of vomiting, diarrhea, or both. In the absence of an obvious history of gastrointestinal fluid losses, several other diagnostic possibilities must be considered. Substantial ECF losses may occur into the abdominal cavity with peritonitis or pancreatitis, and into the bowel lumen with ileus or pseudomembranous colitis. The surreptitious cathartic abuser may present with evidence of ECF volume depletion and no history of gastrointestinal losses. The presence of hypokalemic metabolic acidosis and phenolphthalein in the urine may be a clue to this diagnosis. Loss of haustra on barium enema and melanosis coli on endoscopy are other clues to cathartic abuse. Burns or muscle damage may also lead to a state of hypovolemia and

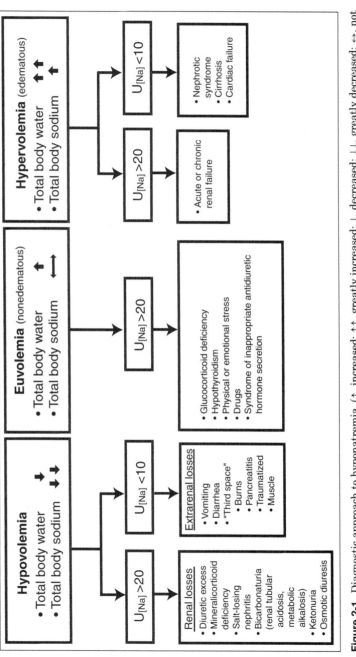

Figure 2-1. Diagnostic approach to hyponatremia. (↑, increased; ↑↑, greatly increased; ↓, decreased; ↓↓, greatly decreased; ↔, not increased or decreased; $U_{[Na]}$ = urinary sodium concentration, in mEq per L.)

hyponatremia secondary to substantial fluid and electrolyte losses from skin or into muscle.

2. In a hypovolemic hyponatremic patient with a **urinary sodium level of greater than 20 mEq per L,** renal losses are occurring, and several different diagnostic possibilities must be considered.

a. **Excessive use of diuretics** is foremost among these diagnoses. It occurs almost exclusively with thiazide diuretics, because these agents, unlike loop diuretics, alter only urinary diluting ability; urinary concentration remains unimpaired. A fall in plasma sodium concentration in a patient receiving diuretics may be the first clue that a diuretic dosage adjustment is needed. In some patients with diuretic abuse, ECF volume depletion is not readily apparent from clinical examination. An important clue, however, to the diagnosis of diuretic-induced hyponatremia is that virtually all these patients have an associated hypokalemic metabolic alkalosis if they are receiving potassium-losing diuretics. If, however, a potassium-sparing diuretic is involved (e.g., triamterene, amiloride, or spironolactone), neither hypokalemia nor metabolic alkalosis may be present. Cessation of use of the diuretic is the best means of confirming the diagnosis of diuretic-induced hyponatremia. However, it must be remembered that restoration of ECF volume also is necessary to correct the hyponatremia. In the hypokalemic patient, potassium replacement also may be necessary for complete correction of the plasma sodium concentration imbalance.

Surreptitious diuretic abuse occurs among premenopausal women who use diuretics for weight loss or other cosmetic reasons (e.g., thick ankles or calves, "puffy" face). These patients may be difficult to distinguish from patients with surreptitious vomiting, because both may present with evidence of ECF volume depletion and hypokalemic metabolic alkalosis. The presence or absence of hyponatremia depends on the patient's water intake. The pivotal diagnostic test to distinguish between the hypovolemic hyponatremic patient with metabolic alkalosis who is a diuretic abuser and the patient who is a surreptitious vomiter is the urinary chloride concentration. Surreptitious vomiters have low (less than 10 mEq per L) concentrations and surreptitious diuretic abusers high (greater than 20 mEq per L) concentrations.

b. **Salt-losing nephritis.** Patients with medullary cystic disease, chronic interstitial nephritis, polycystic kidney disease, analgesic nephropathy, partial urinary tract obstruction, and, rarely, chronic glomerulonephritis may present with hypovolemic hyponatremia secondary to salt-losing nephritis. These patients generally have moderately advanced renal impairment with serum creatinine levels greater than 3 to 4 mg per dL. This diagnosis should virtually never be considered in patients with renal disease that is not associated with elevated serum creatinine. Patients with salt-losing nephritis may need supplemental sodium chloride (NaCl) intake to avoid ECF volume depletion, or they may become very susceptible to ECF volume depletion in association with either decreased intake or extrarenal (e.g., gastrointestinal) sodium and water losses. Because these patients may be pigmented secondary to uremic dermatitis and exhibit hyponatremia and volume depletion, their disease was initially described as mimicking Addison's disease.

c. **Mineralocorticoid deficiency.** The patient with Addison's disease (i.e., primary adrenal insufficiency) generally has associated hyperkalemia; prerenal azotemia generally does not increase serum creatinine to concentrations greater than 3 mg per dL. In patients with mineralocorticoid deficiency, ECF volume repletion may correct both the hyponatremia and the hyperkalemia. During periods of stress, the plasma cortisol level may fall within the normal range. Thus, if adrenal insufficiency is suspected, a 2-hour cosyntropin (Cortrosyn) stimulation test should be performed. In addition to a urinary sodium concentration of greater than 20 mEq per L, a urinary potassium concentration of less than 20 mEq per L may be another clue to mineralocorticoid deficiency. If fluid intake has been restricted, the patient with Addison's disease may not present with hyponatremia, and hyperkalemia may not be present if the ECF volume depletion is not severe. Thus, a high index of suspicion is necessary to make the diagnosis of adrenal insufficiency. These patients may present with nonspecific symptoms such as weight loss, anorexia, abdominal pain, nausea, vomiting, diarrhea, and fever.

   d. Osmotic diuresis obligating anion and cation excretion is another major diagnostic consideration in the hypovolemic hyponatremic patient with a urinary sodium concentration greater than 20 mEq per L.

   (1) Glucose, urea, or mannitol diuresis. The uncontrolled diabetic patient may have substantial glucosuria, causing water and electrolyte losses and, thus, ECF volume depletion. The urea diuresis after the relief of a urinary tract obstruction is another example of an osmotic diuresis that can cause ECF volume depletion. A chronic mannitol infusion without electrolyte replacement can produce a similar situation.

   (2) Bicarbonaturia. Increased anion excretion also can obligate renal water and electrolyte losses. The most frequently encountered example of this is metabolic alkalosis with bicarbonaturia. The bicarbonate anion in the urine is accompanied by cations, including sodium and potassium, which maintain electrical neutrality. Bicarbonaturia may accompany the early development of metabolic alkalosis accompanying postoperative nasogastric suction or vomiting. Proximal renal tubular acidosis (e.g., in Fanconi's syndrome) is another condition in which bicarbonaturia causes renal electrolyte loss. In the absence of a urinary tract infection with urease-producing organisms, a urinary pH (measured by a pH meter) greater than 6.1 indicates the presence of bicarbonate in the urine.

   (3) Ketonuria. Ketoacid anions also can obligate renal electrolyte losses in spite of ECF volume depletion; this may contribute to urinary electrolyte losses in diabetic or alcoholic ketoacidosis or starvation.

C. Euvolemic hyponatremia is a commonly encountered form of hyponatremia in hospitalized patients. The urinary sodium concentration in euvolemic hyponatremia is generally greater than 20 mEq per L. However, if the patient is on a sodium-restricted diet or is volume depleted, the urinary sodium concentration may be less than 10 mEq per L. Refeeding with a normal salt intake or expansion of ECF volume with saline increases urinary sodium concentration to more than 20 mEq per L, but hyponatremia will persist in the patient with euvolemic hyponatremia. These patients show no signs of either an increase or decrease in total body sodium. Although the water retention leads to an excess in total body water, no edema is detected because two-thirds of the water is inside the cell. A limited number of diagnostic possibilities are available with hyponatremic patients who exhibit neither edema nor ECF volume depletion (i.e., euvolemic hyponatremic patients) (Fig. 2-1). Two endocrine disorders must be considered: hypothyroidism and secondary adrenal insufficiency associated with pituitary or hypothalamic disease.

   1. The occurrence of hyponatremia with **hypothyroidism** generally suggests severe disease, including myxedema coma. In some patients, particularly the elderly, the diagnosis may not be readily apparent. Thus, thyroid function must be assessed in the euvolemic hyponatremic patient.

   2. **Glucocorticoid deficiency.** An intact renin-angiotensin-aldosterone system avoids ECF volume depletion in patients with secondary adrenal insufficiency, but it is clear that glucocorticoid deficiency alone can impair water excretion and cause hyponatremia. Although skull films and computed tomographic (CT) scans should always be obtained in the euvolemic hyponatremic patient when the cause of the hyponatremia is not obvious, normal skull films or CT scans do not exclude secondary adrenal insufficiency. A low plasma cortisol level associated with a low adrenocorticotropic hormone level supports the diagnosis of secondary adrenal insufficiency. In this setting, both secondary adrenal insufficiency and secondary hypothyroidism may contribute to the hyponatremia accompanying pituitary insufficiency.
   3. **Emotional or physical stress** must be considered in the euvolemic hyponatremic patient before invoking the diagnosis of the syndrome of inappropriate antidiuretic hormone (SIADH). Acute pain or severe emotional stress (e.g., decompensated psychosis associated with continued water ingestion) may lead to acute and severe hyponatremia. It is likely that a combination of emotional shock and physical pain accounts for the frequently encountered secretion of vasopressin in the postoperative state, which in turn leads to hyponatremia in the face of hypotonic fluid administration.
   4. A number of **pharmacologic agents** either stimulate the release of vasopressin or enhance its action. These include:
      a. Nicotine
      b. Chlorpropamide
      c. Tolbutamide
      d. Clofibrate
      e. Cyclophosphamide
      f. Morphine
      g. Barbiturates
      h. Vincristine
      i. Carbamazepine (Tegretol)
      j. Acetaminophen
      k. Nonsteroidal anti-inflammatory drugs (NSAIDs)
      l. Antipsychotics
      m. Antidepressants
         Thus, determining whether the euvolemic hyponatremic patient is receiving such drugs is an important diagnostic step.
   5. **SIADH** should be considered after exclusion of other diagnoses in the euvolemic hyponatremic patient. In general, the causes of SIADH include:
      a. **Carcinomas,** most frequently but not exclusively of the
         (1) Lung
         (2) Duodenum
         (3) Pancreas
      b. **Pulmonary disorders,** including but not limited to
         (1) Viral pneumonia
         (2) Bacterial pneumonia
         (3) Pulmonary abscess
         (4) Tuberculosis
         (5) Aspergillosis
      c. **Central nervous system (CNS) disorders:**
         (1) Encephalitis (viral or bacterial)
         (2) Meningitis (viral, bacterial, or tubercular)
         (3) Acute psychosis
         (4) Stroke (cerebral thrombosis or hemorrhage)
         (5) Acute intermittent porphyria
         (6) Brain tumor
         (7) Brain abscess

    (8) Subdural or subarachnoid hematoma or hemorrhage
    (9) Guillain-Barré syndrome
    (10) Head trauma
  d. Acquired immunodeficiency syndrome
    Thus, SIADH occurs primarily in association with infections and with vascular and neoplastic processes in the CNS or lung.

III. Signs and symptoms. The level of hyponatremia that may cause signs and symptoms varies with the rate of decline in the plasma sodium concentration and the age of the patient. In general, the young-adult patient appears to tolerate a specific level of hyponatremia better than does the older patient. However, the acute (i.e., within a few hours) development of hyponatremia in a previously asymptomatic young patient may cause severe CNS signs and symptoms, such as depressed sensorium, seizures, and even death, when the plasma sodium concentration has reached only a level between 125 and 130 mEq per L. This is because the capacity of brain cells to extrude osmotically active particles, and thus relieve the brain swelling that accompanies hyponatremia, requires a longer time to be invoked at the beginning of the condition. Conversely, this protective mechanism against brain swelling becomes very effective with the chronic development of hyponatremia over days or weeks, so that an elderly person may present without overt signs or symptoms even with a plasma sodium concentration below 110 mEq per L.

    Gastrointestinal symptoms, including anorexia and nausea, may occur early with hyponatremia. The more severe later signs and symptoms relate to the CNS, because the cell swelling that occurs with hyponatremia is tolerated worst within the rigid encasement of the skull. Severe hyponatremia of rapid onset may lead to brain edema and herniation and thus requires rapid treatment. Cheyne-Stokes respiration may be a hallmark of severe acute hyponatremia. In addition to exposure, uremia, and hypothyroidism, hyponatremia also should be considered in the differential diagnosis of the hypothermic patient.

    In summary, **symptoms** that may be associated with hyponatremia include:
  A. Lethargy, apathy
  B. Disorientation
  C. Muscle cramps
  D. Anorexia, nausea
  E. Agitation
    Signs that may be associated with hyponatremia include:
  F. Abnormal sensorium
  G. Depressed deep tendon reflexes
  H. Cheyne-Stokes respiration
  I. Hypothermia
  J. Pathologic reflexes
  K. Pseudobulbar palsy
  L. Seizures

IV. Therapy
  A. Factors affecting the approach to treatment. The presence or absence of symptoms and the duration of the hyponatremia are the primary guides to treatment strategy. Different time-dependent processes are involved in the adaptation to changes in tonicity, and the presence of cerebral symptoms reflects a failure of the adaptive response. In this regard, hyponatremia developing within 48 hours carries a greater risk of permanent neurologic sequelae from cerebral edema if the plasma sodium concentration is not corrected expeditiously. Conversely, patients with chronic hyponatremia are at risk of osmotic demyelination if the correction is excessive or too rapid.
  B. Cerebral adaptation to hypotonicity. Decreases in extracellular osmolality cause the movement of water into cells, increasing intracellular volume and causing tissue edema. Edema within the cranium raises intracranial pressure, leading to neurologic syndromes. To prevent this complication, a volume-regulatory adaptation occurs. Early in the course of hyponatremia,

within 1 to 3 hours, cerebral ECF volume decreases through the movement of fluid into the cerebrospinal fluid (CSF), which is then shunted into the systemic circulation. Thereafter, the brain adapts by losing cellular potassium and organic solutes, which tend to lower the intracellular osmolality without substantial gain of water. If hyponatremia persists, other organic osmolytes, such as phosphocreatine, myoinositol, and amino acids (e.g., glutamine and taurine) are lost. The loss of these solutes greatly decreases cerebral swelling. Patients in whom this adaptive response fails are prone to severe cerebral edema when they develop hyponatremia. Postoperative menstruant females; elderly women on a thiazide; directic, psychiatric polydipsic patients; and hypoxemic patients are particularly prone to hyponatremia-related encephalopathy. Conversely, as noted earlier, patients who have had the adaptive response are at risk of osmotic demyelination syndrome if the hyponatremia is excessively or too rapidly corrected. For example, a rapid increase in plasma osmolality may cause excessive cerebral water loss in previously adapted brains. Alcoholic subjects, burn victims, and severely hypokalemic patients are at risk for this complication.

C. **Acute symptomatic hyponatremia,** developing in less than 48 hours, is almost inevitable in hospital patients receiving hypotonic fluids. Treatment should be prompt, because the risk of acute cerebral edema exceeds the risk of osmotic demyelination. The aim should be to raise the serum Na^+ by 2 mmol per L per hour until symptoms resolve. Complete correction is unnecessary, although it is not unsafe. Hypertonic saline (3% NaCl) is infused at the rate of 1 to 2 mL per kg per hour, and a loop diuretic, such as furosemide, enhances solute-free water excretion and hastens the return to a normal serum Na^+. If severe neurologic symptoms (seizures, obtundation, or coma) are present, 3% NaCl may be infused at 4 to 6 mL per kg per hour. Even 29.2% NaCl (50 mL) has been used safely. Serum electrolytes should be carefully monitored.

D. **Chronic symptomatic hyponatremia.** If hyponatremia has been present for more than 48 hours or the duration is unknown, correction must be handled carefully. Whether it is the rate of correction of hyponatremia or the magnitude that predisposes to osmotic demyelination is unknown, but in practice dissociating the two is difficult, because a rapid correction rate usually means a greater correction over a given period of time.

The following guidelines are fundamental to successful therapy:

1. Because cerebral water is increased only by approximately 10% in severe chronic hyponatremia, promptly increase the serum Na^+ level by 10%, or by approximately 10 mEq per L.
2. After the initial correction, do not exceed a correction rate of 1.0 to 1.5 mEq per L per hour.
3. Do not increase the serum Na^+ by more than 12 mEq per L per 24 hours.

It is important to take into account the rate of infusion and the electrolyte content of infused fluids and the rate of production and electrolyte content of the urine.

Once the desired increment in serum Na^+ concentration is obtained, the treatment should consist of water restriction.

E. The approach to the **chronic asymptomatic patient with hyponatremia** is different. Initial bedside evaluation includes searching for an underlying disorder. Hypothyroidism and adrenal insufficiency should be sought as possible etiologies, and hormones must be replaced if these deficiencies are found. A careful analysis of the patient's medications should be made and necessary adjustments undertaken.

For patients with SIADH, if the etiology is not identifiable or cannot be treated, the approach should be conservative, because rapid changes in serum tonicity lead to a greater degree of cerebral water loss and possible demyelination. Various approaches can be considered.

1. **Fluid restriction** is an easy and usually successful option, if the patient complies. A calculation must be made of the fluid restriction that will

maintain a specific serum Na^+. The daily osmolar load ingested divided by the minimal urinary osmolality (a function of the severity of the diluting disorder) determines a patient's maximal urine volume. On a normal North American diet, the daily osmolar load is about 10 mOsm per kilogram of body weight; in a healthy person, the minimum urinary osmolality (given no circulating vasopressin) can be as low as 50 mOsm per kg. Thus, the daily urine volume in a 70-kg man can be as high as 14 L (700 mOsm per 50 mOsm per L). If the patient has SIADH, and the urinary osmolality cannot be lowered below 500 mOsm per kg, the same osmolar load of 700 mOsm per day allows for only 1.4 L of urine. Thus, if the patient drinks more than 1.4 L per day, the serum Na^+ will fall. A measurement of urinary sodium (U_{Na}) and potassium concentration (U_K) can guide the degree of water restriction that is required. If $U_{Na} + U_K$ is greater than the serum sodium concentration, water restriction alone may not be sufficient to increase serum sodium concentration.

2. **Pharmacologic agents. Lithium** was the first drug used to antagonize the action of vasopressin in hyponatremic disorders. Lithium may be neurotoxic, and its effects are unpredictable. Therefore, **demeclocycline** has become the agent of choice. This drug inhibits the formation and action of cyclic adenosine monophosphate in the renal collecting duct. The onset of action is 3 to 6 days after treatment is started. The dose must be decreased to the lowest level that keeps the serum sodium concentration within the desired range with unrestricted water intake; this dose is usually 300 to 900 mg daily. The drug should be given 1 to 2 hours after meals, and calcium-, aluminum-, and magnesium-containing antacids should be avoided. However, polyuria tends to make patients noncompliant. Skin photosensitivity may occur; in children, tooth or bone abnormalities may result. Nephrotoxicity also limits the drug's use, especially in patients with underlying liver disease or congestive heart failure, in whom the hepatic metabolism of demeclocycline may be impaired.

3. **Vasopressin antagonists.** Specific antagonists of vasopressin action on the collecting duct may soon supplement these pharmacologic agents. Orally active, nonpeptide vasopressin type 2 (V_2)–receptor antagonists that have shown encouraging results in animal models and humans with hyponatremia are undergoing clinical studies, but these "aquaretic" agents have not yet been approved by the U.S. Food and Drug Administration (FDA).

4. **Increase in solute excretion.** Because urine flow can be significantly increased by obligating the excretion of solutes and thereby allowing a greater intake of water, measures to increase solute excretion have been used. A loop diuretic, when combined with high sodium intake (2 to 3 g additional NaCl), is effective. A single diuretic dose (40 mg furosemide) is usually sufficient. The dose should be doubled if the diuresis induced in the first 8 hours is less than 60% of the total daily urine output. Administration of urea to increase the solute load increases urine flow by causing an osmotic diuresis. This permits a more liberal water intake without worsening the hyponatremia and without altering urinary concentration. The dose is usually 30 to 60 g of urea daily. The major limitations are gastrointestinal distress and unpalatability.

F. **Hypovolemic and hypervolemic hyponatremia.** Symptoms directly related to hyponatremia are unusual in hypovolemic hyponatremia, because loss of both sodium and water limits osmotic shifts in the brain. Restoration of ECF volume with crystalloids or colloids interrupts the nonosmotic release of vasopressin. In patients with hypovolemic hyponatremia from diuretics, the drug must be discontinued and potassium repletion ensured. The treatment of hyponatremia in hypervolemic states is more difficult, because it requires attention to the underlying disorder of heart failure or chronic liver disease. In congestive heart failure, both sodium and water restriction are critical. Refractory patients may be treated with a combination of an angiotensin-converting enzyme (ACE) inhibitor and a diuretic. The resultant increase in cardiac output with ACE inhibitors may increase solute-free water excretion and correct hyponatremia. Loop diuretics diminish the action of vasopressin on the collecting tubules, thereby increasing solute-free water excretion. Thiazide diuretics impair urinary dilution and may worsen hyponatremia. Water and salt restriction are also the mainstay of therapy in cirrhotic patients. For both disorders, V_2- receptor antagonists are under investigation, and these aquaretics may be clinically available to treat hyponatremia in the near future.

Hypernatremia. *Hypernatremia,* defined as a plasma sodium concentration greater than 150 mEq per L, is less common than hyponatremia, probably not because of a more frequent occurrence of disorders of urinary dilution than of urinary concentration, but rather because of drinking behavior. Specifically, if an inability to dilute the urine is present, water intake of 1 to 2 L per day may cause hyponatremia. This amount of fluid intake may be ingested as routine behavior in spite of a hypo-osmolar stimulus to suppress thirst, which may explain the frequency of hyponatremia. Conversely, urinary-concentrating defects that cause renal water losses generally do not cause hypernatremia unless a disturbance in thirst is also present or the patient cannot drink or obtain adequate fluid to drink. The very young, the very old, and the very sick are, therefore, those populations that develop hypernatremia most frequently. In the absence of an inability to drink (e.g., with coma, nausea, and vomiting) or to obtain water (e.g., in infants or severely ill adults), the thirst mechanism is very effective in preventing hypernatremia. Although, as noted, hyponatremia does not always reflect a hypotonic state (i.e., pseudo- or translocation hyponatremia), hypernatremia always denotes a hypertonic state.

I. **Approach to the hypernatremic patient.** As is the case with hyponatremia, hypernatremic patients may have low, high, or normal total body sodium (Fig. 2-2). Such a classification allows the clinician to focus on the most likely diagnosis in each category.

A. **Hypovolemic hypernatremic patient.** The hypernatremic patient may have evidence of ECF volume depletion that has occurred secondary to either renal or extrarenal losses. These patients have sustained water losses that are greater than the sodium losses.

1. **Extrarenal losses.** If the losses have been from an extrarenal site (e.g., in diarrhea), then sodium and water conservation by the kidney should be readily apparent. In such patients, the urine sodium concentration is less than 10 mEq per L, and the urine is hypertonic. In fact, hypotonic diarrhea losses are among the most common causes of hypernatremia in both children and adults, especially in those who are on lactulose for underlying liver disease.

2. **Renal losses.** In contrast, hypotonic electrolyte losses may occur in the urine during osmotic diuresis or use of loop diuretics. In these patients, evidence of renal sodium and water conservation is, of course, not present, because the urine is the source of the losses. Thus, the urine is not hypertonic, and urine sodium concentration is generally greater than 20 mEq per L. In the hyperglycemic diabetic patient with good renal function and profound glucosuria, hypernatremia may be a presenting feature, because hypotonic renal losses may obscure any effect of hyperglycemia to shift water osmotically from cells to ECF. This is particularly true if the patient does not have access to water or is incapable of ingesting fluids (e.g., a comatose, ketoacidotic diabetic patient). In the setting of high-protein tube feedings, the high rate of urea excretion leads to significant renal water losses.

B. **Hypervolemic hypernatremic patient.** Patients with hypernatremia also may have evidence of ECF volume expansion. Generally, these patients have received excessive amounts of hypertonic NaCl or sodium bicarbonate. In such an acute setting, the incidence of ECF volume expansion is most likely to be associated with pulmonary congestion, elevated neck veins, or both, rather than with peripheral edema. This variety of hypervolemic

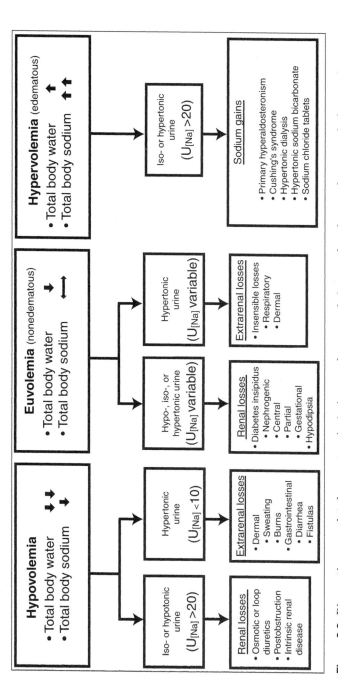

Figure 2-2. Diagnostic approach to hypernatremia. (↑, increased; ↑↑, greatly increased; ↓, decreased; ↓↓, greatly decreased; ↔, not increased or decreased; $U_{[Na]}$ = urinary sodium concentration, in mEq per L.)

hypernatremia is rather infrequent, but may occur with cardiac resuscitation or NaCl tablets taken during exercise in a high temperature, high humidity environment.

C. Euvolemic hypernatremia. Most patients with hypernatremia secondary to water loss appear euvolemic with normal total body sodium, because loss of water without sodium does not lead to overt volume contraction. Water loss in and of itself need not culminate in hypernatremia unless it is unaccompanied by water intake. Because such hypodipsia is uncommon, hypernatremia usually supervenes only in those who have no access to water or who have a neurologic deficit that does not allow them to seek it. Extrarenal water loss occurs from the skin and respiratory tract in febrile or other hypermetabolic states. Urine osmolality is very high, reflecting an intact osmoreceptor-vasopressin-renal response. Thus, the defense against hyperosmolality requires both stimulation of thirst and the ability to respond by drinking water. The urine sodium concentration varies with sodium intake. The renal losses of water that lead to euvolemic hypernatremia are a consequence of a defect in vasopressin production or release (central diabetes insipidus), a failure of the collecting duct to respond to the hormone (nephrogenic), or excessive rapid degradation of vasopressin (gestational).

1. Approximately 50% of instances of **central diabetes insipidus** have no detectable underlying cause and thus are classified as idiopathic. Trauma, surgical procedures in the area of the pituitary or hypothalamus, and brain neoplasms, either primary or secondary (e.g., from metastatic breast cancer), constitute the majority of the remaining causes of central diabetes insipidus. In addition, encephalitis, sarcoidosis, or eosinophilic granuloma may cause central diabetes insipidus. Central diabetes insipidus can be partial, with some preservation of vasopressin release. When the central diabetes is associated with hypothalamic lesions and hypodipsia, these patients present with hypernatremia and a concentrated urine. A congenital form of central diabetes insipidus has also been described.

2. **Nephrogenic diabetes insipidus.** This disorder can be **congenital or acquired.** The congenital form is inherited as an x-linked disorder. The underlying defect resides in the vasopressin receptor that is localized to the x chromosone. A rarer autosomal recessive form is related to a mutation in the vasopressin dependent water channel (AQP2). A number of acquired causes have been described, many of them also associated with decreased AQP2 production:

   a. **Secondary to renal diseases.** Medullary or interstitial renal diseases are particularly likely to be accompanied by vasopressin-resistant renal concentrating defects; the most frequent of these diseases are medullary cystic disease, chronic interstitial nephritis (e.g., analgesic nephropathy), polycystic kidney disease, and partial bilateral urinary tract obstruction. Far-advanced renal disease of any cause is uniformly associated with a renal concentrating defect. However, because of the very low glomerular filtration rate, the renal water loss (i.e., polyuria) is modest (2 to 4 L per day).

   b. **Secondary to hypercalcemia and hypokalemia.** Hypercalcemia secondary to any cause, including primary hyperparathyroidism, vitamin D intoxication, milk-alkali syndrome, hyperthyroidism, and tumor, may also cause nephrogenic diabetes insipidus. Similarly, hypokalemia secondary to any cause, including primary aldosteronism, diarrhea, and chronic diuretic use, may cause nephrogenic diabetes insipidus. However, some of the polyuria accompanying hypercalcemia or hypokalemia may be due to stimulation of thirst and the resultant increase in water intake.

   c. **Drugs, dietary abnormalities, and other causes.** Various drugs impair the end-organ response to vasopressin and thus cause a renal concentrating defect (see section **I.C.2.d.3**). Excess water intake and dietary sodium and protein restriction also have been shown to impair urinary concentration. Other unique causes of nephrogenic diabetes insipidus include multiple myeloma, amyloidosis, Sjögren's syndrome, and sarcoidosis.

d. A **summary** of acquired causes of nephrogenic diabetes insipidus includes:

(1) Chronic renal disease
Polycystic kidney disease
Medullary cystic disease
Pyelonephritis
Urinary tract obstruction
Far-advanced renal failure
Analgesic nephropathy

(2) Electrolyte disorders
Hypokalemia
Hypercalcemia

(3) Drugs
Lithium
Demeclocycline
Acetohexamide
Tolazamide
Glyburide
Propoxyphene
Amphotericin
Methoxyflurane
Vinblastine
Colchicine

(4) Dietary abnormalities
Excessive water intake
Decreased sodium chloride intake
Decreased protein intake

(5) Miscellaneous
Multiple myeloma
Amyloidosis
Sjögren's syndrome
Sarcoidosis
Sickle cell disease

3. Diabetes insipidus secondary to vasopressinase. Central diabetes insipidus and nephrogenic diabetes are not the only causes of polyuria during pregnancy. Vasopressinase is an enzyme, produced in the placenta, that causes *in vivo* degradation of arginine vasopressin during pregnancy. Normally, an increase in vasopressin synthesis and release during pregnancy compensates for the increased degradation of the hormone. In rare cases, however, excessive vasopressinase has been incriminated in causing polyuria during pregnancy. Because vasopressinase cannot degrade deamino-8-D-arginine vasopressin, this is the treatment of choice for pregnancy-related polyuria.

4. Response to fluid deprivation and arginine vasopressin in the diagnosis of polyuric disorder. The various forms of diabetes insipidus must be differentiated from primary polydipsia in patients who present with polyuria. Table 2-1 summarizes the procedure and interpretation of a water deprivation test. Patients with compulsive water drinking may present with polyuria and a blunted response to the fluid deprivation test; on cessation of fluid intake, hypernatremia does not develop in these patients and their renal concentration defect is primarily due to a resistance of the kidney to vasopressin. However, because patients with central or nephrogenic diabetes insipidus may present with polyuria and polydipsia in the absence of hypernatremia, awareness of the diagnosis of compulsive (psychogenic) water drinking is quite important. Menopausal women

Table 2-1. Procedure and interpretation of a water deprivation test

Cause of polyuria	Urinary osmolality with water deprivation (mOsm/kg of water)	Plasma arginine vasopressin (AVP) after dehydration	Increase in urinary osmolality with exogenous AVP
Normal	>800	>2 pg/mL	Little or no increase
Complete central diabetes insipidus	<300	Undetectable	Substantially increased
Partial central diabetes insipidus	300–800	<1.5 pg/mL	Increase of more than 10% after water deprivation
Nephrogenic diabetes insipidus	<300–500	>5 pg/mL	Little or no increase
Primary polydipsia	>500	<5 pg/mL	Little or no increase

Note: Water intake is restricted until the patient loses 3% to 5% of his or her body weight or until three consecutive hourly determinations of urinary osmolality are within 10% of each other. (Caution must be exercised to ensure that the patient does not become excessively dehydrated.) Aqueous AVP (5 units subcutaneously) is given, and urinary osmolality is measured after 60 minutes. The expected responses are given above.
From Lanese D, Teitelbaum I. Hypernatremia. In: Jacobson HR, Striker GE, Klahr S, eds. *The principles and practice of nephrology,* 2nd ed. St. Louis: Mosby, 1995:893–898. Reprinted with permission.

with previous psychiatric problems are particularly prone to compulsive water drinking. Psychoneurosis and psychosis are also frequently associated with increased water intake. Last, the patient with nephrogenic diabetes insipidus may occasionally have vasopressin-resistant hypotonic urine (e.g., hypercalcemic or hypokalemic nephropathy); thus, the temporary absence of fluid intake because of an intercurrent illness can be associated with hypernatremia. In all hypernatremic patients who primarily have water losses without electrolyte losses, the urine sodium excretion concentration merely reflects sodium intake. During any solute-free water diuresis, the urinary sodium concentration declines so that sodium balance is maintained.

II. **Signs and symptoms.** Polyuria and polydipsia may be prominent symptoms in the patient who subsequently develops hypernatremia in association with inadequate water intake.

A. **CNS dysfunction.** Neurologic abnormalities constitute the most prominent manifestations of hypernatremic states. These neurologic manifestations appear to be due primarily to the cellular dehydration and shrinkage of brain cells that are associated with tearing of cerebral vessels. Capillary and venous congestion, subcortical and subarachnoid bleeding, and venous sinus thrombosis all have been described with hypernatremia.

B. **Prognosis of acute versus chronic hypernatremia.** The signs and symptoms of hypernatremia are more severe in acute than in chronic hypernatremia. Indeed, 75% mortality has been reported in association with acute hypernatremia in adults with acute elevations of plasma sodium concentration above 160 mEq per L. These adults, however, frequently have severe primary diseases associated with their hypernatremia, and these primary diseases may largely account for the high mortality. A 45% mortality has been reported in children with acute hypernatremia, and as many as two-thirds of the surviving children may have neurologic sequelae.

C. **Idiogenic osmoles with chronic hypernatremia.** The more benign course of chronic hypernatremia appears to be related to cellular mechanisms that protect against severe brain dehydration. The brain, however, requires some period of time, perhaps days, to adapt. In chronic hypernatremia, brain cells generate idiogenic osmoles, some of which appear to be amino acids; these idiogenic osmoles are osmotically active and restore brain water to near-control levels in spite of persistent hypernatremia. The presence of these idiogenic anions with chronic hypernatremia, although protective against brain dehydration and shrinkage, may predispose to brain edema if the hypernatremia is corrected too rapidly.

D. Correlation of CNS dysfunction with degree of hyperosmolality. The earliest manifestations of hypernatremia are restlessness, increased irritability, and lethargy. These symptoms may be followed by muscular twitching, hyperflexia, tremulousness, and ataxia. The level of hyperosmolality at which these signs and symptoms occur depends not only on the rapidity of the change in the plasma sodium concentration but also on the age of the patient; the very young and the very old exhibit the most severe manifestations. In general, however, these signs and symptoms may occur progressively with plasma osmolality in the range of 325 to 375 mOsm per kg of water. At plasma osmolalities above this level, tonic muscular spasticity, focal and grand mal seizures, and death may occur. The elderly patient with dementia or severe cerebrovascular disease may demonstrate these life-threatening signs and symptoms at a lower level of plasma hyperosmolality.

III. Therapy. Hypernatremia is frequently a preventable electrolyte disorder if water losses are recognized and appropriately replaced. In most cases, hypernatremia can be treated by the judicious administration of water to patients with water-losing disorders who cannot obtain water. The treatment of hypernatremia depends on two important factors: ECF volume status and the rate of development of the hypernatremia.

A. Correction of ECF volume depletion. When hypernatremia is associated with ECF volume depletion, the primary therapeutic goal is to administer isotonic saline until restoration of ECF volume is achieved, as assessed by normal neck veins and absence of orthostatic hypotension and tachycardia. Hypotonic (0.45%) NaCl or 5% glucose solutions can then be used to correct plasma osmolality.

B. Correction of ECF volume expansion. In contrast, if hypernatremia is associated with ECF volume expansion, diuretics (e.g., furosemide) can be used to treat the hypernatremia. In the presence of advanced renal failure, the patient with hypernatremia and fluid overload may need to be dialyzed to treat the hypernatremia.

C. Water-replacement method of calculation. Last, the patient with euvolemic hypernatremia can be treated primarily with water replacement either orally or parenterally with 5% glucose in water. The method of calculation of the necessary water replacement for a 75-kg man with a plasma sodium of 154 mEq per L is as follows:

$$\text{Total body water (TBW)} = \text{body weight} \times 60\% \text{ or}$$
$$\text{TBW} = 75 \times 0.6 = 45 \text{ L}$$

Then,

$$\frac{\text{Actual plasma sodium}}{\text{Desired plasma sodium}} \times \text{TBW} = \frac{154 \text{ mEq/L}}{140 \text{ mEq/L}} \times 45 \text{ L} = 49.5 \text{ L}$$

Therefore, the repletion of 4.5 L (49.5 L – 45 L) positive water balance will correct the plasma sodium concentration. Ongoing water losses should not be overlooked.

D. Rate of correction. The recommended rate of correction of hypernatremia depends on the rate of development of the hypernatremia and the symptoms. More neurologic signs and symptoms are associated with acute hypernatremia; therefore, this biochemical abnormality should be corrected rapidly, over a few hours.

Conversely idiogenic osmoles appear to accumulate in brain cells during periods of chronic hypernatremia, a mechanism that protects against brain shrinkage. Thus, the rapid correction of chronic hypernatremia can create an osmotic gradient between the ECF and intracellular compartments, with osmotic water movement into cells and subsequent brain edema. In general, therefore, chronic hypernatremia is best corrected gradually, at a rate not to exceed 2 mOsm per hour. One-half of the correction can be achieved in 24 hours and the other half in the next 24 hours or longer.

Suggested readings

Berl T, Schrier RW. Disorders of water metabolism. In: Schrier RW, ed. *Renal and electrolyte disorders,* 6th ed. Philadelphia: Lippincott Williams & Wilkins, 2003: 1–63.

Berl T, Verbails S. Pathophysiology of water balance. In: Brenner B, ed. *The kidney,* 7th ed. Philadelphia: WB Saunders, 2003:857–919.

Bichet D. Nephrogenic and central diabetes insipidus. In: Schrier RW, ed. *Diseases of the kidney and urinary tract,* 7th ed. Philadelphia: Lippincott Williams & Wilkins, 2001:2549–2576.

Durr JA, Hoggard JG, Hunt JM, Schrier RW. Diabetes insipidus due to abnormally high circulating vasopressinase activity in a pregnancy. *N Engl J Med* 1987;316:1070–1074.

Furst H, Hallowsk K, Post J, et al. The urine/plasma electrolyte: rate a predictive guide to water restriction. *Am J Med Sci* 2000;319:240–244.

Kumar S, Berl T. Disorders of water metabolism. In: Schrier RW, ed. *Atlas of diseases of the kidney.* Philadelphia: Blackwell, 1999:1–22.

Kumar S, Berl T. Sodium. *Lancet* 1998;352:220–228.

Lanese D, Teitelbaum I. Hypernatremia. In: Jacobson HR, Striker GE, Klahr S, eds. *The principles and practice of nephrology,* 2nd ed. St. Louis: Mosby, 1995:893–898.

Thurman J, Halterman R, Berl T. Therapy of dysnatremic disorders. In: Brady N, Wilcox C, eds. *Therapy of nephrology and hypertension,* Philadelphia: WB Saunders, 2003:335–348.

Verbalis J. The syndrome of inappropriate anti-diuretic hormone secretion and other hypo-osmolar disorders. In Schrier RW, ed. *Diseases of the kidney and urinary tract,* 7th ed. Philadelphia: Lippincott Williams & Wilkins, 2001:2511–2598.

The Patient with Hypokalemia or Hyperkalemia

Catherine L. Kelleher and Stuart L. Linas

Potassium is the most abundant cation in the human body. It regulates intracellular enzyme function and helps determine neuromuscular and cardiovascular tissue excitability. Ninety percent of total body potassium is located in intracellular fluid (ICF; primarily in muscle), 10% in the extracellular fluid (ECF), and less than 1% in plasma. The ratio of extracellular potassium to intracellular potassium determines membrane potential. The acuity of changes in serum potassium concentration and membrane potential determines the severity of clinical symptoms and underlies the clinical findings caused by disorders of potassium metabolism.

I. **Overview of potassium physiology.** The typical Western diet contains between 40 and 120 mEq of potassium a day. Tight contol of the serum potassium between 3.5 and 5.5 mEq per day is primarily accomplished by the kidney, where secretion varies between 40 and 120 mEq per day. Potassium losses in stool and sweat are small (5 to 10 mEq). Although total body potassium declines with aging, and the rate of decline appears to be influenced by sex and race, the clinical significance of these observations is not clear. The internal regulation of potassium involves the interplay of several hormonal systems as well as the internal acid-base enviornment.

A. **Internal balance.** After a meal, potassium is rapidly redistributed between the plasma and intracellular compartments. Several systems interact to regulate the transcellular movement of potassium:

1. **Insulin.** The binding of the insulin hormone to insulin receptors causes a hyperpolarization of cell membranes that facilitates potassium uptake. Insulin also activates sodium-potassium adenosine triphosphatase (ATPase) pumps and causes the cellular uptake of potassium.

2. **Catecholamines.** Activation of the beta$_2$ adrenoreceptor results in cellular potassium uptake. This effect is transduced by cyclic adenosine monophosphate (cAMP) activation of sodium-potassium ATPase pumps, causing an influx of potassium in exchange for sodium. Therapeutic agents such as theophylline potentiate beta$_2$ adrenoreceptor-mediated potassium uptake by inhibiting the degradation of cAMP.

3. **Aldosterone.** Although this mineralocorticoid facilitates potassium uptake into muscle, clear proof of the clinical significance of this effect is lacking.

4. **Acid-base.** Inorganic acidosis (e.g., hydrochloric acid) facilitates potassium movement from ICF to ECF. Protons enter cells, whereas impermeant inorganic ions do not. The resulting increases in ICF positive charge favor the outward movement of potassium. Because organic ions (lactate, ketoacids) are less restricted from entering cells, increases in serum potassium may not occur in organic acidosis.

5. **Tonicity.** Hyperglycemia causes potassium-rich fluid to leave the cell, thus increasing ECF potassium. Under most conditions, increases in insulin modulate and reverse the effect of increased extracellular tonicity. However, when insulin cannot be increased (as in diabetes mellitus) or hyperglycemia occurs rapidly (as with the administration of 50% glucose), hyperkalemia occurs. Rapid infusions of mannitol also may cause hyperkalemia.

B. **External balance.** Urinary potassium excretion is the result of a difference between the potassium secreted and potassium reabsorbed in the distal nephron. Potassium is freely filtered at the glomerulus. More than 50% of filtered potassium is reabsorbed in the proximal convoluted tubule. In the descending limb of Henle's loop, especially in deep nephrons, potassium concentration increases. In the ascending limb of the loop of Henle, the Na-K-2Cl cotransporter leads to the reabsorption of potassium. When the tubular fluid reaches the early distal convoluted tubule, only 10% to 15% of filtered potassium remains. Potassium is secreted by the principal cells of the cortical collecting and outer-medullary collecting duct. Potassium is reabsorbed in the collecting tubule, an effect mediated by intercalated cells. A fall in glomerular filtration rate (GFR) is not generally associated with decreased potassium excretion and hyperkalemia until the GFR is less than 20 mL per minute. The major factors regulating potassium excretion follow.

1. **Distal nephron flow rate and sodium delivery.** Under normal conditions, sodium delivered to the cortical collecting tubule is reabsorbed through apical sodium channels in the principal cells. This increases cell sodium concentration and basolateral sodium-potassium-ATPase activity. The resultant increases in cellular potassium lead to an increased apical potassium transport through specific potassium channels. Increases in sodium delivery facilitate this mechanism of potassium secretion. In addition, increases in tubular flow rate help maintain a low urinary potassium concentration, which favors the movement of potassium from cells into tubular fluid.
2. **Mineralocorticoids.** Aldosterone is the major mineralocorticoid; it increases potassium secretion into the tubular fluid by:
   a. Increasing the number and activity of apical sodium channels
   b. Increasing basolateral sodium-potassium ATPase activity
   c. Increasing the number of apical potassium channels
3. Increases or decreases in **dietary potassium** increase or decrease urinary potassium, respectively. Renal adaptation to high potassium intake is mediated by a potassium-induced increase in aldosterone secretion and by an increase in distal nephron sodium-potassium ATPase activity. In response to potassium restriction, mineralocorticoid activity decreases, thus causing a decline in potassium secretion.
4. Increases in relatively nonresorbable **anions** (e.g., bicarbonate, penicillins) trap secreted potassium in the tubular lumen and limit potassium reabsorption in the medullary collecting duct. The resulting renal potassium losses may lead to severe potassium depletion.

II. **Hypokalemia**
   A. **Diagnosis.** The **initial approach** to hypokalemia is to determine whether it is spurious, secondary to a shift of potassium from the extracellular to intracellular compartments, or a result of a true decreases in total body potassium (Fig. 3-1).
      Spurious hypokalemia occurs in the setting of extreme leukocytosis (*in vitro* white blood cells uptake potassium in the test tube) and is not associated with changes in either internal or external potassium balance.
      Potassium shifts into cells may occur acutely in conditions associated with increases in endogenous insulin or catecholamines. For example, catecholamine release associated with shortness of breath (asthma, chronic obstructive pulmonary disease exacerbations, heart failure, chest pain syndromes including myocardial infarction or angina) or catecholamine release from a drug withdrawal syndrome (alcohol, narcotics, or barbiturates) shifts potassium to inside cells thereby decreasing the serum potassium concentration. Hypokalemia may also be caused by insulin administration (correction of diabetic ketoacidosis, postresuscitation for hyperkalemia) or $beta_2$-adrenoreceptor mimetics ($beta_2$ agonists, theophylline). Other common causes of decreases in serum potassium without decreases in total body potassium include hypokalemic periodic paralysis (familial and hyperthyroid types), treatment of megaloblastic anemias, and refeeding syndromes

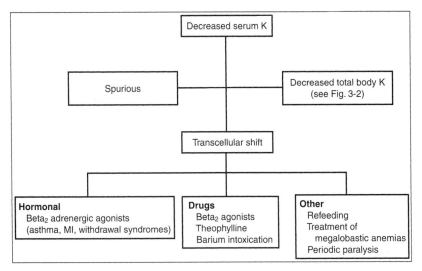

Figure 3-1. Diagnostic approach to hypokalemia. (K, potassium; MI, myocardial infarction.)

(probably insulin mediated). The refeeding syndrome, in which severely malnourished patients are begun on nasogastric feeding, is also seen in older adults in whom the clinical manifestations of malnutrition are less clinically apparent.

Decreases in total body potassium (Fig. 3-2) are caused by either inadequate potassium intake or by excessive renal or extrarenal potassium losses. The measurement of urinary potassium excretion (by 24-hour measurements or "spot" potassium concentrations) is used to distinguish renal versus extrarenal potassium loss. Urinary potassium concentrations less than 20 mEq per L suggest poor potassium intake or extrarenal potassium loss. Serum acid-base status is also helpful in evaluating the site of potassium loss. Metabolic acidosis may suggest gastrointestinal (GI) losses (diarrhea of any cause, e.g., infectious, toxic, laxative abuse). A normal serum pH is less helpful, because hypokalemia can be secondary to both decreases in intake and GI losses. Metabolic alkalosis with urinary potassium of less than 20 mEq per L, although rare, is associated with laxative abuse, villous adenoma, or congenital chloride-losing diarrhea. Hypokalemia with a urinary potassium excretion of greater than 20 mEq per L suggests renal potassium wasting. The serum pH also is used to further evaluate etiologies. Metabolic acidosis suggests renal tubular acidosis (type 1 or type 2), diabetic ketoacidosis (osmotic diuresis), ureterosigmoidostomy, or carbonic anhydrase inhibitor use.

More commonly, renal potassium losses are associated with **metabolic alkalosis.** In this clinical setting, the urinary chloride concentration is helpful. A low urinary chloride concentration (less than 20 mEq per L) suggests potassium losses from upper GI losses, recent diuretic use, or a posthypercapnic syndrome. Hypokalemia with a high urinary chloride concentration is further distinguished on the basis of the presence or absence of hypertension. In normotensive individuals, hypokalemia with metabolic alkalosis and a high urinary chloride occurs with diuretic use (loop or distal convoluted tubule–acting diuretics), in Bartter's and Gitelman's syndrome, and with severe decreases in total body magnesium or potassium.

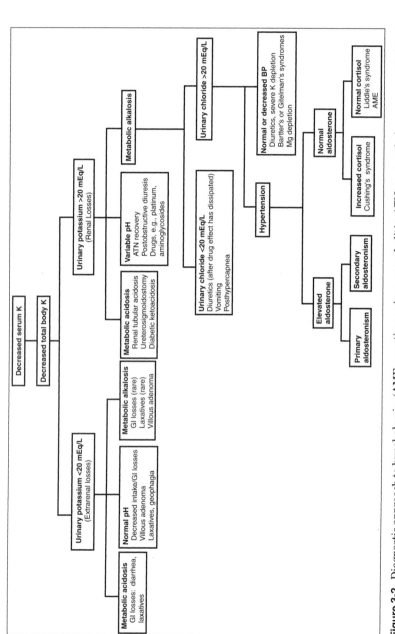

Figure 3-2. Diagnostic approach to hypokalemia. (AME, aseptic meningo-encephalitis; ATN, acute tubular necroses; BP, blood pressure; GI, gastrointestinal; K, potassium.)

Hypokalemia with renal potassium wasting, renal chloride wasting, and hypertension is further evaluated by urinary aldosterone concentrations. An elevated aldosterone level suggests either primary aldosteronism (adenoma, hyperplasia, glucocorticoid remedial) or secondary aldosteronism (renovascular or accelerated hypertension, diuretic use). Conversely, normal aldosterone levels with increases in serum cortisol suggest Cushing's syndrome or exogenous steroid use. Normal cortisol levels indicate Liddle's syndrome (caused by increases in the activity of the cortical collecting tubule sodium channel) or apparent mineralocorticoid excess syndrome [decreases in 11β hydroxy-steroid dehydrogenase activity in kidney tissue (congenital, licorice ingestion) causing the mineralocorticoid receptor to respond to glucocorticoid]. Increases in urinary potassium excretion without a significant acid-base disorder are seen during the recovery phase of acute tubular necrosis, postobstructive diuresis, and magnesium depletion associated with drugs such as aminoglycosides and cis-platinum, or in myelomonocytic leukemia (secondary to lysozymuria).

Finally, hypokalemia is frequently associated with chronic alcoholism. The mechanism behind this electrolyte abnormality is not well defined but is probably multifactorial secondary to poor intake, diarrhea, alcohol withdrawal with respiratory alkalosis, and kaliuresis associated with hypomagnesemia.

Although **cell-shift hypokalemia** and **decreases in total body potassium** do occur as isolated problems, they frequently occur **simultaneously.** Decreases in total body potassium potentiate the effects of drugs and hormones to shift potassium into cells. For example, small changes in potassium during insulin therapy may not cause hypokalemia if total body potassium is normal, but in the setting of total body potassium depletion (e.g., during the treatment of diabetic ketoacidosis or with diuretic use), cellular shifts of potassium during insulin therapy can result in profound hypokalemia.

B. The **manifestations** of hypokalemia are mainly cardiac and neuromuscular (Table 3-1). The most dramatic neuromuscular symptoms are paresis, paralysis, and respiratory failure. Potassium depletion causes supraventricular and ventricular arrhythmias, especially in patients on digitalis therapy. Although severe hypokalemia is more likely to cause complications, even minimal decreases in serum or total body potassium can be arrhythmogenic in patients with underlying heart disease or who are on digitalis therapy.

C. The **treatment** of hypokalemia depends on the underlying cause, the degree of potassium depletion, and the risk of potassium depletion to the patient. In general, hypokalemia secondary to cell shift is managed by treating underlying conditions. For example, hypokalemia in the setting of catecholamine increases, as in chest pain syndromes, is managed with appropriate treatments for the pain. However, when cell-shift hypokalemia is associated with life-threatening conditions such as paresis, paralysis, or hypokalemia in the setting of myocardial infarction, the administration of potassium is indicated. With potassium depletion, replacement therapy depends on the estimated degree of decreases in total body potassium. For example, decreases in total body potassium accompanied by a fall in serum potassium to 3.5 to 3.0 mEq per L are associated with a potassium deficit of 150 to 200 mEq. Decreases in serum potassium from 3 to 2 mEq per L are associated with 200- to 400-mEq additional decreases in total body potassium. Potassium can be administered intravenously, but in limited quantities (10 mEq per hour into a peripheral vein; 15 to 20 mEq per hour into a central vein). Larger potassium requirements can only be accomplished by oral therapy or with dialysis.

III. **Hyperkalemia**

A. The **approach** to hyperkalemia (Fig. 3-3) is to determine whether increases in serum potassium are spurious, caused by shifts of potassium from cellular to extracellular spaces, or represent a true increase in total body potassium.

Table 3-1. Clinical manifestations of hypokalemia

Cardiovascular
  Electrocardiographic abnormalities: U waves, QT prolongation, ST depression
    Predisposition to digitalis toxicity
    Atrial/ventricular arrhythmias
Neuromuscular
  Skeletal muscle
    Weakness
    Cramps
    Tetany
    Paralysis—flaccid
    Rhabdomyolysis
  Smooth muscle
    Constipation
    Ileus
    Urinary retention
Endocrine
  Carbohydrate intolerance
  Diabetes mellitus
  Decreased aldosterone
  Growth retardation
Renal/electrolyte
  Decreased renal blood flow, glomerular filtration rate
  Nephrogenic diabetes insipidus
  Increased ammoniagenesis (hepatic encephalopathy)
  Chloride wasting/metabolic alkalosis
  Cyst formation
  Interstitial nephritis
  Tubular vacuolization

Spurious hyperkalemia is caused by red blood cell hemolysis *in vitro*, ischemic blood draws, extreme thrombocytosis (greater than 1 million mL), or leukocytosis (greater than 50,000 mL). Spurious hyperkalemia is distinguished from true hyperkalemia by the absence of electrocardiographic (ECG) abnormalities. Hyperkalemia caused by **cell shifts** of potassium occurs acutely and results from decreased potassium transfer into cells (with decreases in insulin or beta-adrenergic blocker therapy), increased potassium movement from cells to the extracellular space (with metabolic acidosis), hypertonicity (with hyperglycemia or the administration of mannitol), exercise, muscle breakdown (with rhabdomyolysis), or drug intoxications from digitalis or succinylcholine.

Sustained hyperkalemia is caused by decreases in renal potassium excretion. This usually is not seen until the glomerular filtration rate is less than 20 mL per minute. However, it may be seen with less severe decreases in GFR when the kidney is challenged with a potassium load from potassium ingestion (e.g., diet, salt substitutes, or drugs, including potassium chloride and potassium citrate) and from increases in endogenous potassium production (e.g., GI bleed, resolving hematoma, rhabdomyolysis, catabolic states, tumor lysis). Hyperkalemia with less severe decreases in renal function is also associated with reductions in the distal nephron flow rate or low serum aldosterone levels as, for example, with hyporenin-hypoaldosteronism. Last, hyperkalemia is also associated with less severe decreases in GFR when drugs that alter potassium excretion [e.g., potassium-sparing diuretics, beta-adrenegic blockers, angiotensin-converting enzyme inhibitors, angiotensin receptor blockers, nonsteroidal anti-inflammatory drugs (NSAIDs)] are

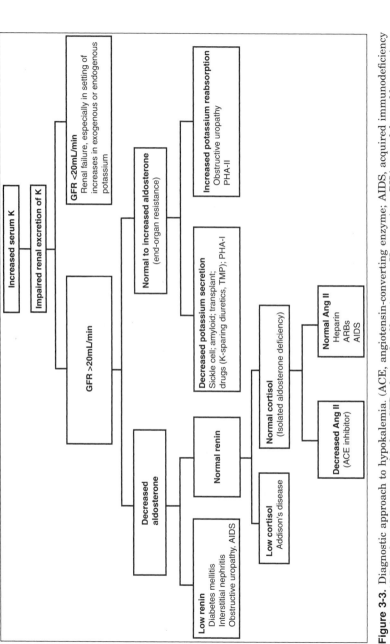

Figure 3-3. Diagnostic approach to hypokalemia. (ACE, angiotensin-converting enzyme; AIDS, acquired immunodeficiency syndrome; ARBs, adrenergic receptor binders; GFR, glomerular filtration rate; K, potassium; PHA, pseudohypoaldosteronism; TMP, trimethoprim-sulfa.)

Table 3-2. Commonly used medications causing hyperkalemia

Medication	Mechanism
Digitalis overdose	Inhibition of the Na-K-ATPase pump
Angiotensin II inhibitors	Decreased aldosterone excretion
NSAIDs	Blocks prostaglandin stimulation of renin
Trimethoprim	A cationic agent that decreases the number of open sodium channels in the luminal membrane of cortical collecting ducts
Pentamidine	Same mechanism as trimethoprim—blocks distal potassium excretion
Spirolactone	Competes for aldosterone receptor in collecting tubule
Amiloride	Blocks sodium channel
Heparin	Decrease aldosterone
Salt substitutes	Contain potassium
Succinylcholine	Moves potassium from intracellular to extracellular fluid
Cyclosporine	Multifactorial, including hyporenin hypoaldosteronism and interference with aldosterone action in the potassium-secreting cells of the cortical collecting duct
Pentamidine	Blocks distal potassium secretion

administered. Clinical studies also suggest that older adults are at increased risk for hyperkalemia. Although no clear explanation exists for this observation, it may be related to an age-associated decline in aldosterone synthesis or possibly a decline in tubular sensitivity to its action. Commonly used medications causing hyperkalemia are shown in Table 3-2.

Hyperkalemia also occurs in the **setting of a relatively well preserved GFR.** The causes of hyperkalemia in this setting are distinguished on the basis of plasma or urinary aldosterone levels. Decreases in aldosterone occur in the setting of normal, increased, or decreased plasma renin activity. Decreased plasma renin activity (hyporeninemic hypoaldosteronism) tends to occur in older adults and is associated with a number of renal diseases, including diabetes, interstitial nephritis (e.g., sickle cell anemia, analgesic use, heavy metal toxicity), obstructive uropathy, systemic lupus erythematosus, and amyloidosis. Decreases in plasma renin activity also are associated with acquired immunodeficiency syndrome (AIDS) nephropathy, transplantation, and medications including cyclosporine and NSAIDs. Hyperreninemic hypoaldosteronism also occurs both with decreases in cortisol production (Addison's disease) and with normal cortisol production when medications such as angiotensin-converting enzyme inhibitors, angiotensin receptor blockers, and heparin are used. Finally, increases in serum potassium can be associated with normal to high levels of aldosterone and endorgan resistance to aldosterone. Aldosterone resistance is caused by decreases in potassium secretion (drugs such as potassium-sparing diuretics, trimethoprim, and pentamidine), interstitial renal diseases (systemic lupus erythematosus, sickle cell anemia), obstructive uropathy, or transplantation. It also occurs in an unusual hereditary disease called *pseudohypoaldosteronism type 1,* in which the etiology is either a decrease in aldosterone receptor number or increases in the activity of the sodium chloride (NaCl) cotransporter in the distal convoluted tubule. With decreased activity of the cotransporter, sodium delivery to the distal tubule is decreased. Hyperkalemia in association with normal potassium secretion and increased potassium reabsorption occurs with obstructive uropathy.

B. Diagnosis. The **urinary potassium excretion rate** or **transtubular potassium gradient (TTKG)** (urine potassium divided by serum potassium divided by the ratio of urine osmolality to plasma osmolality) is used to distinguish renal from extrarenal causes of hyperkalemia (Table 3-2). Extrarenal causes of hyperkalemia (e.g., diet) are associated with increases in potassium excretion (24-hour urinary potassium excretion greater than 80 mEq per day and TTKG greater than 10). In contrast, renal causes of hyperkalemia (for example, Addison's disease) are associated with decreases in urinary potassium excretion (less than 20 mEq per day) and TTKG (less than 3). The administration of a mineralocorticoid (0.05 mg fludrocortisone) results in increases in urinary potassium excretion (greater than 40 mEq per day) and TTKG (greater than 7) in patients with aldosterone deficiency (Addison's disease) but no increases in urinary potassium excretion or in TTKG in patients with aldosterone resistance (e.g., sickle cell anemia).

C. The **clinical manifestations** of hyperkalemia are predominantly cardiac and neuromuscular. It is important to note that patients with hyperkalemia often present with vague GI complaints and nonspecific unwell feelings. Electrocardiogram (ECG) abnormalities include peak T waves, widened QRS interval, and asystole. Neuromuscular abnormalities include weakness, constipation, and paralysis.

D. The **treatment** of hyperkalemia (Fig. 3-4) depends on the presence or absence of ECG and neuromuscular abnormalities. In the absence of symptoms or ECG abnormalities, hyperkalemia is treated conservatively—for example, by decreasing dietary potassium or withdrawing offending drugs.

Figure 3-4. Treatment of hyperkalemia. (GFR, glomerular filtration rate; K, potassium.)

In the presence of ECG abnormalities or symptoms, the goal of therapy is to stabalize cell membranes. First-line therapy includes calcium gluconate, 10 to 30 mL as a 10% solution (onset of action 1 or 2 minutes). Although the mechanism remains undefined, calcium antagonizes the membranes and depolarizes effects of hyperkalemia. Other therapies include sodium bicarbonate, 50 to 150 mEq (onset 15 to 30 minutes) and insulin 5 to 10 units intravenously (onset 5 to 10 minutes), which increases the activity of the Na-K-ATPase pump in skeletal muscle and drives the potassium into cells. Glucose, 25 grams intravenously, is given simultanously to prevent hypoglycemia. Blood sugars should be monitored for approximately 6 hours to identify and treat hypoglycemia from the insulin. Albuterol nebulizer, 20 mg in 4 mL normal saline (onset 15 to 30 minutes), also activates the Na-K-ATPase and drives potassium into cells. Potassium driven intracellularly generally begins to move extracellularly again after approximately 6 hours, increasing the serum potassium concentration. Therefore, therapy to remove potassium from the body should be started simultaneously. Reductions in total body potassium may be achieved through a potassium exchange resin. The primary potassium resin used is sodium polystyrene sulfonate. One gram of this medication binds approximately 1 meq of potassium and releases 1 to 2 meq of sodium back into the circulation. This medication may be given orally (onset 2 hours) or by enema (onset 30 to 60 minutes). Finally, if indicated, hemodialysis is initiated, removing 25 to 30 mEq of potassium per hour.

Suggested readings

Allon M. Hyperkalemia in end stage renal disease: mechanisms and management. *J Am Soc Nephrol* 1995;6:1134–1142.

Ethier JH, Kanel KS, Magner PO, Lemann J, Halperin ML. The transtubular potassium concentration in patients with hypokalemia and hyperkalemia. *Am J Kidney Dis* 1990;15:309–315.

Gennari FJ. Hypokalemia. *N Engl J Med* 1998;339:451–458.

Halperin ML, Kamel SK. Electrolyte quintet: potassium. *Lancet* 1998;352:135–140.

Kamel KS, Halperin ML. Treatment of hypokalemia and hyperkalemia. In: Brady HR, Wilcox CS, eds. *Therapy in nephrology and hypertension.* Philadelphia: WB Saunders, 1999:270–278.

Kellerman PS, Linas SL. Disorders of potassium metabolism. In: Feehally J, Johnson R, eds. *Comprehensive clinical nephrology.* London: Mosby International, 1999.

Osorio FV, Linas SL. Disorders of potassium metabolism. In: Schrier RW, ed. *Atlas of diseases of the kidney,* vol 1. Philadelphia: Blackwell Science, 1998:sec 1.

Oster JR, Singer I, Fishman LM. Heparin-induced aldosterone suppression and hyperkalemia. *Am J Med* 1995;98:575–586.

Perazella MA, Mahnensmith RL. Hyperkalemia in the elderly. *JGIM.* 1997;10:646–656.

Perazella M, Rastegar Asghar. Disorders of potassium and acid–base metabolism in association with renal disease. In Schrier RW, ed. *Diseases of the kidney and urinary tract,* 7th ed. Philadelphia: Lippincott Williams & Wilkins, 2001:2577–2606.

Peterson L, Levi M. Disorders of potassium metabolism. In: Schrier RW, ed. *Renal and electrolyte disorders,* 6th ed. Philadelphia: Lippincott Williams & Wilkins, 2003:171–215.

Moonseong QH, Heshka S, Wang J, et al. Total body potassium differs by sex and age across the adult like span. *Am J Clin Nutri* 2003;78:72–77.

Weiner ID, Linas SL, Wingo CS. Disorders of potassium metabolism. In: Johnson RJ, Feehally JF, ed. *Comprehensive clinical nephrology,* 2nd ed. St. Louis: Mosby, 2003;109–121.

Weiner ID, Wingo CS. Hyperkalemia: a potential silent killer. *J Am Soc Nephrol* 1998;9:1535–1543.

Weiner ID, Wingo CS. Hypokalemia: consequences, causes, and correction. *J Am Soc Nephrol* 1997;8:1179–1188.

The Patient with an Acid-Base Disorder

William D. Kaehny

I. **Acid-base disorders** occur commonly in hospitalized patients and are important markers of an underlying disordered physiology. Occasionally, acid-base disorders disrupt homeostasis sufficiently to move the arterial pH into a dangerous range (less than 7.10 or greater than 7.60). Depending on the overall status of the patient and the response of the cardiovascular system, the pH level may require direct attention. After the clinician is alerted to the presence of an acid-base disorder by clinical and laboratory clues, a logical progression of analysis leads to optimal management of the patient.

   A. **Step 1.** Measure pH. This identifies **acidemia or alkalemia.** The change in bicarbonate and partial pressure of CO_2 (PCO_2) indicates whether the primary process is metabolic or respiratory.

   B. **Step 2.** Check the compensatory or secondary response of the PCO_2 or HCO_3^- to see if the disorder is **simple** or **mixed.**

   C. **Step 3.** Calculate the serum **anion gap** (AG) to screen for an increase in organic anions such as lactate. Add any increase in AG (ΔAG) that is **potential HCO_3^-** to the serum total carbon dioxide (CO_2) content (tCO_2) to screen for a hidden metabolic alkalosis.

   D. **Step 4.** Determine the **cause** of the acid-base disorder from the clinical setting and laboratory tests.

   E. **Step 5. Treat** the underlying disorder, unless the pH is dangerous either acutely or chronically (such as acidosis affecting bone).

II. **When to suspect acid-base disorders**

   A. **Clinical.** The underlying cause of the acid-base disorder is most frequently responsible for a patient's signs and symptoms. Certain clinical settings and findings should alert the clinician to the likelihood of an acid-base disorder. Coma, seizures, congestive heart failure, shock, vomiting, diarrhea, and renal failure generate changes in the PCO_2 or HCO_3^- levels. Marked changes in the pH occasionally may cause direct clinical manifestations. Severe alkalemia causes an irritability of heart and skeletal muscle. Severe acidemia causes a depression of heart pump function and vascular tone. Although central nervous system dysfunction appears frequently with acid-base disorders, changes in pH do not appear responsible. Rather, altered plasma osmolality and PCO_2 appear to be the causative agents.

   B. **Laboratory.** A thoughtful measurement of serum electrolytes in patients with abnormal losses or gains of body fluids is good practice. An abnormal serum tCO_2 is definite evidence of an acid-base disorder; an abnormal serum AG is very suggestive; an abnormal serum potassium is suspicious.

   1. **Serum tCO_2.** The HCO_3^- in blood can be estimated reasonably by measuring the tCO_2 in venous serum. Acid is added to the serum to release CO_2 from HCO_3^- plus dissolved CO_2, carbonate, and carbonic acid. The CO_2 diffuses into a buffer solution and causes the pH to change. This change is translated into tCO_2 in mmol per L. The serum tCO_2 is 1 to 3 mmol per L greater than the arterial HCO_3^- because it is from venous blood, which has more HCO_3^-, and it includes more than HCO_3^-. Normal sea level serum tCO_2 levels average 26 to 27 mmol per L. A value below 24 or above 30 likely marks a clinical acid-base disorder. An acid-base disorder of the mixed type may exist with a normal serum tCO_2.

2. The **serum anion gap** is calculated from the venous serum sodium, chloride, and tCO_2:

$$AG = Na^+ - (Cl^- + tCO_2)$$

The units are mEq per L, because this calculation estimates the charge difference between the so-called unmeasured anions (serum total anions represented by Cl^- and HCO_3^-) and unmeasured cations (total cations represented by Na^+). The average normal value is 9 ± 3 mEq per L, but may vary in a given laboratory. Albumin contributes most to the AG. A fall in serum albumin of 1 g per dL from a normal of 4.5 decreases the AG by 2.5 mEq per L.

   a. **Metabolic acidosis** due to an organic acid such as lactic or acetoacetic acid is marked by an increased AG. An increase in the AG of 8 mEq per L to 17 or higher usually indicates the presence of organic acidosis, although at times the exact anion may not be identified. The anion of the organic acid replaces the HCO_3^- lost in the buffering of the hydrogen ion (H^+) part of the acid and thus increases the unmeasured anions. Importantly, a normal or slightly elevated AG does not rule out the presence of organic metabolic acidosis, such as diabetic ketoacidosis, because a patient with good renal perfusion and ample urine flow may excrete the ketoanions at a rate sufficient to keep the serum AG from rising markedly.

   b. **Metabolic alkalosis.** At times, a metabolic acidosis that increases the AG and lowers the HCO_3^- may coincide with a process that generates a metabolic alkalosis. For example, vomiting that generates a high HCO_3^- may be caused by diabetic ketoacidosis, which lowers the HCO_3^-. In this case, the serum tCO_2 (and arterial HCO_3^-) may be low or normal despite the elevating action of the metabolic alkalosis. The clue to the presence of such hidden metabolic alkalosis is derived in a holmesian fashion by adding the measured serum tCO_2 and the ΔAG (measured AG – 9). If this sum is greater than 30 mEq per L, a hidden metabolic alkalosis is likely present. The ΔAG is a marker of "lost" or potential HCO_3^-, that which was titrated by the H^+ of an organic acid. Pure metabolic alkalosis may directly increase the AG by up to 5 mEq per L due to effects on the albumin concentration and charge.

3. **Serum potassium.** Potassium metabolism is linked to acid-base metabolism at the levels of cell shifts, renal tubular functions, and gastrointestinal transport. Therefore, an abnormal serum potassium concentration alerts the clinician to the likelihood that an acid-base disorder is present also.

III. **Identifying the major acid-base disorders.** When the clinician suspects that an acid-base disorder might be present and that patient management might be adjusted, a set of acid-base variables should be obtained: pH, PCO_2, and HCO_3^-.

A. **Chemistry and physiology** of acid-base. Cellular, tissue, and organ systems apparently function best at an extracellular fluid (ECF) pH of around 7.40. Intracellular fluid (ICF) pH is heterogeneous within the cell, depending on organelles and metabolic activity, but averages around 7.00. ECF pH is a function of the state of available buffers, those molecules that respond to changes in pH by binding or releasing H^+ to keep pH close to 7.40. Thus, buffers prevent extreme shifts in pH in the face of the gain or loss of acids or bases.

   1. **Blood pH** is the mathematical expression of the intensity of acidity or H^+ activity. It can be translated into H^+ concentration in mol per L:

$$pH = -\log[H^+] \text{ or } [H^+] = 10^{-pH}$$

H^+ concentration usually is expressed in nmol per L. H^+ concentration is 100 nmol per L at pH 7.00 and 40 nmol per L at pH 7.40. Within the pH range of 7.26 to 7.45, H^+ concentration is estimated accurately as (80 – the decimal of pH). For example, at pH 7.32, H^+ equals 80 minus 32 or 48 nmol per L. The pH is measured at body temperature with a glass, flow-through electrode.

2. The **partial pressure of carbon dioxide in blood,** PCO_2, represents the respiratory component in blood. The respiratory system determines the level at which the PCO_2 is set. PCO_2 substitutes for the buffer carbonic acid, H_2CO_3, in the acid-base equation. H_2CO_3 is formed from water and CO_2. PCO_2 is measured in whole blood with a pH electrode that detects the change caused by the diffusion of CO_2 from the sample into a buffer solution.

3. HCO_3^- is the metabolic component of the acid-base equation, serving as the base of the H^+-binding partner in the buffer pair. HCO_3^- concentration is controlled by the buffering state, metabolic processes, and the kidneys. HCO_3^- concentration is calculated from the pH and PCO_2 using the Henderson-Hasselbalch equation. The fact that it is calculated makes it no less reliable a value than the serum tCO_2, which is also calculated.

4. The **acid-base equation** allows the determination of the state of ECF acid-base balance, the presence of an acid-base disorder, the nature of the disorder, and the presence of a simple or mixed disorder:

$$pH = \text{constant} \times [HCO_3^-]/PCO_2$$

Thus, the pH level depends on the ratio or mathematical relationship between the HCO_3^- and the PCO_2. An acid-base disorder is generated by an alteration from normal of either of these two factors. The resultant change in pH results in chemical shifts in the buffers, which mitigate the change in pH somewhat. A physiologic response occurs in the respiratory system for a metabolic disorder and in the kidneys for a respiratory disorder. A new steady state ensues, with the new pH set by the new values of the HCO_3^- concentration and PCO_2.

B. **Measurement of acid-base variables.** The determination of the acid-base state usually is based on an analysis of arterial blood, although arterialized venous blood analysis is equally valid. After warming the extremity, blood is drawn without air mixing from an artery or from a forearm vein without tourniquet. Although experimental studies show that ICF pH and mixed venous acid-base measurements correlate with organ function, arterial blood measurements are easily available and provide a readily interpretable view of the metabolic state of organs and their function. Keep in mind that tissue hypoperfusion, as in cardiopulmonary arrest or profound shock, makes tissue acidosis worse than that reflected by arterial blood acid-base values.

1. **Calculation of HCO_3^-** from pH and PCO_2. Arterial HCO_3^- is 1 to 3 mmol per L less than venous tCO_2. To calculate the HCO_3^- or verify the reported value, convert the pH to H^+ and use a simplified form of the Henderson equation:

$$HCO_3^- = 24 \times PCO_2/H^+$$

C. **Identification of a major acid-base disorder.** The basis of this approach is to determine the direction (up or down) in which the measured values differ from the arbitrary normal values for pH (7.40), PCO_2 (40 mm Hg), and HCO_3^- (24 mmol per L). First, determine if acidemia (pH down) or alkalemia (pH up) is present. Then determine if the primary generating change was in the HCO_3^- or in the PCO_2 (Table 4-1). The compensating

Table 4-1. Simple acid-base disorders

	Metabolic acidosis	Metabolic alkalosis	Respiratory acidosis	Respiratory alkalosis
Primary change	$\downarrow HCO_3^-$	$\uparrow HCO_3^-$	$\uparrow Pco_2$	$\downarrow Pco_2$
Compensation	$\downarrow Pco_2$	$\uparrow Pco_2$	$\uparrow HCO_3^-$	$\downarrow HCO_3^-$
Effect on pH	$\downarrow pH$	$\uparrow pH$	$\downarrow pH$	$\uparrow pH$

$\downarrow$ decreased; $\uparrow$ increased.

factor should change in the same direction as the generating factor to yield a simple acid-base disorder.

1. **Example of a simple disorder.** Arterial blood analysis revealed the following values: pH 7.55, HCO_3^- 18 mmol per L, PCO_2 21 mm Hg.
   a. **Step 1.** The pH is up. Thus, alkalemia is present and must be due to an increased HCO_3^- (as in metabolic alkalosis) or to a decreased PCO_2 (as in respiratory alkalosis).
   b. **Step 2.** The HCO_3^- is low and cannot be responsible for an increased pH.
   c. **Step 3.** Because the PCO_2 is low, it can account for the increased pH; this is respiratory alkalosis.
   d. **Step 4.** The HCO_3^- change is in same direction as that of the PCO_2; this is consistent with a simple respiratory alkalosis.
2. **Example of a mixed acid-base disorder.** Sampling of arterial blood yielded the following: pH 7.55, HCO_3^- 30 mmol per L, and PCO_2 35 mm Hg.
   a. **Step 1.** The pH is up. Thus, alkalemia is present.
   b. **Step 2.** The HCO_3^- is increased and may be responsible for the increased pH.
   c. **Step 3.** The PCO_2 is low and it, too, can account for an increased pH.
   d. **Step 4.** The two acid-base determinants are changed from normal in opposite directions. Thus, this is mixed metabolic and respiratory alkalosis. The metabolic alkalosis is dominant because the percent change in HCO_3^- is 6/24 or 25% whereas the percent change in PCO_2 is 5/40 or 12.5%.
IV. **Judging whether an acid-base disorder is simple or mixed.** When an underlying process generates an acid-base disorder by perturbing one member of the $HCO_3^- - PCO_2$ buffer pair (remember that PCO_2 represents H_2CO_3), the other partner is adjusted by the physiologic response of the body and changes in the same direction as the primary partner in order to reduce the magnitude of the change in pH. The time-honored term for this physiologic response is *compensation*. However, the physiologic response mechanisms may be activated by stimuli other than pH and actually may contribute to the maintenance of the abnormal pH. Thus, some have termed these responses maladaptive, because they are not always truly compensatory. For example, a low PCO_2 in response to metabolic acidosis actually causes the kidneys to reduce HCO_3^- reabsorption. Importantly, compensation does not restore the pH to normal, because that would shut off the stimulus for the compensatory mechanism.
   A. **Steps in judging whether an acid-base disorder is simple.** After the major disorder is identified, determine whether the compensation for the primary event is appropriate.
      1. **Check directions of changes from normal of HCO_3^- and PCO_2.** The acid-base buffer pair change from normal in the same direction in all simple acid-base disorders. If they change in opposite directions, the disorder must be mixed. This step was discussed in section **III.C.2.d.**
      2. **Compare the magnitude of the compensation of the PCO_2 or HCO_3^- with the primary change in the HCO_3^- or PCO_2.** In metabolic disorders,

Table 4-2. Appropriate compensations in the acid-base disorders

	Change in PCO_2 per change in HCO_3^-	Change in pH per change in HCO_3^-
Metabolic acidosis	1.0–1.5 per 1	0.010 per 1
Metabolic alkalosis	0.25–1.00 per 1	0.015 per 1

	Change in HCO_3^- per change in PCO_2	Change in pH per change in PCO_2
Respiratory acidosis		
Acute	1 per 10	0.08 per 10
Chronic	4 per 10	0.03 per 10
Respiratory alkalosis		
Acute	1 per 10	0.08 per 10
Chronic	4 per 10	0.03 per 10

the primary change occurs in the HCO_3^-, with the compensation occurring in the PCO_2. The opposite is true in the respiratory disorders. Table 4-2 contains guidelines or rules that can be used to judge whether compensation is appropriate. The respiratory disorders have two stages of compensation: acute, when only tissue buffering slightly changes the HCO_3^-, and chronic (after 24 hours), when the kidneys cause major changes in the HCO_3^- concentration. If the measured change in the compensating factor does not approximate the change predicted, a mixed disorder is likely. Two methods of predicting compensation appear in Table 4-2. One describes the expected changes in the buffer partner for a given change in the generating partner. For example, a fall in HCO_3^- of 10 mmol per L in metabolic acidosis is expected to result in hyperventilation that drops the PCO_2 by 10 to 15 mm Hg to 25 to 30 mm Hg. The other method relates the primary, generating factor change to a change in pH. For example, a fall in HCO_3^- of 10 mmol per L in metabolic acidosis is expected to decrease the pH by 0.1 to 7.30.

3. **Check the anion gap for evidence of a hidden metabolic disorder.** An increase in the AG of more than 8 mEq per L to greater than 17 suggests the presence of metabolic acidosis due to an organic acid. Also if the ΔAG is added to the measured serum tCO_2, the theoretical maximum serum tCO_2 can be estimated. A value greater than 30 mmol per L suggests metabolic alkalosis.

B. **Application of the rules**

1. The **primary event in metabolic acidosis** is a fall in HCO_3^-; the **compensation** is a fall in the PCO_2, due to the stimulation of central nervous system receptors by the low pH. Hyperventilation increases the excretion of CO_2, and PCO_2 falls. For example, if the HCO_3^- falls from 24 mmol per L by 10 to 14 mmol per L, the PCO_2 should fall by 1.0 to 1.5 times as much, or 10 to 15 mm Hg, to a level of 25 to 30 mm Hg ($40 - 10 = 30$; $40 - 15 = 25$).

2. The **primary event in metabolic alkalosis** is a rise in HCO_3^-. The respiratory system responds to the rise in pH with hypoventilation, which reduces carbon dioxide excretion and results in a rise in PCO_2. For example, if HCO_3^- rises by 16 mmol per L from 24 to 40 mmol per L, the PCO_2 should rise by 0.25 to 1.00 multiplied by the rise in HCO_3^- of 16, or by 4 to 16 mm Hg, to a level of 44 to 56 mm Hg ($40 + 4 = 44$; $40 + 16 = 56$). This response is tempered by the body's response to the concomitant hypoxemia resulting from hypoventilation.

3. The **primary event in respiratory acidosis** is a rise in PCO_2. During the acute phase (up to 24 hours), only buffering contributes measurably

to the response. The HCO_3^- should increase, but not to as high as 30 mmol per L. In contrast, the kidneys respond to chronic elevations of PCO_2 by generating sufficient HCO_3^- to prevent the pH from falling to less than 7.20, even in the most severe cases of chronic respiratory acidosis.

4. The **primary event in respiratory alkalosis** is a fall in PCO_2. Initially, buffering occurs as a result of the release of H^+ from cells; later (hours) the kidneys dump HCO_3^- into the urine, with a resultant fall in blood HCO_3^-, as defined in Table 4-2.

C. **Effects of respiratory responses to metabolic disorders.** The kidneys respond to changes in PCO_2 regardless of the pH. A fall in PCO_2 causes renal HCO_3^- loss; a rise in PCO_2 causes renal HCO_3^- generation. Thus, in chronic metabolic acidosis (lasting days), some of the reduction in bicarbonate actually is due to the compensatory fall in PCO_2 and not directly to the process causing the metabolic acidosis. Similarly, the increase in PCO_2 in chronic metabolic alkalosis contributes to the hyperbicarbonatemia.

D. **Examples of mixed acid-base disorders.** Four combinations of the "double" mixed acid-base disorders are possible. Two are important because they cause drastic changes in pH: metabolic and respiratory acidosis and metabolic and respiratory alkalosis. The other two disorders tend to be associated with pH values close to normal and are not dangerous per se; however, they are important markers of underlying disease. Two other mixed disorders, so-called *triple disorders,* also have been described. The anion gap points to both metabolic acidosis and alkalosis developing simultaneously or sequentially in these. The imposition of a respiratory disorder yields the infamous triple acid-base disorder.

1. **Metabolic acidosis and respiratory acidosis.** A patient with emphysema and carbon dioxide retention (chronic respiratory acidosis) develops diarrhea (metabolic acidosis). Note how the reduction in HCO_3^- to normal results in severe acidemia (Table 4-3).

2. **Metabolic alkalosis and respiratory acidosis.** The same emphysematous patient is given a diuretic for cor pulmonale. The bicarbonate level rises from 40 to 48 mmol per L, which, with the PCO_2 at 80 mm Hg, sets the pH at 7.40. Although this is a normal pH, some believe it is better for carbon dioxide-retaining patients to be mildly acidemic to keep ventilation stimulated.

3. **Triple acid-base disorder.** A more common mixture of disorders involves metabolic acidosis developing in a patient with metabolic alkalosis and superimposed respiratory alkalosis. For example, a patient with metabolic alkalosis (HCO_3^- 32) from nasogastric suction becomes septic, which generates both lactic acidosis and pronounced hyperventilation, thus causing independent respiratory alkalosis due to endotoxin (Table 4-4). Note that both the metabolic and respiratory alkaloses should cause only small increases in the anion gap. The lactic acidosis of septic shock results in a fall of from 32 to 24 mmol per L in the HCO_3^- with a reciprocal increase in anion gap. The anion gap of 33 is diagnostic of organic acidosis. The ΔAG of 26 (35–9) added to the serum tCO_2 of 9 yields 35 mmol per L, an estimate of the value before acidosis, indicative of metabolic alkalosis. The evidence for the presence of respiratory

Table 4-3. Example of a mixed acid-base disorder

	Health	Emphysema	Emphysema and diarrhea
pH	7.40	7.32	7.10
PCO_2	40	80	80
HCO_3^-	24	40	24

Table 4-4. Example of a triple mixed acid-base disorder

	Health	Nasogastric suction	Septic shock	Endotoxemia
pH	7.40	7.49	7.14	7.44
Pco_2	40	44	24	12
HCO_3^-	24	32	8	8
Anion gap	9	11	33	35
Venous total carbon dioxide	26	35	9	9
Disorder		Metabolic alkalosis	Metabolic alkalosis	Metabolic alkalosis
			Metabolic acidosis	Metabolic acidosis
				Respiratory alkalosis

alkalosis is the high pH and low PCO_2 due to the hyperventilation caused by endotoxemia.

V. Identify the underlying cause of an acid-base disorder. Usually, the cause of an acid-base disorder is obvious from the history, examination, and clinical course. However, on occasion, careful review of a thoughtful differential diagnosis is necessary to identify a remote causative disorder.

A. Causes of metabolic acidosis. The anion gap is used to divide the causes of metabolic acidosis into those with influx of organic acid into plasma (increased anion gap) and those with external losses of bicarbonate (normal anion gap; hyperchloremic). Some disorders belong to both groups at different stages (diabetic ketoacidosis) or are generated by mechanisms other than those described (renal failure). A list of causes is given in Table 4-5.

1. Metabolic acidosis with increased anion gap. Severe metabolic acidosis is caused by only three broad groups of disorders: ketoacidosis, lactic acidosis, and poisonings. In addition, renal failure may cause mild to moderate acidosis. This yields the mnemonic KlaPR (pronounced clapper) for **k**etoacidosis, **l**actic **a**cidosis, **p**oisonings, **r**enal failure.

a. Ketoacidosis arises when glucose is not available to cells because of insulin lack, cell dysfunction, or glucose depletion, and fatty acids are oxidized to yield energy, acetone (not an acid), and the two ketoacids (acetoacetic and beta-hydroxybutyric). The H^+ produced are consumed (buffered) by HCO_3^-, producing carbonic acid, which dehydrates into water and carbon dioxide. The ketoanions accumulate in the serum in place of the HCO_3^-, further increasing the anion gap. The diagnostic test for ketoacidosis consists of testing the serum with a nitroprusside reagent, which only reacts with the acetoacetate. In diabetic ketoacidosis, the beta-hydroxybutyrate-acetoacetate ratio averages 5 to 2, whereas in alcoholic ketoacidosis, it may reach as high as 20 to 1. In these cases, only urine, a concentrate of serum, may have a concentration of acetoacetate high enough to give a positive purple reaction with the reagent. **Diabetic ketoacidosis** occurs because of insulin deficiency. Hyperglycemia may be corrected by volume re-expansion, but insulin is needed to stop ketogenesis. Volume expansion enhances the renal excretion of ketoanions, thus correcting the increased anion gap. However, the kidneys take time to generate new HCO_3^- to replace that lost earlier in buffering H^+. Thus, early in diabetic ketoacidosis, the anion gap usually is increased; during correction, the anion

Table 4-5. Causes of metabolic acidosis

High anion gap type
Ketoacidosis
  Diabetic
  Alcoholic
  Starvation
Lactic acidosis
  Type A
  Type B
  D-Lactic acidosis
Poisonings
  Ethylene glycol
  Methanol
  Salicylate
Advanced renal failure
Normal anion gap type
Gastrointestinal HCO_3^- loss
  Diarrhea
  External fistulae
Renal HCO_3^- loss
  Acetazolamide
  Proximal renal tubular acidosis (RTA)
  Distal RTA
  Hyperkalemic RTA
Miscellaneous
  NH_4Cl ingestion
  Sulfur ingestion
  Toluene inhalation
  Pronounced dilution

gap may return to normal despite a low HCO_3^-. Chloride replaces the ketoanions, and this stage is therefore called hyperchloremic or normal anion gap metabolic acidosis. **Alcoholic ketacidosis** occurs because of volume depletion, which causes the α-adrenergic suppression of insulin release. The patient relates a story of severe vomiting following recently increased alcohol intake. Urine ketones are usually positive. Blood glucose ranges between 50 and 250 mg per dL. **Starvation** ketoacidosis occurs because of the use of fatty acids for energy maintenance. The degree of acidosis is mild, with arterial HCO_3^- not less than 18 mmol per L.

  b. **Lactic acidosis** arises when oxygen delivery to cells is inadequate for the demand (type A) or cell processes cannot use oxygen (type B). In this situation, glucose is metabolized via anaerobic glycolysis to pyruvate and then to the dead-end metabolite lactate. The H^+ produced from nicotinamide adenine dinucleotide (NADH) (one per lactate) are buffered by HCO_3^-, which is replaced in the blood by lactate. Thus, the anion gap is increased. **Type A lactic acidosis** is caused by the primary inadequate delivery of oxygen to tissues. Shock is the most common mechanism. Hypovolemia, heart failure, and sepsis cause shock. Because carbon monoxide binds more avidly to hemoglobin than does oxygen, carbon monoxide poisoning can cause varying degrees of lactic acidosis. **Type B lactic acidosis** occurs when tissue oxygenation is normal but tissues cannot use the oxygen normally or need excessive amounts of oxygen. Causes of type B lactic acidosis include hepatic failure, malignancy drugs, and seizures. Metformin is a biguanide hypoglycemic agent that rarely (8 per 100,000) causes lactic acidosis in contrast to its relative, phenformin. Renal, liver, and heart failure are risk factors. Reverse transcriptase inhibitors for AIDS also are rare causes of lactic acidosis due to injury to cell mitochondria. Lactic acidosis has been seen in patients receiving large intravenous doses of lorazepam and diazepam due to the propylene glycol solvent. **D-lactic acidosis** is generated when colon bacteria metabolize malabsorbed sugars into both L- and D-lactate, which accumulates in the blood. The clinical manifestation is metabolic encephalopathy. At least two dozen inborn errors of metabolism result in pediatric lactic acidosis. The diagnosis is usually established by exclusion of ketoacidosis, intoxications, and advanced renal failure as causes for a high anion gap metabolic acidosis. L-lactate can be measured by an automated assay, but measurement is often unnecessary.

c. Three modern **poisonings** cause high anion gap metabolic acidosis: **ethylene glycol ingestion, methanol ingestion**, and **salicylate intoxication.** Methanol and ethylene glycol are low-molecular-weight alcohols that readily enter cells. Metabolism generates H^+ that cause acidosis and formate (with methanol) or glycolate (with ethylene glycol) that causes a high anion gap. A clue to the presence of early stages of acidosis with elevated alcohol levels is an increased osmolal gap. This gap is the difference between the measured serum osmolality and the calculated osmolality (calc Sosm).

$$\text{Calc Sosm} = 2 \times [Na^+] + [\text{glucose}]/18 + [\text{urea nitrogen}]/2.8$$
$$+ [\text{ethanol}]/4.6$$

If this difference is greater than 25 mOsm per kg of serum, the presence of a toxic alcohol is likely. Needlelike or envelope-shaped calcium oxalate crystals in the urine suggest ethylene glycol ingestion. The combination of high anion gap metabolic acidosis and a high osmolal gap is an indication for specific analysis for methanol and ethylene glycol. The decision to measure levels of these alcohols, of course, must be tempered by the clinical setting. Salicylate intoxication is an important frequent unintentional chronic or intentional acute overdose that causes metabolic acidosis, respiratory alkalosis, or a mixed disorder. It should be suspected at the extremes of age.

d. **Renal failure.** Failure to excrete the daily acid load of 1 mmol per kg of body weight that is generated by metabolism results in metabolic acidosis. Bone buffers take up some hydrogen ions during chronic renal failure, and, thus, the degree of acidosis is moderated until the end stages of disease. Arterial bicarbonate usually remains above 15 mmol per L. In acute renal failure, venous tCO_2 or arterial HCO_3^- falls by about 0.5 mmol per L per day unless hypercatabolism increases daily acid production. The anion gap increases less than the HCO_3^- falls, resulting in hyperchloremic metabolic acidosis in early and middle stages of chronic renal failure. In advanced chronic renal failure, the serum anion gap rises about 0.5 mEq per L for each 1.0 mg per dL rise in serum creatinine. Retention of sulfate, phosphate, and organic anions causes the increase in anion gap.

2. **Metabolic acidosis with normal anion gap (hyperchloremic)** can be caused by three groups of disorders: gastrointestinal HCO_3^- loss, renal HCO_3^- loss or acid retention, and inorganic acid intake.

a. **Gastrointestinal bicarbonate loss.** The gastrointestinal tract distal to the stomach has the capacity to absorb chloride and secrete bicarbonate. Thus, diarrhea and external drainage of pancreatic, biliary, or small-bowel juices can cause external losses of bicarbonate-rich fluid. Relatively chloride-rich fluid remains behind. This generates hyperchloremic metabolic acidosis (normal anion gap). An interesting variety of this disorder occurs when normal urine, rich in sodium chloride (NaCl) from dietary sources, is drained into the gut via ureterosigmoidostomy or ileal loop conduit (both bladder replacement constructions). If contact time with mucosa is excessive, the gut reabsorbs the chloride in exchange for bicarbonate, resulting in hyperchloremic metabolic acidosis.

b. Renal bicarbonate loss. The proximal renal tubule reabsorbs the bulk (85%) of filtered HCO_3^-. The carbonic anhydrase inhibitor **acetazolamide** blocks much of this reabsorption, resulting in urinary bicarbonate losses until arterial HCO_3^- falls to 16 to 18 mmol per L. The filtered load of HCO_3^- at this concentration can be completely reabsorbed by the distal nephron. Thus, the urine becomes bicarbonate-free, with an acidic pH, in this new steady state. **Proximal renal tubular acidosis** (old type II RTA), a defect in proximal tubular HCO_3^- reabsorption, has identical features. Proximal RTA is unusual but may occur with Wilson's disease, multiple myeloma, transplant rejection, and in other disease states. **Distal RTA** (old type I) differs in that it is a defect of the collecting duct, in which the daily metabolic acid load is not excreted totally and a small HCO_3^- leak occurs every day. This leads to a mild-to-moderate normal anion gap, hyperchloremic metabolic acidosis, and hypercalciuria with calcium stones or nephrocalcinosis. Two varieties occur: **hypokalemic distal RTA and hyperkalemic distal RTA.** Hypokalemic distal RTA occurs when collecting duct potassium secretion is intact and in fact enhanced by the small amount of bicarbonaturia. Hyperkalemic distal RTA occurs due to two distinct mechanisms when collecting duct hydrogen ion and potassium secretion are impaired: hypoaldosteronism (old type IV RTA) or tubular defect. Hypokalemic distal RTA occurs with amphotericin B toxicity, cirrhosis of the liver, medullary sponge kidney, and many other diseases. Chronic obstruction of the kidney, lupus erythematosus, and sickle cell disease can cause the tubular defect type of hyperkalemic distal RTA. Diabetes mellitus, mild chronic renal failure, and old age are associated with the hyporeninemic hypoaldosteronism type of hyperkalemic distal RTA. Diagnosis of RTA is made by eliminating non-renal causes for a normal anion gap metabolic acidosis (e.g., diarrhea). Proximal RTA is characterized by urinary wasting of more than 5% to 15% of the filtered load of HCO_3^- when serum levels are maintained close to normal. Hypokalemic distal RTA is characterized by the inability to decrease urine pH to less than 5.4 with an oral acid load of ammonium chloride. Hyperkalemic normal ion gap metabolic acidosis almost always is due to distal RTA. The tubular defect type is marked by an inability to acidify maximally (urine pH usually above 6.0), in contrast to the hypoaldosteronism type, in which the intensity of acidification is intact (urine pH can fall lower than 5.5). In both types, renal ammonium excretion is reduced, and the urine anion gap often is positive (see section **V.A.2.d**).

c. Inorganic acid intake. The ingestion of ammonium chloride to reduce appetite or acidify urine produces hyperchloremic metabolic acidosis. Inorganic sulfur, such as flowers of sulfur cathartic, is oxidized to form H_2SO_4. The hydrogen ions titrate the HCO_3^- down, and the sulfate is excreted rapidly with sodium. This leaves a low HCO_3^- with a normal anion gap. A similar process happens with toluene inhalation from paint or glue sniffing. Toluene is metabolized to hippuric acid, and the hippurate is excreted rapidly.

d. On occasion, the **urinary anion gap** (UAG) may help to distinguish gastrointestinal from renal loss of HCO_3^- as the cause of hyperchloremic metabolic acidosis:

$$UAG = (Na^+ + K^+) - Cl^-.$$

The UAG is an estimate of urinary ammonium that is elevated in gastrointestinal HCO_3^- loss but low in distal RTA. UAG is a negative value if urine ammonium is high (as in diarrhea; average, -20 mEq per L), whereas it is positive if urine ammonium is low (as in distal RTA; average, $+23$ mEq per L).

B. Causes of metabolic alkalosis. Metabolic alkalosis is characterized by a low urine Cl^-, indicating the avidity of the kidney for solute, largely NaCl. During the generation phases of metabolic alkalosis, bicarbonaturia may occur and necessitate Na^+ and K^+ excretion. Thus, urine Cl^- is a better marker than urine Na^+ of the stimulation of renal salt reabsorption by volume depletion. During the maintenance stage of metabolic alkalosis, bicarbonaturia is minimal, urine pH is acid, and urine Na^+ is low. Volume-depleted metabolic alkalosis is due to external losses of hydrogen ion or chloride. Volume-replete metabolic alkalosis is characterized by spot urine Cl^- of usually well over 20 mmol per L. The kidney is not avid for salt because of volume expansion (mild) and thus excretes the daily Na^+ and Cl^- load without difficulty. This group of disorders is due to hypermineralocorticoidism or profound potassium depletion.

1. **Metabolic alkaloses of the volume-depleted variety** have in common the external loss of fluids rich in H^+ or Cl^-. The stomach, kidney, or skin may be the culprit (Table 4-6).

2. **Metabolic alkaloses of the volume-replete variety** are characterized by enhanced renal H^+ secretion despite normal or increased ECF volume. The stimulus for this sustained H^+ secretion is aldosterone (or a relative) or major cellular potassium depletion (see Table 4-6). Gitelman's syndrome is an autosomal recessive disorder usually appearing in adults as hypokalemic, hypomagnesemic metabolic alkalosis. The distal convoluted tubule Na^+Cl^- cotransporter is defective. In contrast, Bartter's syndrome appears in childhood as hypokalemic metabolic alkalosis. In this syndrome, defects in loop of Henle Na^+Cl^- reabsorption lead to normotensive secondary hyperaldosteronism. Diuretic abuse resembles these disorders.

Table 4-6. Causes of metabolic alkalosis

Volume-depleted type
 Gastric acid loss
 Vomiting
 Gastric suction
 Renal chloride loss
 Diuretics
 Post-hypercapnia
 Cystic fibrosis

Volume-replete type
 Mineralocorticoid excess
 Hyperaldosteronism
 Gitelman's syndrome
 Bartter's syndrome
 Cushing's syndrome
 Licorice excess
 Profound potassium depletion

Table 4-7. Causes of chronic respiratory acidosis

Abnormal respiratory drive
  Obesity hypoventilation syndrome
  Sleep apnea
  Brainstem infarcts
  Myxedema
Abnormal nerve conduction
  Poliomyelitis
  Multiple sclerosis
  Amyotrophic lateral sclerosis
  Phrenic nerve injury
  Guillain-Barré syndrome
Thoracic cage problems
  Kyphoscoliosis
  Ankylosing spondylitis
  Muscular dystrophy
  Polymyositis
Pleural disease
  Fibrothorax
  Hydrothorax
Pulmonary disease
  Advanced interstitial fibrosis
  Chronic obstructive lung disease

C. **Causes of respiratory acidosis.** Two ventilatory abnormalities allow CO_2 retention and increased PCO_2: alveolar hypoventilation and severe ventilation–perfusion mismatching. Hypoxemia occurs in both settings. Causes according to level of respiratory system affected are listed in Table 4-7. Renal compensation for chronic respiratory acidosis produces very high HCO_3^- levels. If the PCO_2 is reduced by artificial ventilation, the high HCO_3^- may persist if not enough chloride is provided to replace it. This results in post-hypercapnic metabolic alkalosis. Acetazolamide may be useful in this setting.

D. **Causes of respiratory alkalosis.** Disorders that drive ventilation independent of PCO_2 can cause hyperventilation and hypocapnia. Inflammatory and mass lesions of the brain, psychiatric disorders, and certain central-acting drugs and chemicals increase central respiratory drive and produce hypocapnia. Importantly, salicylates, endotoxin, and progesterone are among this group of drugs and chemicals. Disorders that cause hypoxemia are common causes of the hyperventilation that causes hypocapnia. Disorders that reduce lung or chest compliance, such as mild pneumonia or pulmonary edema; vascular disorders, such as emboli; and mixed disorders, such as hepatic cirrhosis or failure, can cause hypocapnia. Volume depletion is a primary stimulus to hyperventilation and hypocapnia.

VI. **Treating acid-base disorders.** As discussed, acid-base disorders are markers of underlying diseases, and these diseases should be the targets of treatment.

A. **Step 1.** Correct volume and electrolyte deficiencies.

B. **Step 2.** Direct specific treatment at the underlying cause.

C. **Step 3.** Manipulate the bicarbonate or PCO_2 only if the pH is adversely affecting organ function or if pH is less than 7.10 or greater than 7.60.

D. **Treatment of metabolic acidosis** with alkali has not been shown to be efficacious in acute situations, including cardiopulmonary resuscitation, possibly because the HCO_3^- reaction with H^+ generates CO_2 at the tissue level and lowers cell pH. However, a mixture of carbonate and bicarbonate that produces less CO_2 has not been shown to be of clinical benefit. At present, we cannot recommend alkali therapy for any acute metabolic acidosis. In chronic distal renal tubular acidosis, alkali therapy reduces bone loss, hypercalciuria, and nephrocalcinosis. Oral alkali can be given as sodium bicarbonate tablets, 500 mg or 6 mmol, or as sodium or potassium citrate solution, 1 mmol per mL. Usually 3 mmol per kilogram of body weight is the starting dose. Oral HCO_3^- is accompanied by a sodium or potassium load that must be watched for adverse effects.

1. Insulin is the specific **treatment for diabetic ketoacidosis.** HCO_3^- and phosphate administration are unnecessary, but potassium repletion is important. Volume and electrolyte repletion, plus glucose and thiamine, suffice to correct alcoholic ketoacidosis. Starvation requires only calories. Note that metabolism of ketoanions, as with all organic anions, produces HCO_3^-; metabolism corrects about half of the HCO_3^- deficit. If alkali is given unwisely, an overshoot metabolic alkalosis may result.

2. In the **treatment of lactic acidosis,** the restoration of tissue perfusion and oxygenation is desirable, but often difficult to attain. Attention to potassium and calcium levels is important.

3. **Treatment of poisonings.** Ethylene glycol and methanol poisoning require immediate fomepizole infusion to retard metabolism of the alcohol to toxic products. Hemodialysis is started if renal failure is present. An alternative approach is to infuse ethanol to maintain a blood level of 100 mg per dL to compete for alcohol dehydrogenase activity. The loading dose of ethanol is 0.6 to 1.0 g per kg of body weight followed by a maintenance infusion of 10 to 20 g per hour. Blood alcohol levels must be monitored frequently. Salicylate intoxication should be treated with urinary alkalinization by infusing a 5% glucose solution containing $NaHCO_3$, 150 mmol added per liter, at 375 mL per hour, for 4 or more hours. Hemodialysis should be used to remove salicylate in patients with prominent renal failure, worsening mental status, recalcitrant acidosis, or general deterioration.

E. **Correction of metabolic alkalosis** very rarely requires the administration of acid. If renal failure prohibits renal excretion of HCO_3^-, the patient usually requires dialysis for other reasons. A low-bicarbonate dialysate can be used. If heart failure precludes the use of NaCl, then acetazolamide, 500 mg by mouth or intravenously, consistently reduces the serum tCO_2 by about 6 mmol per L. Rarely, dilute hydrochloric acid, 150 mmol per L, can be infused at 250 mL per hour into a central venous catheter or, preferably, in parenteral nutrition solution. Acid infusion is fraught with the potential complications of hemolysis and vascular necrosis and is best avoided. Ammonium chloride can be substituted for hydrochloric acid, but it causes gastric distress even when given intravenously and may cause ammonia intoxication.

1. **Volume-depletion metabolic alkalosis is corrected** by providing ample chloride with sodium or potassium. Prevention, however, is preferable. Proton-pump inhibitors minimize gastric acid loss in patients with nasogastric suction. Use of the potassium-sparing diuretics spironolactone, triamterene, and amiloride reduces the frequency and severity of diuretic-induced alkalosis.

2. **Treatment of volume-replete metabolic alkalosis.** If possible, the cause of increased mineralocorticoid production should be removed. For example, a functioning adrenal adenoma should be surgically excised. In the interim, the use of spironolactone in doses up to 400 mg per day with large amounts of potassium chloride may be effective. Indomethacin may be beneficial in Bartter's syndrome.

F. **Respiratory acidosis per se does not require direct treatment.** Even at chronic PCO_2 levels above 100 mm Hg, the kidneys generate and maintain HCO_3^- levels sufficient to keep the pH above 7.20. However, adequate oxygenation is the critical issue in both acute and chronic respiratory acidosis.

    G. Definitive treatment of respiratory alkalosis again requires the correction of the underlying condition causing hyperventilation. The provision of oxygen is essential for the hypoxemic patient.

    H. Treatment of mixed acid-base disorders

        1. Metabolic acidosis and respiratory acidosis. The most rapid treatment is to provide assisted or controlled ventilation. The administration of base is not warranted. The correction of the cause of metabolic acidosis is a priority.

        2. In **metabolic alkalosis and respiratory acidosis,** the pH is often alkalemic. Acetazolamide given daily or every other day may be used to keep the pH near 7.35 to 7.40, which is a good level to avoid respiratory suppression.

        3. Metabolic alkalosis and respiratory alkalosis in combination may produce severe alkalemia with dangerous arrhythmias. The most expedient treatment consists of intravenous morphine and a benzodiazepine, with immediate access to airway intubation and mechanical ventilation.

Suggested readings

Adrogué HJ, Madias NE. Management of life-threatening acid-base disorders. *N Engl J Med* 1998;338:26–34,107–111.

Alpern RJ, Preisig PA. Renal acid-base transport. In: Schrier RW, ed. *Diseases of the kidney and urinary tract,* 7th ed. Philadelphia: Lippincott Williams & Wilkins: 2001;203–216.

Batlle DC, Hizon M, Cohen E, et al. The use of the urinary anion gap in the diagnosis of hyperchloremic metabolic acidosis. *N Engl J Med* 1988;318:594–599.

DuBose TD Jr. Hyperkalemic hyperchloremic metabolic acidosis: pathophysiologic insights. *Kidney Int* 1997;51:591–602.

Gabow PA, Kaehny WD, Fennessey PV, et al. Diagnostic importance of an increased serum anion gap. *N Engl J Med* 1980;303:854–858.

Galla JH. Metabolic alkalosis. *J Am Soc Nephrol* 2000;11:369–375.

Kaehny W. Pathogenesis and management of respiratory and mixed acid-base disorders. In: Schrier RW, ed. *Renal and electrolyte disorders,* 6th ed. Philadelphia: Lippincott Williams & Wilkins: 154–170.

Kassirer JP, Bleich HL. Rapid estimation of plasma carbon dioxide tension from pH and total carbon dioxide content. *N Engl J Med* 1965;272:1067–1068.

Kraut JA, Kurtz I. Use of base in the treatment of severe acidemic states. *Am J Kidney Dis* 2001;38:703–727.

Rodriguez-Soriano J. Renal tubular acidosis. The clinical entity. *J Am Soc Nephrol* 2002;13:2160–2170.

Shapiro J, Kaehny W. Pathogenesis and management of metabolic acidosis and alkalosis. In: Schrier RW, ed. *Renal and electrolyte disorders,* 6th ed. Philadelphia: Lippincott Williams & Wilkins: 115–153.

The Patient with Disorders of Serum Calcium and Phosphate

Robert F. Reilly

DISORDERS OF SERUM CALCIUM

The majority of calcium in the body is in the form of hydroxyapatite in bone (99%). Although a small fraction of total body calcium is contained in the extracellular fluid (ECF), only the concentration of ionized calcium in the ECF is physiologically active and regulated. Approximately 60% of calcium in the ECF is ultrafiltrable and exists either free in solution as ionized calcium (50%) or complexed to anions such as citrate, phosphate, sulfate, and bicarbonate (10%). The remaining 40% is bound to proteins (primarily albumin).

Figure 5-1 illustrates calcium fluxes between the ECF, intestine, kidney, and bone. Net intestinal absorption of calcium amounts to about 200 mg of the normal dietary intake of 800 to 1,000 mg. In the steady state, this net intestinal absorption is matched by urinary excretion. As a result, 10,600 mg of the approximately 10,800 mg (98%) of calcium that is filtered daily is reabsorbed.

  I. Calcium regulation. Plasma-ionized calcium is regulated through a complex and coordinated interplay of parathyroid hormone (PTH) and $1,25(OH)_2$ vitamin D_3 (calcitriol) in intestine, bone, and kidney. The parathyroid gland senses the ECF ionized calcium concentration via a calcium-sensing receptor. High concentrations of ECF calcium stimulate the receptor and activate second messenger pathways that, in turn, inhibit the release of PTH. Low concentrations of ECF calcium stimulate PTH secretion and production and increase parathyroid gland mass. The parathyroid gland responds quickly (within minutes) to alterations in ionized calcium concentration. An inverse sigmoid relationship exists between ECF calcium concentration and PTH secretion, with a nonsuppressible component present even at high plasma calcium concentration. The amount of hormone stored is enough to support basal secretion for 6 hours and stimulated secretion for 2 hours.

       In bone, PTH in the presence of permissive amounts of calcitriol stimulates reabsorption by increasing osteoclast number and activity. In intestine, PTH enhances calcium and phosphate absorption indirectly by promoting the formation of calcitriol. In kidney, PTH augments distal tubular reabsorption of calcium, stimulates the formation of calcitriol in the proximal tubule, and decreases proximal tubular reabsorption of phosphate and bicarbonate.

       Calcitriol is produced in proximal tubule via $1\text{-}\alpha$ hydroxylation of $25(OH)$vitamin D_3 (calcidiol). The calcitriol biosynthetic pathway is illustrated in Figure 5-2. Principal stimulators of $1\text{-}\alpha$ hydroxylase are PTH and hypophosphatemia. The major function of calcitriol is to enhance the availability of calcium and phosphate for new bone formation and the prevention of symptomatic hypocalcemia and hypophosphatemia. In intestine and kidney, calcitriol increases the production of calcium-binding proteins (calbindins) that aid in the transcellular movement of calcium; this may be the rate-limiting step in transepithelial calcium flux. In bone, calcitriol potentiates the actions of PTH, stimulates osteoclastic reabsorption, and induces the differentiation of monocytes into osteoclasts.

       In the parathyroid gland, calcitriol binds to its receptor, leading to a decrease in PTH production. The PTH gene promoter contains regions that bind the calcitriol receptor. Binding results in a dramatic decrease in PTH expression. Calcitriol is the most potent suppressor of PTH gene transcription.

Figure 5-1. Calcium homeostasis.

II. Hypercalcemia
A. Etiology. Three basic pathophysiologic mechanisms contribute to hypercalcemia: increased calcium absorption from the gastrointestinal tract, decreased renal calcium excretion, and increased bone resorption of calcium. The most common etiologies of hypercalcemia are listed in Table 5-1.
1. **Increased calcium absorption from the gastrointestinal tract** plays a primary role in the hypercalcemia of the milk-alkali syndrome, vitamin D intoxication, and granulomatous disorders.
   a. **Milk-alkali syndrome** is the result of the ingestion of excess amounts of calcium and alkali. In the past, the most common sources of calcium and alkali were milk and sodium bicarbonate, respectively. Today this syndrome most often occurs in elderly women consuming excess amounts of calcium carbonate or citrate for the treatment of osteoporosis. Patients present with the classic triad of hypercalcemia, metabolic alkalosis, and renal insufficiency. Treatment of hypercalcemia in these patients is often complicated by hypocalcemia resulting from sustained PTH suppression.
   b. **Hypercalcemia in renal failure** is uncommon, except in patients treated with calcium and vitamin D supplements. This disorder and the milk-alkali syndrome illustrate the important concept that hypercalcemia from ingestion of excessive amounts of dietary calcium alone does not occur in the absence of renal impairment.
   c. **Vitamin D intoxication** also results in hypercalcemia. Calcium is

Figure 5-2. Vitamin D metabolism. (PTH, parathyroid hormone; UV, ultraviolet.)

absorbed primarily in the small intestine, and this process is stimulated by calcitriol.

  d. Hypercalcemia may also be secondary to **granulomatous disorders,** such as sarcoidosis. Activated macrophages produce calcitriol, which leads to increased intestinal absorption of dietary calcium. Hypercalciuria is seen more commonly than hypercalcemia. Lymphomas occasionally cause hypercalcemia via the same mechanism.

Table 5-1. Etiologies of hypercalcemia

Hyperparathyroidism
Malignancy
Vitamin A and D intoxication
Milk-alkali syndrome
Thyrotoxicosis
Granulomatous disease
Immobilization
Paget's disease
Thiazide diuretic intake
Addison's disease
Pheochromocytoma
Lithium intake
Renal failure
Post renal transplant
Familial hypocalciuric hypercalcemia

2. **Increased calcium resorption from bone** plays a primary role in hypercalcemia resulting from primary and secondary hyperparathyroidism, malignancy, hyperthyroidism, immobilization, Paget's disease, and vitamin A toxicity.

a. **Primary hyperparathyroidism** is the most frequent cause of hypercalcemia, with an estimated prevalence of 1 per 10,000. The underlying pathology is most often a solitary adenoma (80%). Among the remainder, 15% to 20% have diffuse hyperplasia, and approximately one-half of these have a familial syndrome [multiple endocrine neoplasia (MEN) type I, associated with pituitary adenomas and islet cell tumors, or MEN type II, associated with medullary carcinoma of the thyroid and pheochromocytoma]. Multiple adenomas are uncommon, and parathyroid carcinoma is rare (occurring in less than 1%). Hypercalcemia results from increased calcium reabsorption from bone, increased calcium absorption from intestine mediated by calcitriol, and increased distal tubular renal calcium reabsorption. In primary hyperparathyroidism, the hypercalcemia is often mild, asymptomatic, and identified on routine blood chemistries in the outpatient setting. Patients most commonly present in the fifth and sixth decades. Women are affected two to three times more frequently than men, and two-thirds of all cases occur in postmenopausal women.

b. **Secondary hyperparathyroidism** leads to hypercalcemia after renal transplantation when plasma phosphate, vitamin D metabolism, and renal function improve, but PTH secretion remains high secondary to increased parathyroid mass. In most patients, the hypercalcemia resolves during the first year following transplantation.

c. **Malignancy** is the second most common cause of hypercalcemia. Hypercalcemia of malignancy results from several pathophysiologic mechanisms: the overproduction of PTH-related peptide (PTHrP), local reabsorption of bone around sites of tumor infiltration (mediated via a variety of cytokines and osteolytic prostaglandins), and the production of calcitriol (e.g., with lymphomas). Patients with squamous cell cancer of the lung, breast cancer, multiple myeloma, and renal cell carcinoma are at highest risk. Hypercalcemia due to tumoral production of PTHrP is often referred to as humoral hypercalcemia of malignancy (HHM). PTHrP has 70% amino acid identity to the first 13 amino acids of PTH, binds to the PTH receptor, and has biological activity similar, but not identical to PTH. HHM often presents with severe hypercalcemia (calcium concentration greater than 14 mg per dL) in a patient with either a known history of malignancy or evidence of malignancy at initial presentation. PTHrP is immunologically distinct from PTH and is not detected by standard PTH assays, but specific assays for PTHrP are commercially available. Assays that measure the C-terminal fragment of PTHrP may show an increase when used in pregnant patients or patients with chronic kidney disease. Median survival from the onset of hypercalcemia with HHM is only 3 months. Squamous cell tumors, renal cell carcinomas, and most breast neoplasms produce PTHrP. The diagnoses of primary hyperparathyroidism and malignancy are not mutually exclusive. An increased incidence of primary hyperparathyroidism has been reported in patients with malignancy.

Multiple myeloma is associated with hypercalcemia and localized osteolytic lesions in the skeleton. Approximately 30% of myeloma patients experience hypercalcemia at some time during the course of their disease. Bone destruction occurs as a consequence of the release of interleukin-6, interleukin-1, and tumor necrosis factor–β by malignant plasma cells. Bony lesions demonstrate a marked increase in osteoclastic resorption without manifestations of increased bone formation, in contrast to metastatic lesions of breast and prostate cancer, which generally show some increase in bone formation and radionuclide uptake at sites of increased osteoblastic activity.

d. Hyperthyroidism results in mild hypercalcemia in 10% to 20% of patients as a result of increased bone turnover.

e. Immobilization and Paget's disease also cause hypercalcemia, although this is more likely in children. In adults, hypercalciuria is more common than hypercalcemia.

f. Rare causes of hypercalcemia include lithium use (mild; interferes with the calcium sensing receptor); thiazide diuretic use (occult primary hyperparathyroidism should be suspected); pheochromocytoma; primary adrenal insufficiency; and a rare genetic disorder, familial hypocalciuric hypercalcemia (FHH).

FHH is an autosomal dominant disorder caused by a mutation in the calcium-sensing receptor. It presents with mild hypercalcemia early in life, hypocalciuria, and a normal or slightly increased PTH concentration in the absence of signs or symptoms of hypercalcemia. As a result of the mutation, the calcium-sensing receptor is less sensitive to plasma calcium concentration, and a higher than normal calcium concentration is required to suppress PTH. One should be aware of FHH, because this condition is often misdiagnosed as primary hyperparathyroidism, and patients may be inappropriately subjected to neck exploration. FHH may account for a small percentage of patients who undergo surgery for primary hyperparathyroidism in whom no adenoma is found.

B. Signs and symptoms of hypercalcemia are related to the severity and rate of rise in plasma-ionized calcium concentration. Mild hypercalcemia is generally asymptomatic and often incidentally discovered on routine blood chemistries, as is the case in many patients with primary hyperparathyroidism. In contrast, severe hypercalcemia is often associated with neurologic and gastrointestinal symptoms. The patient may present with a wide range of central nervous system symptoms, from mild mental status changes to stupor and coma. Gastrointestinal symptoms include constipation, anorexia, nausea, and vomiting. Abdominal pain may result from hypercalcemia-induced peptic ulcer disease or pancreatitis. As discussed in Chapter 2, Hypernatremia (section I.C.2.a), hypercalcemia results in polyuria and secondary polydipsia that leads to ECF volume contraction, a reduction in the glomerular filtration rate (GFR), and an elevation in blood urea nitrogen (BUN) and creatinine concentrations. Hypercalcemia also potentiates the cardiac effects of digitalis toxicity.

C. Diagnosis. The most common causes of hypercalcemia are primary hyperparathyroidism and malignancy. These two disorders make up more than 90% of all cases. Initial evaluation includes a history and physical examination. Use of calcium supplements, antacids, vitamin preparations, and over-the-counter medications should be determined. A chest x-ray should be obtained to rule out pulmonary malignancies and granulomatous disorders.

1. Initial laboratory examination includes measurement of electrolytes, BUN, creatinine, and phosphorus; serum protein electrophoresis; and a 24-hour urine test for calcium and creatinine. The presence of a high serum chloride concentration and a low serum phosphorus concentration in a ratio greater than 33 to 1 is suggestive of primary hyperparathyroidism resulting from PTH's effect of decreasing proximal tubular phosphate reabsorption. A low serum chloride concentration, a high serum bicarbonate concentration, and elevated BUN and creatinine concentrations are characteristic of milk-alkali syndrome. A monoclonal spike on either serum protein electrophoresis or urine protein electrophoresis is suggestive of multiple myeloma or light chain disease. A low serum phosphorus concentration is found in primary hyperparathyroidism and HHM. The 24-hour urinary calcium excretion is low in hypercalcemia caused by the milk-alkali syndrome, use of thiazide diuretics, or FHH.

As a general rule, primary hyperparathyroidism is the etiology in asymptomatic outpatients with a serum calcium concentration of less than or equal to 11 mg per dL, whereas malignancy is often the cause in symptomatic patients with an abrupt onset of disease and serum calcium concentration of greater than or equal to 14 mg per dL.

2. **Intact PTH concentration** is obtained after the initial evaluation is completed. The most common cause of an elevated PTH concentration is primary hyperparathyroidism, although an elevated PTH concentration may also be seen with lithium use and FHH. Occasionally, in primary hyperparathyroidism, the PTH concentration will be inappropriately within the normal range compared to the increase in serum calcium. In all other conditions, PTH will be suppressed by hypercalcemia.

3. If no obvious malignancy is present and the PTH concentration is not increased, then the possibility of vitamin D intoxication or granulomatous disease should be evaluated further with an analysis of **calcidiol and calcitriol** concentration. An increased calcidiol concentration is seen with the ingestion of either vitamin D or calcidiol. An elevated calcitriol concentration is observed with calcitriol ingestion, granulomatous disease, lymphoma, and primary hyperparathyroidism.

4. As a final step, if the calcitriol concentration is increased without apparent cause, occult granulomatous disease can be evaluated with a **hydrocortisone suppression test.** After the administration of 40 mg of hydrocortisone every 8 hours for 10 days, the hypercalcemia will resolve if it is the result of granulomatous disease.

D. **Treatment** of hypercalcemia varies depending on the severity of the serum calcium elevation. It is directed at increasing urinary calcium excretion, inhibiting bone resorption, and decreasing intestinal calcium absorption.

1. **Urinary calcium excretion is increased** by expanding the ECF volume and, subsequently, administering loop diuretics. Calcium reabsorption in the proximal tubule is passive and parallels sodium reabsorption. ECF volume contraction, therefore, increases proximal sodium reabsorption and helps maintain hypercalcemia. Patients with hypercalcemia are often volume contracted. Hypercalcemia decreases sodium reabsorption in the thick ascending limb of the loop of Henle via the activation of the calcium sensing receptor, and it also antagonizes the effects of antidiuretic hormone. In the setting of a reduced GFR, higher doses of loop diuretics may be required. In the presence of little or no renal function and severe hypercalcemia, hemodialysis is indicated. If hypercalcemia is moderate, volume expansion and loop diuretics may be the only therapy required.

2. **An agent that inhibits bone resorption** is often required when hypercalcemia is moderate or severe. In the acute setting, calcitonin is often helpful because of its rapid onset of action (2 to 4 hours). Calcitonin inhibits osteoclastic bone resorption and increases renal calcium excretion. It reduces serum calcium concentration, however, by only 1 to 2 mg per dL, and tachyphylaxis often develops with repeated use. For these reasons, calcitonin should not be used as the sole agent to inhibit bone resorption.

a. **Bisphosphonates** are the agents of choice for the management of hypercalcemia due to bone resorption. These analogues of inorganic pyrophosphate are selectively concentrated in bone, where they interfere with osteoclast attachment and function. Bisphosphonates have a slow onset (2 to 3 days) and a long duration of action (several weeks). Etidronate was the first bisphosphonate approved for the treatment of hypercalcemia. The serum calcium concentration begins to fall on day 2 with etidronate and reaches a nadir on day 7. The hypocalcemic effect may be prolonged for several weeks. If serum calcium falls rapidly within the first 48 hours, the drug should be discontinued to avoid hypocalcemia. Etidronate can be given intravenously at a dosage of

7.5 mg per kg over 4 hours for 3 consecutive days. A single intravenous dose of 30 mg per kg as an infusion over 24 hours in 1 L of normal saline, however, may be more effective.

Pamidronate is more potent than etidronate and is the most widely used bisphosphonate in the treatment of hypercalcemia. It is given at a dose of either 60 or 90 mg intravenously over 4 hours. If serum calcium concentration is less than or equal to 13.5 mg per dL, 60 mg is given. If serum calcium concentration is greater than 13.5 mg per dL, 90 mg is administered. Serum calcium concentration gradually falls over the ensuing 2 to 4 days. A single dose is usually effective for 1 to 2 weeks. In most patients, serum calcium concentration normalizes after 7 days. The dose of both etidronate and pamidronate must be adjusted for renal function.

b. **Plicamycin (mithramycin)** can be used except in patients with severe hepatic, renal, and marrow disorders. Its effect begins in 12 hours and peaks at 48 hours. The dose can be repeated at 3- to 7-day intervals. Its side-effect profile (nausea, hepatotoxicity, proteinuria, and thrombocytopenia) has led to decreased enthusiasm for its use.

c. **Gallium nitrate** inhibits bone resorption by unknown mechanisms and is an additional agent that can be employed to treat hypercalcemia of malignancy. It is administered as a continuous infusion at a dose of 100 to 200 mg per m^2 for 5 consecutive days. Gallium nitrate should not be administered to patients wih serum creatinine concentrations above 2.5 mg per dL, and it is probably best reserved for patients who have not responded to more conventional agents. A summary of treatment options is shown in Table 5-2.

3. **Measures to decrease intestinal absorption** of calcium are often employed in outpatients with mild disease. Corticosteroids may be helpful in vitamin D intoxication, granulomatous disease, and certain neoplasms (lymphoma, myeloma). Alternatives to corticosteroids include ketoconazole and hydroxychloroquine. Oral phosphate can be administered, providing the patient does not have an elevated serum phosphorus concentration or renal failure. Oral phosphate, however, often causes diarrhea and only lowers the serum calcium concentration by about 1 mg per dL.

4. Whether to **surgically remove** a solitary parathyroid adenoma remains a difficult management issue. The following criteria for surgical intervention were suggested at a 1991 National Institutes of Health consensus conference: a total serum calcium concentration that is greater than 1 mg per dL above the upper limit of the normal range; evidence of overt bone disease; cortical bone mineral density that is more than 2 standard deviations (SD) below the adjusted mean for age, sex, and race; reduction in renal function by more than 30%; a history of nephrolithiasis or nephrocalcinosis; urinary calcium excretion greater than 400 mg per day; and

Table 5-2. Treatment of hypercalcemia

Drug	Dosage
Normal saline	2–4 L/d initially
Furosemide	20–160 mg i.v. q8h after volume expansion
Salmon calcitonin	4 IU/kg s.c. q12h
Etidronate disodium	7.5 mg/kg i.v. over 4 hr q.d. for 3–7 d, 30 mg/kg i.v. over 24 hrs single dose
Pamidronate disodium	60–90 mg i.v. over 4 hr
Plicamycin	25 μg/kg i.v. over 4 hr q.d. for 3–4 d
Corticosteroids	200–300 mg hydrocortisone i.v. q.d. for 3–5 d
Gallium nitrate	100–200 mg/m^2 for 5 d

an episode of acute symptomatic hypercalcemia. It is estimated that approximately 50% of patients meet these criteria.

With the advent of minimally invasive parathyroid surgery, these criteria are likely to be liberalized. The adenoma is initially localized with sestaMIBI scanning. If a solitary hot spot is identified, the adenoma is resected under local anesthesia. Parathyroid hormone concentration is measured intraoperatively. Its concentration should fall within minutes if the adenoma is successfully resected, given the short half-life of PTH (4 minutes). If the PTH concentration remains elevated, then the patient is placed under general anesthesia and the opposite side of the neck explored. The combination of sestaMIBI scanning and intraoperative PTH concentration measurement results in the successful removal of solitary adenomas in the vast majority of cases.

III. Hypocalcemia

A. Etiology.

True hypocalcemia is the result of decreased calcium absorption from the gastrointestinal tract or decreased calcium resorption from bone. Given that 98% of total body calcium is contained within the skeleton, sustained hypocalcemia cannot occur without an abnormality of either PTH or calcitriol action in bone.

Total plasma calcium is composed of three components: ionized calcium (50%), complexed calcium (10%), and protein-bound calcium (40%). True hypocalcemia is present only when the ionized calcium concentration is reduced. The reference range for ionized calcium concentration is 4.2 to 5.0 mg per dL (1.05 to 1.25 mmol per L). Therefore, whenever a low total serum calcium concentration is observed, this value must be compared with the serum albumin concentration. For every decrease of 1 g per dL in serum albumin concentration from its normal concentration of 4 g per dL, a decrease of 0.8 mg per dL in total serum calcium concentration can be expected. Thus, for each fall of 1 g per dL in serum albumin concentration, 0.8 mg per dL must be added to the total serum calcium concentration. The binding of calcium to albumin is affected by ECF pH. Acidemia increases and alkalemia decreases the ionized calcium concentration. Ionized calcium concentration increases approximately 0.2 mg per dL for each 0.1 decrease in pH. These correction factors are only general guidelines and should not be used as a substitute for the direct measurement of serum-ionized calcium concentration if clinical suspicion warrants.

True hypocalcemia is caused by decreased PTH secretion, end-organ resistance to PTH, or disorders of vitamin D metabolism. Occasionally, hypocalcemia occurs acutely as a result of either the extravascular deposition of calcium or the intravascular binding of calcium. The most common etiologies of true hypocalcemia are illustrated in Table 5-3.

1. Hypoparathyroidism is caused by a wide variety of acquired and inherited diseases that result from the impaired synthesis and release of PTH or from peripheral tissue resistance to PTH.

a. The most common cause of idiopathic hypoparathyroidism is **polyglandular autoimmune syndrome type I,** characterized by chronic mucocutaneous candidiasis and primary adrenal insufficiency. Occasionally, pernicious anemia, diabetes mellitus, vitiligo, and autoimmune thyroid disease also are associated. Mucocutaneous candidiasis often presents first in early childhood and is followed several years later by hypoparathyroidism. Adrenal insufficiency appears in adolescence. The combination of hypoparathyroidism, adrenal insufficiency, and mucocutaneous candidiasis is referred to as the "HAM syndrome."

b. Familial hypocalcemia results from activating mutations in the calcium-sensing receptor that increase its sensitivity to calcium.

c. Parathyroid and radical neck surgery can result in a loss of glandular tissue. Surgical removal of parathyroid tissue in secondary or tertiary hyperparathyroidism is often complicated by severe hypocalcemia

Table 5-3. Etiologies of hypocalcemia

Hypoparathyroidism
   Idiopathic—HAM syndrome
   Familial
   Post surgery—hungry bone syndrome
   Infiltrative disorders
   Pseudohypoparathyroidism 1A, 1B, 2
   Hypomagnesemia
Defects in vitamin D metabolism
   Nutritional
   Malabsorption
   Drugs
   Liver disease
   Renal disease
   Vitamin D-dependent rickets
Miscellaneous
   Tumor lysis syndrome
   Osteoblastic metastases
   Acute pancreatitis
   Toxic shock syndrome
   Sepsis

HAM, hypoparathyroidism, adrenal insufficiency, and mucocutaneous candidiasis.

     due to the remineralization of bone, the so-called "hungry bone syndrome."

  d. Hypocalcemia also occurs after **thyroid surgery** (5% of cases); in approximately 0.5% of these patients, the hypocalcemia is permanent. Risk factors for the development of permanent hypocalcemia include removal of three or more parathyroid glands; postoperative PTH concentration of less than or equal to 12 pg per mL; total serum calcium concentration of less than or equal to 8 mg per dL after 1 week of oral calcium supplementation; and a serum phosphorus concentration of less than or equal to 4 mg per dL after 1 week of calcium supplementation.

  e. Transient hypoparathyroidism may occur after the **removal of a parathyroid adenoma.**

  f. **Infiltrative disorders** such as hemochromatosis, Wilson's disease, and infection with human immunodeficiency virus (HIV) can also decrease PTH secretion.

  g. **Severe hypomagnesemia** is the most common cause of hypoparathyroidism. Magnesium deficiency results in end-organ resistance to PTH and a decrease in PTH secretion. Patients with hypocalcemia as a result of hypomagnesemia do not respond to calcium or vitamin D replacement until the magnesium deficit is replaced.

 2. A variety of rare genetic disorders cause **end-organ resistance to PTH,** including pseudohypoparathyroidism types I and II. Patients with pseudohypoparathyroidism are classified on the basis of the response of nephrogenous cyclic adenosine monophosphate to PTH administration. A decreased response is indicative of type I, and a normal response is indicative of type II.

 3. **Defects in vitamin D metabolism** also cause hypocalcemia. Etiologies include decreased intake of vitamin D, malabsorption, drugs, liver disease, kidney disease, and vitamin D–dependent rickets. Nutritional vitamin D deficiency is uncommon in the United States as a result of the supplementation of milk and other food products. It can occur, however, in poorly nourished patients with little sun exposure. Because vitamin D is fat-soluble, vitamin D deficiency can be seen in gastrointestinal malabsorption from any cause. Anticonvulsants induce vitamin D deficiency through mechanisms that are not clear; this generally occurs in patients with additional predisposing factors, such as poor nutrition and decreased sun exposure. Phenobarbital enhances the hepatic metabolism of vitamin D and calcidiol. Vitamin D deficiency can result from hepatocellular disease if the disease is severe enough to impair the 25-hydroxylation of vitamin D to calcidiol. Chronic kidney disease impairs the 1-α hydroxylation of calcidiol to calcitriol. Vitamin D-dependent rickets is a result of either the impaired hydroxylation of calcidiol to calcitriol (type I) or end-organ resistance to calcitriol (type II). Type I patients respond to physiologic doses of calcitriol. Patients with type II disease have dramatically increased concentrations of calcitriol, respond poorly to calcitriol therapy, and have mutations in the vitamin D receptor.

4. **Less common causes** of hypocalcemia include the tumor lysis syndrome, osteoblastic metastases, acute pancreatitis, toxic shock syndrome, and sepsis. The acute addition or release of phosphate into the extracellular space may cause hypocalcemia via a variety of mechanisms. Calcium and phosphate may precipitate in tissues, although the exact tissue in which the deposition occurs has never been identified. In addition, phosphate infusion increases the rate of bone formation and inhibits PTH-induced bone resorption, which then decreases calcium concentration.

B. As is the case for hypercalcemia, the **signs and symptoms** of hypocalcemia depend not only on the degree of hypocalcemia, but also on the rate of decline of the serum calcium concentration. The threshold at which symptoms develop also depends on the serum pH and whether concomitant hypomagnesemia, hypokalemia, or hyponatremia is present. Symptoms of neuromuscular excitability predominate. The patient may complain of circumoral and distal extremity paresthesias or of carpopedal spasm. Central nervous system manifestations include mental status changes, irritability, and seizures. On physical examination, hypotension, bradycardia, laryngeal spasm, and bronchospasm may be present. Chvostek's and Trousseau's signs should be checked. Chvostek's sign is a facial twitch elicited by tapping on the facial nerve just below the zygomatic arch with the mouth slightly open. A positive sign is occasionally observed in normal patients. Trousseau's sign is the development of wrist flexion, metacarpophalangeal joint flexion, hyperextended fingers, and thumb flexion after a sphygmomanometer cuff is inflated around the arm to 20 mmHg above systolic pressure for a duration of 3 minutes.

C. **Diagnosis.** The differential diagnosis of true hypocalcemia is often straightforward, and a diagnostic algorithm is shown in Figure 5-3. The most common causes are magnesium deficiency, kidney failure, and complications of parathyroid surgery.

1. The first step in the evaluation of the patient with a decreased total serum calcium concentration is to **examine the serum albumin** and, if necessary, measure the ionized serum calcium concentration. If true hypocalcemia is documented, then blood analysis should be obtained for BUN, creatinine, magnesium, and phosphorus concentration, and a 24-hour urine sample should be collected to test phosphorus and creatinine excretion.

2. The second step is to **evaluate the serum magnesium concentration.** Hypomagnesemia is the most common cause of hypocalcemia in hospitalized patients. A high index of suspicion should be present in patients with a history of steatorrhea, diarrhea, or chronic alcoholism. These patients generally have severe hypomagnesemia, and the hypocalcemia does not correct until magnesium losses are replaced. It frequently requires several days for the serum calcium concentration to correct after magnesium deficiency is reversed.

3. **Serum and urinary phosphorus concentrations** are evaluated next. Hyperphosphatemia in the absence of kidney failure suggests a diagnosis of either hypoparathyroidism or pseudohypoparathyroidism. Measuring

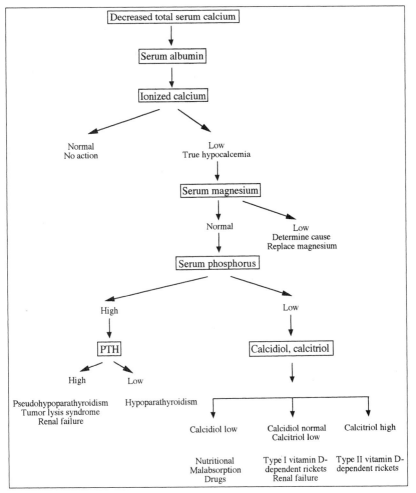

Figure 5-3. Evaluation of hypocalcemia. (PTH, parathyroid hormone.)

the PTH concentration can differentiate these disorders. In primary hypoparathyroidism, PTH is low; in pseudohypoparathyroidism, PTH is increased. A decrease in serum phosphorus concentration indicates a defect in vitamin D metabolism. Hypocalcemia results in secondary hyperparathyroidism that, in turn, reduces proximal tubular reabsorption of phosphate and thus results in phosphate wasting. Therefore, the fractional excretion (FE) of phosphate is expected to be high (more than 5%). In hypophosphatemia, the kidney has an extraordinary ability to conserve phosphate, and, in extrarenal disorders, the FE of phosphate is below 1%. If phosphaturia is noted, then calcidiol and calcitriol concentration should be measured. Calcidiol concentration is reduced with malabsorption, liver disease, and phenobarbital. Calcitriol concentration is reduced in kidney failure and increased in type II vitamin D-dependent rickets.

D. The **management of hypocalcemia** is dependent on both its severity and cause.

In an **emergency situation in which hypocalcemia is suspected and seizures, tetany, hypotension, or cardiac arrhythmias are present,** intravenous calcium should be administered (100 to 300 mg over 10 to 15 minutes) before the results of the serum calcium concentration return from the clinical laboratory. Patients with symptomatic hypocalcemia or a total serum calcium concentration corrected for albumin of less than or equal to 7.5 mg per dL should be initially managed with parenteral calcium. Chronic, mild hypocalcemia, as seen in the outpatient setting, can be treated with oral calcium supplements, to which a vitamin D preparation may be added if necessary.

1. **Acute symptomatic hypocalcemia** is treated with intravenous calcium. In the absence of seizures, tetany, or cardiac arrhythmias, an infusion of 15 mg per kg of elemental calcium given over 4 to 6 hours raises the total serum calcium by 2 to 3 mg per dL. Calcium gluconate (10%) is supplied in 10-mL ampules and contains 94 mg of elemental calcium. The first ampule can be administered over several minutes, followed by a constant infusion begun at a rate of 0.5 to 1.0 mg per kg per hour, with adjustment in the rate based on serial determinations of serum calcium concentration. Calcium glucceptate (10%) provides 90 mg of elemental calcium in a 5-mL ampule. Calcium chloride has higher bioavailability, and 272 mg of elemental calcium is contained in each 10-mL ampule. Treatment of hypocalcemia is ineffective in the presence of hypomagnesemia. In the setting of metabolic acidosis, hypocalcemia should be corrected before acidosis is reversed.

   Patients with **hypoparathyroidism** are managed with calcium and vitamin D supplements. The serum calcium concentration should be maintained at the lower limit of normal. Oral elemental calcium, 1 to 3 g per day, is usually sufficient. A variety of oral calcium preparations are available, some of which are shown in Table 5-4. Calcium is best absorbed when taken between meals. Calcium citrate is more soluble than calcium carbonate, especially in patients who require H_2 blockers or proton pump inhibitors. In the presence of severe hyperphosphatemia, calcium supplementation should be delayed, if possible, until the serum phosphorus concentration is reduced below 6 mg per dL using phosphate binders. Severe hypocalcemia, however, may need to be treated despite hyperphosphatemia.

2. **Calcitriol** is the most potent of the **vitamin D preparations** and has the fastest onset and shortest duration of action, but is also the most expensive. A dose of 0.5 to 1.0 μg per day is usually required. As one moves back up the metabolic pathway to calcidiol, cholecalciferol, and ergocalciferol, cost decreases and duration of action increases. These agents, however, may be less efficacious in the presence of kidney or liver disease.

   Patients with hypoparathyroidism have decreased distal tubular calcium reabsorption as a result of a lack of PTH. Therefore, the increase

Table 5-4. Oral calcium preparations

Preparation	Formulation	Elemental calcium per tablet
Calcium carbonate	Tums 500 mg	200 mg
	Rolaids 550 mg	220 mg
	Os-cal 1,250 mg	500 mg
Calcium citrate	Citracal 950 mg	200 mg
Calcium lactate	650 mg	85 mg
Calcium gluconate	1,000 mg	90 mg

in filtered calcium load that results from calcium and vitamin D replacement can lead to hypercalciuria, nephrolithiasis, and nephrocalcinosis. If urinary calcium excretion exceeds 350 mg per day despite a serum calcium concentration in the low normal range, sodium intake should be restricted; if this is not effective, a thiazide diuretic should be added.

DISORDERS OF SERUM PHOSPHORUS

I. **Overview.** Approximately two-thirds of total plasma phosphorus is organic phosphorus (phospholipids), and one-third is inorganic. Clinical chemistry laboratories assay only the inorganic fraction. The reference range is 2.8 to 4.5 mg per dL (0.89 to 1.44 mmol per L). Approximately 85% of inorganic phosphorus is free and circulates as either $HPO_4(-2)$ or $H_2PO_4(-1)$. The ratio of these two ions depends upon ECF pH. Of the remainder, 10% is protein-bound, and 15% is complexed with either calcium or magnesium.

   As is the case for calcium, the majority of total body phosphate is contained within the skeleton (80%). Of the remainder, about 10% is within skeletal muscle and viscera. Only a small fraction of the phosphate pool is inorganic and available for the synthesis of adenosine triphosphate (ATP). The average Western diet contains 800 to 1,400 mg of phosphate per day, of which approximately 80% is absorbed in small intestine. The majority is absorbed passively, but an active calcitriol-regulated component exists. PTH and calcitriol, through their effects in bone, intestine, and kidney, regulate phosphorus concentration. The major regulator of serum phosphorus concentration is renal phosphate excretion. In kidney, phosphate is reabsorbed primarily in the proximal tubule (80%), where it is cotransported with sodium across the luminal membrane. The sodium-phosphate cotransporter is upregulated in response to phosphate depletion, and, under these circumstances, the kidney is capable of reducing the FE of phosphate to very low levels.

II. **Phosphate regulation.** PTH acts directly in bone to increase phosphate entry into the ECF and indirectly in intestine by stimulating the production of calcitriol. The majority of dietary phosphate is reabsorbed in the small intestine, but a component of unregulated secretion is present in the colon (100 to 200 mg per day). PTH reduces the proximal tubular reabsorption of phosphate in the kidney. The net effect is to increase plasma calcium concentration while keeping serum phosphorus concentration constant. Calcitriol's major roles are to enhance the availability of calcium and phosphate for new bone formation and to defend the ECF from hypocalcemia and hypophosphatemia. PTH and hypophosphatemia stimulate calcitriol production in proximal tubule; although, the kidney is the primary regulator of serum phosphorus concentration. Hypophosphatemia causes the insertion of sodium-phosphate cotransporters into the luminal membrane of the proximal tubule, whereas PTH results in their removal. The ability of PTH to remove sodium-phosphate cotransporters from apical membrane is blunted in chronic phosphate depletion.

III. **Hyperphosphatemia**

   A. **Etiology.** Hyperphosphatemia can result from renal failure, an acute phosphate load from either exogenous or endogenous sources, or increased proximal tubular reabsorption of phosphate. Etiologies are shown in Table 5-5.

      1. **Renal failure** is the underlying cause in 90% or more of cases. As GFR begins to decline, the FE of phosphate increases. Once GFR falls below 30 mL per minute, however, phosphorus reabsorption is maximally suppressed, and the FE cannot increase further. As a result, renal excretion can no longer keep pace with dietary intake, and the serum phosphorus concentration rises. A new steady state is eventually established, albeit at a higher serum phosphorus concentration.

      2. **A sudden, massive phosphate load** may result in an increase in serum phosphorus concentration. Phosphate may be released from either the

Table 5-5. Etiologies of hyperphosphatemia

Decreased renal excretion
  Acute renal failure
  Chronic renal failure
Acute phosphate load
  Tumor lysis syndrome
  Rhabdomyolysis
  Bowel infarction
  Severe hemolysis
Vitamin D intoxication
Increased renal phosphate reabsorption
  Hypoparathyroidism
  Acromegaly
  Thyrotoxicosis
  Drugs—bisphosphonates
  Tumoral calcinosis
Pseudohyperphosphatemia

intracellular space, as is the case in tumor lysis syndrome or rhabdomyolysis, or it can be ingested and absorbed, as in vitamin D intoxication. Tumor lysis syndrome most commonly is seen with the treatment of rapidly growing malignancies such as leukemias and lymphomas. It can occur after the treatment of solid tumors such as small cell carcinoma, breast cancer, and neuroblastoma. Risk factors for tumor lysis syndrome in patients with solid tumors include pretreatment renal impairment, an increased lactate dehydrogenase level, and hyperuricemia. Increased lactate dehydrogenase levels and hyperuricemia are indicators of a large tumor burden.

   3. **Primary increases in tubular phosphate reabsorption** are less common. They can occur in hypoparathyroidism; in acromegaly, as a result of direct stimulation of insulin-like growth factor (IGF) on phosphate transport; with bisphosphonates, via a direct effect on renal phosphate reabsorption; and in tumoral calcinosis. Tumoral calcinosis is caused by an abnormality in the proximal tubule that leads to an increase in phosphate reabsorption.

  B. Many of the **signs and symptoms** of an acute rise in serum phosphorus are secondary to concomitant hypocalcemia due to the deposition of calcium in soft tissues and a resultant fall in ECF ionized calcium concentration. Hyperphosphatemia can also cause hypocalcemia by decreasing the activity of 1-α hydroxylase and calcitriol formation.

  C. **Diagnosis.** Clinically unexplained, persistent hyperphosphatemia should raise the suspicion of pseudohyperphosphatemia, the most common cause of which is paraproteinemia. No consistent relationship of immunoglobulin type or subclass has been identified. This is a method-dependent artifact, and paraprotein interference may be a general problem in spectrophotometric assays. If paraproteinemia is absent, the cause is generally acute or chronic renal failure.

  D. **Treatment** of hyperphosphatemia is aimed at reducing the intestinal absorption of phosphate. This is accomplished through the use of oral phosphate-binding drugs such as calcium carbonate, calcium acetate, sevelamer hydrochloride, and aluminum hydroxide. These agents should be administered with meals. Aluminum hydroxide may be used in the short term, but chronic use in patients with kidney disease should be avoided because of the potential for aluminum toxicity. In patients with coexistent hypocalcemia, it is preferable to lower the serum phosphorus below 6 mg per dL, if

Table 5-6. Etiologies of hypophosphatemia

Decreased dietary intake
   Alcoholism
   Phosphate-binding agents
Shift of phosphate into the intracellular fluid
   Respiratory alkalosis
   Refeeding
   Diabetic ketoacidosis
   Hungry bone syndrome
Increased renal excretion
   Hyperparathyroidism
   Vitamin D deficiency
   X-linked hypophosphatemic rickets
   Autosomal dominant hypophosphatemic rickets
   Fanconi's syndrome
   Drugs—acetazolamide
   Osmotic diuresis
   Oncogenic osteomalacia

possible, before treating the hypocalcemia to avoid the potential complication of metastatic calcification from calcium phosphate coprecipitation.

IV. Hypophosphatemia

  A. Etiology. Hypophosphatemia may result from the redistribution of phosphate from the extracellular to the intracellular space, a decrease in intestinal absorption of phosphate, or a decrease in renal reabsorption of phosphate. The differential diagnosis is presented in Table 5-6.

    1. Respiratory alkalosis and the refeeding syndrome are the most common causes of a **shift of phosphate from the ECF to the ICF** in hospitalized patients. Respiratory alkalosis causes a rise in intracellular pH that stimulates phosphofructokinase, the rate-limiting step in glycolysis. This results in severe hypophosphatemia with serum phosphorus concentrations of less than 0.5 to 1.0 mg per dL. Intracellular shifts are also seen with the treatment of diabetic ketoacidosis and in "hungry bone syndrome," which occurs after parathyroidectomy for secondary hyperparathyroidism. In "hungry bone syndrome," serum calcium and phosphorus concentration fall dramatically in the postoperative period, although clinically, hypocalcemia is more of a management issue than hypophosphatemia.

    2. Decreased dietary intake is an unusual cause of hypophosphatemia because oral intake almost always exceeds gastrointestinal losses, and the kidney is capable of reclaiming nearly all the filtered load of phosphate. In general, decreased intake must be combined with increased gastrointestinal losses (e.g., diarrhea) or the use of phosphate binders for hypophosphatemia to result.

    3. Increased urinary phosphate excretion occurs in primary hyperparathyroidism, secondary hyperparathyroidism due to defects in vitamin D metabolism, Fanconi's syndrome, osmotic diuresis, acetazolamide use, and oncogenic osteomalacia. Oncogenic osteomalacia is a rare disorder associated with mesenchymal tumors; it is characterized by hypophosphatemia, phosphaturia, decreased calcitriol concentration, normal calcidiol concentration, and clinical and histologic evidence of osteomalacia. A considerable delay may occur between the presentation of the syndrome and the discovery of the tumor. The tumor produces a humoral factor that interferes with the proximal tubular reabsorption of phosphate and the production of calcitriol; this interference resolves on removal of the tumor. The humoral factor was identified as fibroblast growth factor 23 (FGF23).

FGF23 is present in the circulation of normal individuals, consistent with a physiologic role in regulating serum phosphorus. Animal studies have shown that FGF23 is phosphaturic. When administered *in vivo*, it induces hypophosphatemia, suppresses 1,25(OH)$_2$ vitamin D$_3$ concentration and leads to osteomalacia. Two inherited renal phosphate wasting disorders, autosomal dominant hypophosphatemic rickets (ADHR) and X-linked hypophosphatemia (XLH), are the result of defects in FGF23 metabolism. Missense mutations in FGF23 cause ADHR.

ADHR is characterized by hypophosphatemia, renal phosphate wasting, short stature, and bony deformities. In ADHR, mutations at a proteolytic cleavage site prevent its cleavage and inactivation. *In vivo* studies showed that biologic activity is limited to full-length FGF23 (251 amino acids). The enzyme responsible for the cleavage of FGF23 has not been identified. One report suggested that Phex, a cell surface metalloprotease, may cleave FGF23, but this has not been confirmed.

XLH is characterized by renal phosphate wasting, hypophosphatemia, growth retardation, defective calcification of cartilage and bone, and resistance to phosphate and vitamin D repletion. Inactivating mutations of Phex cause XLH. Phex is a member of a family of zinc-dependent cell surface proteases that cleave small peptides such as endothelin. It is expressed predominantly in cartilage, bone, and teeth. Its physiologically relevant substrate has yet to be identified. Although it has been postulated that Phex cleaves and inactivates FGF23, the large size of FGF23—251 amino acids—makes this less likely. Other intermediate small-molecular-weight substrates likely link Phex function to FGF23.

B. Signs and symptoms. Hypophosphatemia results in a variety of clinical sequelae. The correction of moderate hypophosphatemia improves diaphragmatic function in patients with acute respiratory failure. In patients with severe hypophosphatemia, failure to wean from mechanical ventilation until repletion of phosphate was demonstrated. *In vitro* hypophosphatemia causes a leftward shift in the oxygen dissociation curve. Neuromuscular symptoms include paresthesias, tremor, muscle weakness, and altered mental status; severe hypophosphatemia increases red cell fragility, which can lead to hemolysis and decreases chemotaxis, phagocytosis, and bacterial killing by white cells, with an increased susceptibility to infection as the possible result.

C. Diagnosis. FE of phosphate or 24-hour urinary phosphate excretion can be used to distinguish among the pathophysiologic mechanisms of hypophosphatemia. If the kidney is responding appropriately to decreased intestinal absorption or redistribution of phosphate into cells, FE of phosphate is below 5%, and the 24-hour urine phosphate excretion is less than 100 mg per day. When the kidney is the cause of hypophosphatemia, the FE of phosphate is greater than 5% and the 24-hour urine excretion contains more than 100 mg of phosphate per day. In this case, a urinalysis for glycosuria, PTH concentration to rule out hyperparathyroidism, and the measurement of calcidiol and calcitriol concentrations are indicated.

D. Treatment is indicated for severe hypophosphatemia (less than or equal to 1 mg per dL) or symptoms. It is complicated by the fact that phosphate is largely an intracellular ion, and that serum phosphorus concentration is not a reliable indicator of total body phosphate stores. Hypophosphatemia is often associated with potassium and magnesium depletion. Phosphate repletion should be undertaken with extreme caution in the rare patient with renal insufficiency; the safest mode of therapy is oral, and hypophosphatemia usually can be corrected with 1,000 mg of phosphate per day. Alternative forms of oral phosphate replacement are listed in Table 5-7. Diarrhea is the most common complication.

Intravenous replacement carries the risk of hypocalcemia and hyperphosphatemia and is only warranted in patients with severe symptomatic hypophosphatemia. Sodium phosphate should be used unless the serum

Table 5-7. Oral phosphate preparations

Preparation	Dosage	Contents
K-phos-neutral	2 tablets, b.i.d. or t.i.d.	250 mg phosphate, 12 mEq sodium, 2 mEq potassium per tablet
Fleets Phospho-Soda	5 mL b.i.d.	149 mg phosphate, 6 mEq sodium per mL
Neutra-Phos-K	1–2 capsules, b.i.d. or t.i.d.	250 mg phosphate, 14 mEq potassium per capsule
K-phos	2 tablets, t.i.d. or q.i.d.	114 mg phosphate, 3.68 mEq potassium per tablet

potassium is less than 4 mEq per L. Serum concentrations of phosphorus, calcium, magnesium, potassium, and urine output should be carefully monitored during intravenous replacement. Once serum phosphorus concentration has increased to more than 1 mg per dL, the patient should be switched to an oral preparation. The administration of doses larger than 0.32 mmol per kg over a 12-hour period is rarely warranted.

Suggested readings

Brooks MJ, Melnik G. The refeeding syndrome: an approach to understanding its complications and preventing its occurrence. *Pharmacotherapy* 1995;15:713–726.

Bugg NC, Jones JA. Hypophosphatemia. *Anaesthesia* 1998;53:895–902.

Bushinsky DA. Calcium. *Lancet* 1998;352:306–311.

Crook M. Phosphate: an abnormal anion? *Br J Hosp Med* 1994;52:200–203.

Econs MJ, Francis F. Positional cloning of the PEX gene: new insights into the pathophysiology of X-linked hypophosphatemic rickets. *Am J Physiol* 1997;273:F489–F498.

Fiaschi-Taesch NM, Stewart AF. Minireview: parathyroid hormone-related protein as an intracrine factor—trafficking mechanisms and functional consequences. *Endocrinology* 2003;144:407–411.

Fiorino AS. Hypercalcemia and alkalosis due to the milk-alkali syndrome: a case report and review. *Yale J Biol Med* 1996;69:517–523.

Guise TA, Mundy GR. Evaluation of hypocalcemia in children and adults. *J Clin Endocrinol Metab* 1995;80:1473–1478.

Lourwood DL. The pharmacology and therapeutic utility of bisphosphonates. *Pharmacotherapy* 1998;18:779–789.

Mundy GR, Guise TA. Hypercalcemia of malignancy. *Am J Med* 1997;103:134–145.

Potts JT Jr., Fradkin JE, Aurbach JD, Bilezikian JP, Raisz LG. Proceedings of the NIH consensus development conference on diagnosis and management of asymptomatic primary hyperparathyroidism. *J Bone Miner Res* 1991;6:S1–S165.

Quarles, LD. FGF23, PHEX, and MEPE regulation of phosphate homeostasis and skeletal mineralization. *Am J Physiol Endocrinol Metab* 2003;285:E1–E9.

Tenenhouse HS, Murer H. Disorders of renal tubular phosphate transport. *J Am Soc Nephrol* 2003;14:240–248.

Reber PM, Heath HH III. Hypocalcemic emergencies. *Med Clin North Am* 1995;79:93–106.

Weisinger JR. Magnesium and phosphorus. *Lancet* 1998;352:391–396.

Zahrani AA, Levine MA. Primary hyperparathyroidism. *Lancet* 1997;349:1233–1236.

The Patient with Kidney Stones

Robert F. Reilly

Nephrolithiasis is a common disorder in the United States, with an annual incidence of 7 to 21 per 10,000 patients. Kidney stones account for approximately 1 in every 100 hospital admissions, with men affected three to four times more frequently than women. It is estimated that, by the age of 70, as many as 20% of all Caucasian men and 7% of all Caucasian women will form a stone. African Americans and Asians are affected less often. The peak incidence occurs between the ages of 20 and 30 years.

Kidney stones are a major cause of morbidity due to associated renal colic, urinary tract obstruction, urinary tract infection (UTI), and renal parenchymal damage. In the United States, calcium-containing stones make up approximately 90% of all stones; they contain primarily calcium oxalate, either alone or in combination with calcium phosphate. The remaining 10% are composed of uric acid, struvite-carbonate, and cystine.

A kidney stone can form only when urine is supersaturated with respect to a stone-forming salt. Interestingly, the urine in many normal subjects is often supersaturated with respect to calcium oxalate, calcium phosphate, or uric acid, yet stone formation does not occur. At least two other factors play a role in the pathogenesis of stone formation: heterogeneous nucleation and the presence in the urine of inhibitors of crystallization. The crystallization of a salt requires much less energy when a surface is present on which it can precipitate (heterogeneous nucleation), as opposed to crystallization that occurs in the absence of such a surface (homogeneous nucleation). In addition, normal urine contains a variety of inorganic and organic substances that act as inhibitors of crystallization. The most clinically important of these are citrate, magnesium, and pyrophosphate.

Sufficient energy must be generated for a crystal to form in solution. Once a crystal forms, it must either grow to sufficient size to occlude the tubular lumen or anchor itself to the urinary epithelium, which in turn provides a surface upon which it can grow. The typical transit time of a crystal in the nephron is on the order of 3 minutes, and this is too short a period for a crystal to nucleate, grow, and occlude the tubular lumen. A recent study of 19 stone formers shed additional light on how stones form in kidney. In 15 patients with idiopathic hypercalciuria the initial site of crystal formation, surprisingly, was in the basement membrane of the thin limb of the loop of Henle. The stone core was made up of calcium phosphate surrounded by calcium oxalate. The crystal deposit then eroded into the renal pelvis where it could be bathed in urine supersaturated with stone forming constituents. Why calcium phosphate would precipitate at the basolateral surface of the thin limb of the loop of Henle remains a mystery. Four of the 19 patients formed stones after intestinal bypass for obesity. In these patients, the mechanism for stone formation was different. Calcium phosphate crystals initially attached to the inner medullary collecting duct. The calcium phosphate core then acted as a nidus for calcium oxalate precipitation that resulted in luminal occlusion and growth along the inner medullary collecting duct out into the renal pelvis.

I. **Initial presentation.** A kidney stone most commonly presents with severe flank pain, sudden in onset, and often associated with nausea and vomiting. The radiation of the pain may provide some clue as to where in the urinary tract the stone is lodged. Stones in the ureteropelvic junction cause flank pain that may radiate to the groin, whereas stones lodged in the narrowest portion of the ureter, where it enters the bladder, are associated with signs of bladder irritation (dysuria, frequency, and urgency). Struvite-carbonate stones are, on occasion, incidentally discovered on abdominal radiograph. A careful abdominal examination and, in women, a pelvic examination, are important to rule out other potential causes of abdominal pain.

A. Laboratory evaluation should include a complete blood cell count, serum chemistries, and urinalysis. The white blood cell count may be mildly elevated but is generally less than 15,000 per mm^3. A white blood cell count greater than 15,000 per mm^3 is suggestive of another intraabdominal cause or an associated infection behind an obstructing calculus. An elevation of the blood urea nitrogen (BUN) and creatinine indicates prerenal azotemia, parenchymal renal disease, or obstruction of a solitary functioning kidney. A urinalysis should be performed routinely in any patient with abdominal pain. Microscopical hematuria is observed in approximately 90% of patients with nephrolithiasis.

B. Once the diagnosis is suspected based on the history, physical examination, and preliminary laboratory studies, **establishing a definitive diagnosis** is the focus of the next stage of the evaluation.

1. A **flat radiographic plate of the abdomen** is often obtained and is capable of identifying radiopaque stones (calcium oxalate, calcium phosphate, struvite-carbonate, and cystine) that are greater than or equal to 2 mm in size. It will miss radiolucent stones, the most common of which are composed of uric acid, and stones that overlie the bony pelvis. For these reasons, an abdominal flat plate is most valuable in ruling out other intraabdominal processes.

2. An **ultrasound examination of the genitourinary tract** often identifies stones in the renal pelvis; however, the majority of stones are lodged in the ureter, and the ultrasound examination often misses these.

3. The **intravenous pyelogram** (IVP) was formerly considered the gold standard for the diagnosis of nephrolithiasis and is still of considerable value in the acute setting. Although the stone itself may not be visualized on an IVP, the site of the obstruction is regularly identified. Structural or anatomic abnormalities that may be present in the urinary tract, and renal or ureteral complications can be recognized. Disadvantages of the IVP include the need for intravenous contrast and the prolonged waiting time often required to visualize the collecting system on the side of the obstruction.

4. **Spiral computed tomography** (CT), when available, is the test of choice in the patient with suspected nephrolithiasis. The advantages of spiral CT include higher sensitivity, faster scan times, and the lack of need for contrast.

C. Management. After the diagnosis is established, subsequent management is determined by; (a) the presence or absence of associated pyelonephritis; (b) whether parenteral narcotics are required for pain control; and (c) the likelihood of spontaneous passage of the stone. Obstructing calculi can be managed with observation alone if pain can be controlled with oral analgesics and spontaneous passage is likely. Extracorporeal shock wave lithotripsy may need to be employed for stones lodged in the upper ureter. Calculi in the lower ureter can be removed via cystoscopy and ureteroscopy. Hospital admission is necessary if there is evidence of infection of the renal parenchyma; when nausea, vomiting, or severe pain preclude the use of oral analgesics; or the stone is unlikely to pass spontaneously. The likelihood of spontaneous passage is determined by the size of the stone and its location in the ureter (see Table 6-1). Small stones in the distal ureter will likely pass, whereas large stones in the upper ureter will likely require urologic consultation and intervention.

II. Types of stones

A. Calcium-containing stones make up 90% of all stones and are generally composed of a mixture of calcium oxalate and calcium phosphate. In mixed stones, calcium oxalate usually predominates, and pure calcium oxalate stones are more common than pure calcium phosphate stones. Calcium

Table 6-1. Likelihood of spontaneous passage

	Likelihood of spontaneous passage
Size	
>6 mm	25%
4–6 mm	60%
<4 mm	90%
Location	
Upper ureter, >6 mm	1%
Upper ureter, <4 mm	81%
Lower ureter, <4 mm	93%

phosphate tends to precipitate in alkaline urine, as occurs with renal tubular acidosis (RTA), whereas the precipitation of calcium oxalate does not vary greatly with pH. Because urine is acidic in most patients, calcium oxalate stones are more common. The major risk factors for the formation of calcium-containing stones include hypercalciuria, hypocitraturia, hyperuricosuria, hyperoxaluria, low urine volume, and medullary sponge kidney. These risk factors can occur either alone or in combination. Their relative frequency is shown in Table 6-2.

1. **Hypercalciuria** is defined as urinary calcium excretion greater than 250 mg per 24 hours in women and greater than 300 mg per 24 hours in men. Hypercalciuria is present in about two-thirds of patients with calcium-containing stones and may result from an increased filtered load, decreased proximal reabsorption, or decreased distal reabsorption of calcium. The proximal reabsorption of calcium parallels sodium reabsorption. Any situation that decreases proximal reabsorption of sodium such as extracellular fluid (ECF) volume expansion also decreases proximal reabsorption of calcium. Distal tubular reabsorption of calcium is stimulated by parathyroid hormone (PTH), thiazides, and amiloride, and inhibited by acidosis and phosphate depletion.

   Hypercalciuria may be idiopathic or secondary to primary hyperparathyroidism, RTA, sarcoidosis, immobilization, Paget's disease, hyperthyroidism, milk-alkali syndrome, and vitamin D intoxication. The idiopathic group makes up 90% of all hypercalciuria. This category of patients is characterized by increased $1,25(OH)_2$ vitamin D_3 concentration, suppressed PTH, and reduced bone mineral density. Three potential pathophysiologic mechanisms are postulated: increased intestinal absorption of calcium, decreased renal reabsorption of calcium or phosphorus, and enhanced bone demineralization. On the basis of a fast-and-calcium-load study, some authors advocate subdividing idiopathic hypercalciuria into absorptive hypercalciuria types I, II, and III, and renal leak hypercalciuria. The rationale for this approach is that the physiologic mechanism identified will help guide specific therapy. In practice, however, this is

Table 6-2. Risk factors for calcium-containing kidney stones

Risk factor	Alone	Combined
Hypercalciuria	60%	80%
Low urine volume	10%	50%
Hypocitraturia	10%	50%
Hyperuricosuria	10%	40%
Hyperoxaluria	2%	15%

often unnecessary. In the past, increased intestinal absorption of calcium was treated with a low-calcium diet. This is no longer the case. Patients with idiopathic hypercalciuria often have reduced bone mass and are in negative calcium balance, which will be further exacerbated by a low-calcium diet. In addition, a reciprocal relationship exists between free calcium and free oxalate in the intestinal lumen. Calcium acts to bind oxalate in the intestine and reduce oxalate absorption. If oral intake of calcium is reduced, oxalate remains free in the intestinal lumen and its absorption increases. A recent study of recurrent stone formers comparing a low-calcium diet to a diet normal in calcium but low in sodium and protein showed that urinary oxalate and the risk for recurrent stone formation were increased in patients on the low-calcium diet. Finally, as shown in Table 6-3, the majority of randomized controlled studies showing that a given pharmacologic intervention reduces the risk of stone disease did not subdivide patients based on the results of a calcium load study.

In primary hyperparathyroidism, the filtered load of calcium is increased as a result of calcium release from bone and increased intestinal calcium absorption mediated by $1,25(OH)_2$ vitamin D_3. An increase in the filtered calcium load overcomes the distal actions of PTH to increase tubular calcium reabsorption. In RTA, the decreased systemic pH results in increased calcium release from bone. In addition, acidosis directly inhibits distal nephron calcium reabsorption.

Macrophages in sarcoidosis produce $1,25(OH)_2$ vitamin D_3, which leads to the increased intestinal absorption of calcium. Immobilization, Paget's disease, and hyperthyroidism cause hypercalciuria by releasing calcium from bone and increasing the filtered calcium load.

2. **Hypocitraturia.** Citrate combines in the tubular lumen with calcium to form a nondissociable but soluble complex. As a result, less free calcium is available to combine with oxalate. Citrate also prevents the nucleation and aggregation of calcium oxalate. Chronic metabolic acidosis from any cause enhances proximal tubular citrate reabsorption and decreases citrate concentration in urine; this is the mechanism whereby chronic diarrhea, RTA, and increased dietary protein load result in hypocitruria. Another important cause of hypocitruria is hypokalemia, which increases the expression of the sodium-citrate cotransporter present in the luminal membrane of the proximal tubule.

3. **Hyperuricosuria.** Uric acid and monosodium urate can act through several mechanisms to decrease the solubility of calcium oxalate in urine. They can act as a nidus upon which calcium salts can precipitate. Uric acid also binds naturally occurring macromolecular inhibitors and attenuates their activity. Finally, the addition of increasing concentrations of sodium urate to normal human urine can induce the precipitation of calcium oxalate via a poorly understood physiologic phenomenon known as "salting out."

4. **Hyperoxaluria.** The etiologies of hyperoxaluria include enteric hyperoxaluria from inflammatory bowel disease, small bowel resection, or jejuno-ileal bypass; dietary excess (e.g., spinach, Swiss chard, rhubarb); and the rare genetic disorder primary hyperoxaluria. Urinary oxalate is derived from two major sources: 80% to 90% comes from endogenous production in liver, and the remainder is obtained from dietary oxalate or ascorbic acid. In enteric hyperoxaluria, the intestinal hyperabsorption of oxalate occurs via two mechanisms. First, free fatty acids complex with calcium and limit the amount of free calcium available to complex oxalate, thereby increasing the oxalate pool available for absorption. Second, bile salts and fatty acids increase the permeability of the colon to oxalate. Additional risk factors for stone formation in these patients include intestinal fluid losses that decrease urine volume, and intestinal bicarbonate and potassium losses that result in hypocitraturia.

Table 6-3. Randomized trials in calcium-containing nephrolithiasis

Author	Treatment	Dose	Condition	No. of patients; length of follow-up	Risk reduction
Borghi	Water		First stone	199; 5 yr	55%
Laerum	Hydrochlorothiazide	25 mg b.i.d.	Noncategorized, recurrent	50; 3 yr	54%
Ettinger	Chlorthalidone	25–50 mg	Noncategorized, recurrent	54; 3 yr	48%
Ettinger	Allopurinol	100 mg t.i.d.	Hyperuricosuria, recurrent	60; 3 yr	45%
Barcelo	Potassium citrate	30–60 mEq	Hypocitraturia, recurrent	57; 3 yr	65%
Ettinger	Potassium-magnesium-citrate	42/21/63 mEq	Noncategorized, recurrent	64; 3 yr	81%
Ettinger	Potassium phosphate	1.4 g	Noncategorized, recurrent	71; 3 yr	None
Ettinger	Magnesium hydroxide	650–1,300 mg	Noncategorized, recurrent	52; 3 yr	None

5. **Low urinary volume.** This is perhaps the most intuitively obvious of the risk factors for calcium-containing kidney stones. The lower the volume of solvent, the more likely that a given amount of salt will be supersaturating. This risk factor is particularly prominent in warm climates with low humidity.

6. **Medullary sponge kidney** should be suspected in women, or in men with no other risk factors for calcium-containing stones. Studies have shown that as many as 3% to 12% of patients with calcium-containing stones have this disorder. It has a prevalence of about 1 in 5,000 and affects males and females equally. The anatomic abnormality is an irregular enlargement of the medullary and inner papillary collecting ducts. The diagnosis is usually established in the fourth or fifth decade by an IVP that reveals radial, linear striations in the papillae or cystic collections of contrast media in ectatic collecting ducts. Patients present with stones or recurrent UTI, often associated with a distal RTA. Malformations of the terminal collecting duct result in urinary stasis that promotes crystal precipitation and attachment to the tubular epithelium.

   In one report, nanobacteria were isolated from 30 of 30 calcium-containing stones. Nanobacteria are members of the Proteobacterium family, and they grow in protein- and lipid-free environments. They are capable of nucleating carbonate apatite directly on their surfaces at physiologic pH. This finding awaits confirmation from other laboratories. A subsequent study failed to culture nanobacteria from 10 upper urinary tract stones.

B. **Uric acid stones** represent approximately 5% of all cases of nephrolithiasis in Western countries. The highest incidence has been reported from Israel and the Middle East, where as many as 75% of all kidney stones consist solely of uric acid. This may be the result of the arid climate and reduced urinary volume. Uric acid is the major metabolic end product of purine metabolism in humans. Unlike most other mammals, humans do not express uricase, which degrades uric acid into the much more soluble allantoin. Uric acid stones are the most common radiolucent stone.

1. **Pathophysiology.** The principal determinant of uric acid crystallization is its relative insolubility at acidic pH. Uric acid is a weak organic acid with two dissociable protons. The first has a pK_a of 5.5, and the second a pK_a of 10. As a result, only the first proton is dissociated in urine. At a pH of less than 5.5, the undissociated acid predominates, and it is more likely to crystallize (solubility 80 mg/L). As pH increases, uric acid dissociates into the more soluble sodium urate (solubility 1 gm/L). Because of the great increase in solubility with increasing pH, uric acid stones are the only kidney stones that can be completely dissolved with medical therapy. The main determinants of uric acid solubility are pH, concentration, and other cations present in urine. A higher sodium concentration decreases, whereas an increased potassium concentration increases, uric acid solubility. This may explain the complication of calcium-containing stone formation that can develop during sodium alkali therapy but not during treatment with potassium alkali. Sodium-containing alkalis also increase urinary calcium excretion secondary to ECF volume expansion.

2. **Signs and symptoms.** Patients with uric acid stones exhibit a lower mean urinary pH and ammonium ion excretion rate. As many as 75% demonstrate a mild defect in renal ammoniagenesis in response to an acid load. Urinary buffers other than ammonia are titrated more fully than in unaffected individuals, with a resultant urine pH approximating 4.5.

   Those with defects in ammoniagenesis, such as the elderly and patients with polycystic kidney disease, are at increased risk for uric acid lithiasis. The second most important risk factor is decreased urine volume. Hyperuricosuria is the least important risk factor and is seen in less than 25% of patients with recurrent uric acid stones.

3. A **definitive diagnosis** is established through stone analysis. The diagnosis is suggested by the presence of a radiolucent stone, although xanthine and 2,8-dihydroxyadenosine stones can also be radiolucent, or by the presence of uric acid crystals in unusually acidic urine.

C. Struvite-carbonate stones are also known as infection stones and are composed of a mixture of magnesium ammonium phosphate (struvite: $MgNH_4PO_4 \cdot 6H_2O$) and carbonate apatite $[Ca_{10}(PO_4)_6CO_3]$. Of all stones, 10% to 15% are estimated to be struvite-carbonate stones. This is likely an overestimate, however, given that these figures are based on reports from chemical stone analyses, and a greater proportion of stones chemically analyzed are obtained from surgical specimens. It is likely that struvite-carbonate stones make up no more than 5% of kidney stones. Their presence is also known as "stone cancer" because, before more recent therapeutic advances, they were the cause of numerous operations, renal failure, and death. Struvite-carbonate stones are the most common cause of staghorn calculi, although cystine, calcium oxalate, and urate stones may occasionally form staghorns. Struvite-carbonate becomes supersaturating in urine only in one circumstance: infection by urea-splitting organisms that secrete urease. The most common urease-producing bacteria include *Proteus, Morganella, Providencia, Pseudomonas,* and *Klebsiella. Escherichia coli* and *Citrobacter* do not produce urease.

1. Risk factors. Women with recurrent UTI and patients with spinal cord injury, other forms of neurogenic bladder, or ileal diversions of the ureter are most prone to the formation of struvite-carbonate stones. Men with indwelling bladder catheters and complete spinal cord transection are at highest risk.

2. Signs and symptoms. Struvite stones may present in a variety of ways, including fever, hematuria, flank pain, recurrent UTI, and septicemia. They can grow to a very large size and fill the renal pelvis as a staghorn calculus. The carbonate apatite component makes them radio-opaque. Rarely, if ever, do they pass spontaneously, and 25% are discovered incidentally. If untreated, they result in loss of the affected kidney in 50% of cases.

3. Pathophysiology. For struvite-carbonate stones to form, the urine must be alkaline, with a pH greater than 7.0 and supersaturated with ammonium hydroxide. Bacterial urease hydrolyzes urea to ammonia and carbon dioxide. The ammonia then hydrolyzes spontaneously to form ammonium hydroxide; the carbon dioxide hydrates to form carbonic acid and, subsequently, bicarbonate. At high pH, the bicarbonate loses its proton to become carbonate. UTI with a urease-producing organism is the only situation in which urinary pH, ammonium, and carbonate are elevated simultaneously. The bacteria produce supersaturation in their own immediate environment. Crystals form around clusters of bacteria, and bacteria permeate every crevice of a struvite-carbonate stone. The stone itself is an infected foreign body.

D. Cystine stones. Cystinuria is the result of an autosomal recessive defect in the proximal tubular and jejunal reabsorption of the dibasic amino acids cysteine, ornithine, lysine, and arginine. Excessive amounts of these amino acids are excreted in urine, but clinical disease is due solely to the poor urinary solubility of cystine. Cystine is a dimer of cysteine. Cystine stones make up less than 1% of all calculi in adults but may constitute as many as 5% to 8% of all kidney stones in children. The prevalence of cystinuria is approximately 1 per 15,000 in the United States. Pure cystine stones form only in homozygotes. A normal adult excretes less than 19 mg of cystine per gram of creatinine in 24 hours. Cystine stones are radio-opaque due to the sulfhydryl moiety of cysteine.

1. Pathophysiology. The solubility of cystine is approximately 250 mg per L, and this rises with increasing urinary pH. The pK_a of cysteine is 6.5; therefore, a gradual increase in solubility occurs as urinary pH rises from 6.5 to 7.5. Supersaturation occurs at cystine concentrations greater than 250 mg per L. If the cystine concentration can be maintained below 200 mg per L, cystine stones should not form. Because homozygotes excrete 800 to 1,000 mg of cystine per day, at least 4 L of urine is required at normal urinary pH to keep the cystine concentration within the soluble range.

2. **Signs and symptoms.** Cystine stones begin to form in the first to fourth decades. Patients tend to have bilateral obstructive staghorn calculi with associated renal failure. Characteristic hexagonal crystals may be identified, particularly in the first morning urine, which is usually acidic. Heterozygotes can form stones either with no cystine or with cystine as only a minor component, given that cystine can act as a nidus for the crystallization of both calcium oxalate and calcium phosphate.

E. **Drug-related stones.** A variety of drugs can precipitate in urine, including sulfonamides, triamterene, acyclovir, and the antiretroviral agent indinavir. Microscopic hematuria occurs in up to 20% of patients on indinavir. Nephrolithiasis develops in 3%, and 5% experience either dysuria or flank pain that resolves when the drug is discontinued. Reports show that patients with flank pain may have abnormal CT scans with a decrease in contrast excretion in the medullary rays.

Approximately 1 in 2,000 stones are ephedrine stones. These can result from either abuse of over-the-counter cold formulations or the ingestion of *Ma-huang*. *Ma-huang* is prepared from the dried stems of ephedra and is rich in ephedrine, norephedrine, pseudoephedrine, and norpseudoephedrine. It is contained in a variety of health food store preparations. The FDA has recently banned the sale of ephedrine-containing products.

III. **Evaluation of the patient**

A. **Calcium-containing stones.** The first question to be addressed in the patient with calcium-containing stones is whether the stone disease is simple or complicated. Simple disease is defined as a single stone in the absence of an associated systemic disorder. Complicated calcium-containing stone disease is present if the patient has multiple stones, evidence of the formation of new stones, enlargement of old stones, or the passage of gravel. This distinction is made based on the initial evaluation. A history should be obtained, looking for a family history of stone disease, skeletal disease, inflammatory bowel disease, and UTI. Environmental risk factors are evaluated, such as fluid intake, urine volume, immobilization, diet, medications, and vitamin ingestion. A physical examination is performed. Initial laboratory evaluation includes blood chemistries, urinalysis, and a flat radiographic plate of the abdomen to assess stone burden. Stone analysis should always be carried out if the patient has saved the stone. Stone analysis is inexpensive. It is also the only way to establish the diagnosis of a specific disorder and often helps to direct therapy. In addition, it was shown that in 15% of cases, analyses of 24-hour urines would not have predicted the chemical composition of the stone.

In the patient with complicated disease, two to three measurements of serum calcium should be performed. If any of these serum calcium levels is above 10 mg per dL, PTH concentration should be evaluated. Blood chemistries are examined. An IVP may be indicated to rule out structural abnormalities that predispose to stone formation. A first morning void urine should be examined for cystine crystals. At least two 24-hour urine collections should be obtained on the patient's usual diet for calcium, citrate, uric acid, oxalate, sodium, phosphate, volume, pH, and creatinine. Further therapeutic intervention depends on the results of these collections. Normal values for 24-hour urine collection are shown in Table 6-4. If a therapeutic intervention is undertaken, a 24-hour urine collection should be repeated in 6 to 8 weeks to verify its expected effect and then repeated on a yearly basis.

B. **Uric acid stones.** The etiologies of **uric acid stones** can be subdivided into three pathophysiologic groups based on risk factors. Low urine volume

Table 6-4. Normal values for 24-hour urine collection

Substance	Male (mg/24 hr)	Female (mg/24 hr)
Calcium	<300	<250
Uric acid	<800	<750
Citrate	>200	>400
Oxalate	<40	<40

contributes to uric acid stones in gastrointestinal disorders such as Crohn's disease, ulcerative colitis, diarrhea, ileostomies, and dehydration. Acidic urinary pH plays an important role in primary gout and gastrointestinal disorders. Hyperuricosuria is divided into those with hyperuricemia (primary gout, enzyme disorders, myeloproliferative diseases, hemolytic anemia, and uricosuric drugs) and those without hyperuricemia (dietary excess).

Primary gout is an inherited disorder most likely transmitted in an autosomal dominant fashion with variable penetrance. It is associated with hyperuricemia, hyperuricosuria, and a persistently acid urine. In affected patients 10% to 20% have uric acid stones, and in 40% kidney stones precede the first attack of articular gout. Because the urine is always acidic, the risk of uric acid lithiasis varies directly with serum and urine uric acid concentration.

Uric acid stones are typically round and smooth and are more likely to pass spontaneously than calcium-containing stones, which are often jagged. They are also radiolucent, as are xanthine, hypoxanthine, and 2,8-dihydroadenine stones. Xanthine, hypoxanthine, and 2,8-dihydroadenine stones should be suspected if a radiolucent stone fails to dissolve with alkali therapy.

C. Struvite-carbonate stones. Seventy-five percent of all staghorn calculi are composed of struvite-carbonate. Struvite-carbonate stones are large and less radiopaque than calcium-containing stones. As with any kidney stone, the definitive diagnosis can only be established on chemical analysis, but a diagnosis of struvite-carbonate stones should be strongly suspected in any patient with an infected alkaline urine. In the presence of an infected acid urine and a staghorn calculus, one should consider the possibility that the two are unrelated and that the calculus may be either calcium-containing or a uric acid stone. Stone analysis and culture should be carried out in all patients after either percutaneous nephrolithotomy or extracorporeal shock wave lithotripsy. Some patients, especially ambulatory men, have stones that contain a mixture of struvite-carbonate and calcium oxalate. These patients should always undergo a complete metabolic evaluation, because virtually all of them have an underlying metabolic defect, and they are probably at higher risk for stone recurrence, even with complete removal of the stone.

Proteus mirabilis accounts for more than one-half of all urease-producing infections. Stone culture, when possible, is important, because culture of the urine is not always completely representative of the organisms present in the stone. If no organisms are cultured, then the possibility of infection with *Ureaplasma urealyticum*, which is often difficult to culture, should be considered.

D. Cystine stones. The presence of characteristic hexagonal crystals in a first morning void urine is diagnostic of cystinuria, although this is a very infrequent finding. The simplest and most rapid screening test for cystinuria is the sodium-nitroprusside test, which has a lower limit of detection of 75 mg per gram of creatinine. The nitroprusside complex binds to sulfide groups and may yield a false positive result in patients taking sulfur-containing drugs. Phosphotungstic acid has also been used as an alternative screening test. Patients with a positive screening test should undergo 24-hour urine cystine quantitation. Cystine stones are usually less radiodense on radiography than calcium-containing or struvite-carbonate stones. They typically have a homogeneous structure without striation.

IV. Treatment

A. Calcium-containing stones. The treatment of calcium-containing stones is determined by whether the patient has simple or complicated disease. The American College of Physicians advises that the patient with a single, isolated stone and no associated systemic disease be managed with nonspecific forms of therapy alone, including increased fluid intake and a diet normal in calcium. This approach is approporiate in patients at low risk of recurrence. One may consider, however, performing more extensive studies in those patients at high risk for recurrence (Caucasian males; 63% will form a second stone within 8 years) or in those who may experience substantial morbidity with a recurrence (kidney transplant patient).

The patient with complicated disease is managed with both nonspecific and specific treatment. Specific therapy varies depending on the assessment of risk factors derived from the analysis of 24-hour urines.

1. Nonspecific therapeutic options include manipulation of fluid intake and diet. Increasing fluid intake is the cheapest way to reduce urinary supersaturation with calcium oxalate and phosphate. In a prospective randomized trial of 199 first-time stone formers followed for a 5-year period, the risk of recurrent stone formation was reduced from 27% to 12% by raising urinary volume to more than 2 L per day with water ingestion. The average increase in urine volume in patients advised to increase fluid intake is approximately 300 mL per day.

Before 1993, the majority of patients with calcium-containing stones were advised to restrict dietary calcium. More recent studies, however, in both men and women suggest that a low-calcium diet may actually increase the risk of forming calcium-containing stones. The postulated mechanism is that ingested calcium aids in complexing dietary oxalate, and a reduction in dietary calcium results in a reciprocal increase in the intestinal absorption of oxalate. As a result, urinary supersaturation of calcium oxalate increases. In these studies, however, the ingestion of a diet high in calcium was also associated with an increased intake of magnesium, potassium, and phosphate, which may have acted as a confounding variable in reducing stone risk. A recent prospective, randomized, controlled trial compared patients on a low-calcium diet to those on a normal calcium, low-sodium, low-protein diet. The relative risk for kidney stone formation was reduced by 51% in those on the normal calcium diet. As predicted, urinary oxalate increased in the low-calcium group, compatible with the reciprocal relationship hypothesis.

Another study examined the effects of the Atkins diet on risk factors for calcium-containing stone disease. Net acid excretion increased by 56 mEq per day, urinary citrate decreased from an average of 763 mg to 449 mg, urinary pH fell from 6.09 to 5.67, and urinary calcium increased from 160 mg to 248 mg. Patients with a history of kidney stones should avoid this highly lithogenic diet.

Based on these findings, the most prudent approach is to consume a diet that is normal in calcium. The question of whether supplemental calcium increases the risk of nephrolithiasis in women is controversial. One report has suggested that any use of supplemental calcium raises the relative risk of stone disease approximately 20%. The risk in this study, however, did not increase with increasing dose. Although the relative risk of kidney stone formation is increased by supplemental calcium, one should bear in mind that women, in general, are at low risk for kidney stone formation.

2. Specific forms of treatment are directed by the results of the 24-hour urine studies. Therapy is focused around agents shown to reduce the relative risk of stone formation in randomized, placebo-controlled clinical trials with greater than 1 year of follow up (results shown in Table 6-3).

This is important because of the "stone clinic effect." After patients present for evaluation of nephrolithiasis, the subsequent period is often associated with a reduced risk for new stone formation (the "stone clinic effect"). This is the result of at least two factors: (a) regression to the mean and (b) increased adherence to nonspecific forms of treatment. Trials with less than 12 to 24 months of follow up should be viewed with skepticism if no effect is detected. At the start of treatment, patients at high risk for recurrence may have stones that are too small to be detected radiographically but that grow and subsequently are identified as new stones. Because calcium-containing stones are often difficult to prevent from increasing in size once a nidus is established, this could minimize the treatment effect in high-risk patients. Agents that were shown to be effective in randomized, placebo-controlled trials with a long duration of follow up include thiazides, allopurinol, potassium citrate, and potassium magnesium citrate.

a. **Hypercalciuria** is managed initially with thiazide diuretics. Thiazides act directly to increase distal calcium reabsorption and indirectly to increase calcium reabsorption in the proximal tubule by inducing a state of mild volume contraction. Volume contraction must be maintained and hypokalemia avoided in order for thiazide diuretics to remain maximally effective. Thiazides generally reduce urinary calcium by approximately 50%. The doses used in studies that show an effect are high, 25 mg of hydrochlorothiazide twice a day or 50 mg of chlorthalidone once a day. If they are ineffective, noncompliance with the low-sodium diet is usually the reason. This can be monitored with a 24-hour urine for sodium. Amiloride acts independently of thiazides at a more distal site and can be added if required. Two randomized, controlled trials in recurrent stone formers demonstrated a reduction in the risk of new stone formation with thiazide diuretics. Although all patients in these trials were calcium-containing stone formers, the minority were actually hypercalciuric. This suggests that thiazides may have additional effects beyond reducing urinary calcium or that the reduction of urinary calcium, even in the absence of hypercalciuria, may reduce the risk for recurrent kidney stone formation. Some have argued that the effect of thiazide diuretics may diminish with time, but this does not appear to be the case.

In patients who cannot tolerate thiazide diuretics, other potential therapies include sodium cellulose phosphate and orthophosphate. These are often poorly tolerated. Slow-release neutral phosphate appears to be better tolerated and may become the second-line agent of choice. Randomized, controlled trials of potassium acid phosphate and magnesium hydroxide showed no benefit when compared to placebo.

b. **Hypocitraturia** is managed with potassium citrate or potassium-magnesium citrate. Each of these agents reduced the relative risk of stone formation in randomized controlled trials. Potassium-magnesium citrate may be especially beneficial in patients receiving thiazide diuretics, because potassium and magnesium losses induced by the diuretic are repleted. Patients with struvite-carbonate stones should not be given citrate, because it may increase the deposition of magnesium ammonium phosphate and carbonate apatite. Citrate may also increase the intestinal absorption of aluminum in patients with renal failure. Potassium-magnesium citrate is not currently clinically available. Citrate preparations are often difficult for patients to tolerate secondary to diarrhea. Slow release preparations such as Urocit®-K are well tolerated but are relatively expensive. In patients with urinary citrate levels of less than 150 mg per 24 hours, 60 mEq should be administered daily in divided doses with meals. If the urinary citrate is greater than 150 mg per 24 hours, the dose is 30 mEq per day.

c. Hyperuricosuria is probably best managed with allopurinol. Whether alkalinization is of benefit is unclear, because heterogeneous nucleation and "salting out" can both be initiated by sodium urate. Citrate may reduce calcium oxalate precipitation in this setting, but this remains to be proven.

d. Hyperoxaluria is managed with a low-oxalate diet. Enteric hyperoxaluria should be initially treated with a low-fat, low-oxalate diet. If this is unsuccessful, calcium carbonate, cholestyramine, or both can be added.

e. Urinary volume should be increased to at least 2 L per day. This is best accomplished by drinking water, which is the only liquid shown to reduce the rate of stone formation in randomized, controlled clinical trials. If the patient will not drink water, lemonade is a sensible, although unproven, alternative. Lemon juice is high in citrate and low in oxalate.

This approach, directed at both specific and nonspecific risk factor reduction for calcium-containing stone disease, was shown to decrease the frequency of recurrent stone formation and reduce the number of cystoscopies, surgeries, and hospitalizations.

B. Uric acid stones. Therapy for uric acid stones is directed at the three major risk factors for uric acid lithiasis (decreased urine pH, decreased urine volume, hyperuricosuria). First, urine volume should be increased to 2 to 3 L per day. Second, the urine should be alkalinized to a pH of 6.5 using potassium citrate. The starting dose is 30 mEq b.i.d., to be titrated upward according to urinary pH. More than 80 to 100 mEq is rarely required. Sodium alkali therapy should be avoided, because it may result in hypercalciuria. In one study of 12 patients, alkali therapy resulted in a dissolution of stones within a period of 3 weeks to 5 months. Increases in urinary pH above 6.5 should be avoided. If the first morning void urine remains acidic, acetazolamide (250 mg) can be added at bedtime.

If hyperuricosuria is present, dietary purine consumption should be reduced. Allopurinol should only be used when stones recur despite fluid and alkali administration, or if uric acid excretion is above 1,000 mg per day. When allopurinol is administered for massive uric acid overproduction, adequate hydration must be maintained to avoid the precipitation of xanthine crystals.

C. Struvite-carbonate stones. Open surgical removal was formerly the treatment of choice for staghorn struvite-carbonate calculi. The recurrence rate, however, 6 years after surgery is 27%, and UTI persists in 41%. A second pyelolithotomy carries substantial morbidity. More recently, the combination of percutaneous nephrolithotomy and extracorporeal shock wave lithotripsy has decreased morbidity substantially and is now the treatment modality of choice. Total elimination of the stone remains a challenge, because of the inability to remove small, bacteria-containing particles that act as nidi for further crystal growth. After complete removal, chronic culture-specific antimicrobial agents are indicated as prophylaxis against recurrent infection. If a struvite-carbonate stone is not removed in its entirety, the patient will continue to have recurrent UTI, and the stone will regrow. Stone growth in the majority of patients with residual fragments progresses despite antibiotic treatment. It can be slowed by reducing the bacterial population, but the chance of cure with antibiotics alone is remote. Urease inhibitors, such as acetohydroxamic acid, reduce urinary saturation of struvite-carbonate and prevent stone growth and may, on occasion, cause dissolution of existing stones. These agents, however, are associated with a variety of severe complications including hemolytic anemia, thrombophlebitis, and nonspecific neurologic symptoms (e.g., disorientation, tremor, headache).

D. Cystine stones. Water is the hallmark of treatment for cystinuria. The required dose should be based on the patient's urinary cystine excretion.

The goal is to reduce the urinary cystine concentration below 250 mg per L. This often requires a urine output of at least 4 L per day. Two 8-oz glasses of water should be ingested every 4 hours. When patients void during the night, they should drink two glasses of water. The urine can be periodically examined for cystine crystals to assess the adequacy of fluid intake.

Urinary alkalinization may be of some benefit. The dissociation constant of cystine is 6.5. As a result, a pH of 7.5 is required for 90% of cystine to take the ionized form. At this pH, the risk of calcium phosphate stones is increased. As a result, alkalinization should be viewed as an ancillary measure. Potassium citrate is the agent of choice and is preferable to sodium-containing alkali because ECF volume expansion increases cystine excretion.

If these measures are ineffective, then either D-penicillamine, alpha-mercaptopropionylglycine, or captopril can be tried. These compounds are thiols that bind preferentially to cysteine, forming compounds that are more soluble than cysteine-cysteine dimers (cystine). Alpha-mercaptopropionylglycine causes fewer complications than D-penicillamine. D-Penicillamine also binds pyridoxine, and thus pyridoxine (50 mg per day) should be administered to prevent deficiency. Zinc supplements can usually prevent the anosmia and loss of taste that often occurs with D-penicillamine. Captopril has fewer side effects than either D-penicillamine or alpha-mercaptopropionylglycine, but may be less effective in reducing urinary cystine.

Suggested readings

Borghi L, Schianchi T, Meschi T, Guerra A, Allegri F, Maggiore U, Novarini A. Comparison of two diets for the prevention of recurrent stones in idiopathic hypercalciuria. *N Engl J Med* 2002;346:77–84.

Coe FL, Favus MJ, Pak CYC, Parks JH, Preminger GM, eds. *Kidney stones: medical and surgical management.* Philadelphia: Lippincott–Raven, 1996.

Delvecchio FC, Preminger GM. Medical management of stone disease. *Curr Opin Urol* 2003;13:229–233.

Evan AP, Lingeman JE, Coe FL, Parks JH, Bledsoe SB, Shao Y, Sommer AJ, Paterson RF, Kuo RL, Grynpas M. Randall's plaque of patients with nephrolithiasis begins in basement membranes of thin loops of Henle. *J Clin Invest* 2003;111:607–616.

Frick KK, Bushinsky DA. Molecular mechanisms of primary hypercalciuria. *J Am Soc Nephrol* 2003;14:1082–1095.

Gettman MT, Segura JW. Struvite stones: diagnosis and current treatment concepts. *J Endourol* 1999;13:653–658.

Low RK, Stoller ML. Uric acid-related nephrolithiasis. *Urol Clin North Am* 1997; 24:135–148.

Pak CYC. Medical prevention of renal stone disease. *Nephron* 1999;81:S60–S65.

Pak CYC. Southwestern internal medicine conference: medical management of nephrolithiasis—a new, simplified approach for general practice. *Am J Med Sci* 1997;313:215–219.

Parks JH, Coe FL. Pathogenesis and treatment of calcium stones. *Semin Nephrol* 1996;16:398–411.

Renner C, Rassweiler J. Treatment of renal stones by extracorporeal shock wave lithotripsy. *Nephron* 1999;81:S71–S81.

Rodman JS. Struvite stones. *Nephron* 1999;81:S50–S59.

Rutchik SD, Resnick MI. Cystine calculi: diagnosis and management. *Urol Clin North Am* 1997;24:163–171.

Shekarriz B, Stoller ML. Cystinuria and other noncalcareous calculi. *Endocrinol Metab Clin North Am* 2002;31:951–977.

Zerwekh JE, Reed-Gitomer BY, Pak CY. Pathogenesis of hypercalciuric nephrolithiasis. *Endocrinol Metab Clin North Am* 2002;31:869–884.

The Patient with Urinary Tract Infection

Marilyn E. Levi,
Jay Redington, and
L. Barth Reller

Urinary tract infections (UTIs) are some of the most common infections experienced by humans, exceeded in frequency among ambulatory patients only by respiratory and gastrointestinal infections. Indeed, bacterial infections of the urinary tract are the most common cause of both community-acquired and nosocomial infections for patients admitted to hospitals in the United States. The prognosis and management of UTIs, however, depend on the site of infection and any predisposing factors.

I. **Definitions.** Some definitions are necessary, because infection of the urinary tract may result from microbial invasion of any of the tissues extending from the urethral orifice to the renal cortex. Although the infection and resultant symptoms may be localized at one site, the presence of bacteria in the urine (bacteriuria) places the entire urinary system at risk of invasion by bacteria.

   A. **Significant bacteriuria** is defined as the presence of 100,000 or more colony-forming units (CFU) of bacteria per mL of urine, although smaller colony counts can be of diagnostic importance, particularly in young women, where 1,000 bacteria per CFU may be associated with cystitis or acute uretheral syndrome.

   B. **Anatomic location.** The first useful distinction is between upper (kidney) and lower (bladder, prostate, and urethra) UTIs. Infections confined to the bladder (cystitis), the urethra (urethritis), and the prostate (prostatitis) commonly cause dysuria, frequency, and urgency. Pyelonephritis is the nonspecific inflammation of the renal parenchyma; acute bacterial pyelonephritis is a clinical syndrome characterized by chills and fever, flank pain, and constitutional symptoms caused by the bacterial invasion of the kidney. Chronic pyelonephritis has a histopathology that is similar to tubulointerstitial nephritis, a renal disease caused by a variety of disorders, such as chronic obstructive uropathy, vesical ureteral reflux (reflux nephropathy), renal medullary disease, drugs and toxins, and possibly chronic or recurring renal bacteriuria.

   C. **Recurrence of UTI** is the result of either relapse or reinfection; making this distinction is clinically important. Reinfection is a recurring infection due to a different microorganism, which is usually drug-susceptible. Most recurring episodes of cystourethritis are due to reinfection. Relapse is a return of infection due to the same microorganism, which often is drug-resistant. Most relapses occur after treatment of acute pyelonephritis or prostatitis. Finally, asymptomatic bacteriuria is an important clue to the presence of parenchymal infection somewhere in the urinary tract; however, the importance of the infection and the need for treatment depend on the age, sex, and underlying condition of the patient.

   D. **Complicated and uncomplicated UTIs.** For the clinician, another important distinction is made between uncomplicated and complicated infections. An uncomplicated infection is an episode of cystourethritis following bacterial colonization of the urethral and bladder mucosae in the absence of upper tract disease. This type of infection is considered *uncomplicated* because sequelae are rare and exclusively due to the morbidity associated with reinfections in a subset of women. Complicated UTIs may also occur with pregnancy, diabetes, immunosuppression, structural abnormalities of the urinary tract, symptoms lasting for greater than 2 weeks, and previous pyelonephritis. Young women constitute a subset of patients with pyelonephritis (acute uncomplicated pyelonephritis) who often respond well to therapy and may also have a low incidence of sequelae. In contrast, complicated infections include those involving parenchyma (pyelonephritis or prostatitis) and frequently occur in the setting of obstructive uropathy or after instrumentation. Episodes may be refractory to therapy, often resulting in relapses, and occasionally leading to significant sequelae such as sepsis, metastatic abscesses, and, rarely, acute renal failure.

   E. Several authors have proposed a **clinical classification** for the practicing clinician (1).
      1. **Asymptomatic bacteriuria**
      2. **Acute uncomplicated cystitis in women**
      3. **Recurrent infections in women**
      4. **Acute uncomplicated pyelonephritis in women**
      5. **Complicated UTIs in both sexes**
      6. **Catheter-associated UTIs**

II. **Risk factors and pathogenesis.** Early recognition and possible prevention depend on an understanding of the pathogenesis and epidemiology of UTIs. Figure 7-1 shows the major risk periods of life for symptomatic UTIs; the increasing prevalence of asymptomatic bacteriuria that accompanies aging is apparent. Much has been learned about the risk factors for UTIs (2). Associations have been established between UTI and age; pregnancy; sexual intercourse; use of diaphragms, condoms, and spermicides, particularly Nonoxynol-9; delayed postcoital micturition; menopause; and a history of recent UTI. Factors that do not seem to increase the risk include diet, use of tampons, clothing, and personal hygiene, including directions of cleansing after defecation and

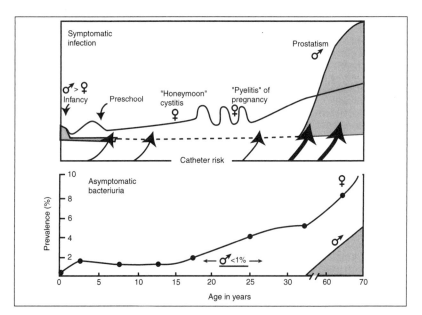

Figure 7-1. Frequency distribution of symptomatic urinary tract infections and prevalence of asymptomatic bacteriuria by age and sex (male, *shaded area;* female, *line*). (Modified from Jawetz's original concept. From Kunin CM. *Detection, prevention and management of urinary tract infections,* 4th ed. Philadelphia: Lea & Febiger, 1987. Reprinted with permission.)

bathing practices. Studies on pathogenesis have elucidated specific interactions between the host and microbes that are causally related to bacteriuria. Bacteria in the enteric flora periodically gain access to the genitourinary tract. How such bacteria actually migrate from the gastrointestinal tract to the periurethra is not known; close proximity of the anus in women is a likely factor. The subsequent bacterial colonization of uroepithelial cells is the biological phenomenon that sets the stage for persistent bacteriuria. The colonization of the periurethra often precedes the onset of bladder bacteriuria. P-fimbriated strains of *Escherichia coli* adhere to uroepithelial cells, in which glycolipids function as receptors in women who secrete blood group antigens. *E. coli* that encode for the type 1 pilus, which contains the adhesin FimH, recognizes multiple cell types associated with cystitis, sepsis, and meningitis. Immunocompromised patients may become infected with less virulent *E. coli* strains. Opposing colonization are several host factors, most notably acid pH, normal vaginal flora, and type-specific cervicovaginal antibodies.

After periurethral colonization, uropathogens gain access to the bladder via the urethra, to the kidneys via the ureters, and to the prostate via the ejaculatory ducts. The urethra and ureterovesical junction are mechanical barriers that prevent ascension. Aside from instrumentation and mechanical obstruction, however, factors promoting ascent of bacteria are not as well understood. In the bladder, organisms multiply, colonize the bladder mucosa, and invade the mucosal surface. Although urine adequately supports the growth of most uropathogens, the bladder has several mechanisms that prevent bacteriuria: (a) a mucopolysaccharide (urine slime) layer covers the bladder epithelium and prevents colonization; (b) Tamm-Horsfall protein, which is a component of uromucoid, adheres to P fimbriae and prevents colonization; and (c) urine flow and bladder contraction serve to prevent stasis and colonization. Bladder bacteriuria sets the stage for subsequent migration to the kidneys, where organisms such as P-fimbriated *E. coli* adhere to renal tubular cells. In fact, outside the setting of obstructive nephropathy, this strain of *E. coli* is the most common cause of pyelonephritis. With obstruction, however, bacterial adherence is ostensibly unimportant. Other host factors that prevent a renal infection are a high urine osmolality, high ammonium concentration, phagocytes, and increased urine flow rate.

III. **Clinical setting**

A. **Asymptomatic bacteriuria** is especially common in women, as evidenced by a minimum prevalence of 2% to 4% in young and 10% in elderly women and a 3 to 4 times higher prevalence of asymptomatic bacteriuria in diabetic women compared to their nondiabetic counterparts. The cumulative prevalence of asymptomatic bacteriuria in women increases about 1% per decade throughout life. Of note, this phenomenon has been observed in different ethnic groups and geographic locations. In contrast to women, the occurrence of asymptomatic bacteriuria in men is rare until after the age of 60 years, at which time the prevalence increases per decade and often approaches the rate in elderly women. For example, in noncatheterized, institutionalized elderly men, the prevalence of bacteriuria exceeds 20%. Prostatic hypertrophy and increased likelihood of instrumentation are thought to account for the bacteriuria of older men. Moreover, differences between men and women in the rates of bacteriuria have been attributed to the shorter female urethra and its proximity to the vaginal and rectal mucosae and the abundant microbial flora of these areas.

B. **Symptomatic UTIs** occur in all age groups. Among newborns and infants, boys are affected more often than girls. When the urinary tract is the source of neonatal sepsis, serious underlying congenital anomalies are frequently present. During childhood, persistent bacteriuria, with or without repeated symptomatic episodes, occurs in a small group (less than 2%) of school-aged girls. Such girls, and also school-aged boys with bacteriuria, should have a urologic evaluation to detect correctable structural abnormalities when UTIs are documented. Sexually active women have a markedly increased risk of episodes of cystitis. *E.coli* is the predominant organism in 75% to 90% of cases, whereas *Staphylococcus saprophyticus* is found in 5% to 15%, primarily in young women. The remainder of cases are due to enterococci and aerobic gram-negative rods, such as *Klebsiella* species and *Proteus mirabilis.*

In the absence of prostatitis, bacteriuria and symptomatic UTIs are unusual in men. In fact, asymptomatic prostatitis is very common in men presenting with febrile UTIs. More recently, uropathogenic strains of *E. coli* have been recognized as causes of cystitis in young men at risk because of homosexuality and anal intercourse, lack of circumcision, or having a partner with vaginal colonization with such P-fimbriated *E. coli.* At any age, both sexes may develop symptomatic infections in the presence of risk factors that alter urinary flow.

1. **Obstruction to urine flow**
   a. **Congenital anomalies**
   b. **Renal calculi**
   c. **Ureteral occlusion (partial or total)**
2. **Vesicoureteral reflux**
3. **Residual urine in bladder**
   a. **Neurogenic bladder**
   b. **Urethral stricture**
   c. **Prostatic hypertrophy**
4. **Instrumentation of urinary tract**
   a. **Indwelling urinary catheter**
   b. **Catheterization**
   c. **Urethral dilation**
   d. **Cystoscopy**

IV. **Clinical features**

A. **Acute urethral syndrome.** The cardinal symptoms of frequency and dysuria occur in more than 90% of ambulatory patients with acute genitourinary tract infections. One-third to one-half of all patients with frequency and dysuria, however, do not have significant bacteriuria, although most have pyuria. These patients have acute urethral syndrome, which can mimic both bladder and renal infections. Vaginitis, urethritis, and prostatitis are common causes of the acute urethral syndrome. Although certain signs and symptoms help to differentiate these clinical entities, a classic UTI can be definitively diagnosed only by quantitative cultures of urine.

1. **Vaginitis.** Approximately 20% of women in the United States have an episode of dysuria each year, and one-half of these seek medical care. The presence of an abnormal vaginal discharge (leukorrhea) and irritation makes vaginitis the likely cause of dysuria, unless a concomitant UTI can be confirmed by culture. *Candida albicans*, the most common specific cause of vaginitis, can be demonstrated readily by culture or by finding yeast cells in a Gram-stained smear of vaginal secretions or in a saline preparation with potassium hydroxide added. Trichomoniasis can be documented with a saline preparation that shows the motile protozoa of *Trichomonas vaginalis.* Nonspecific vaginitis most often is associated with *Gardnerella vaginalis.* A clue to this diagnosis is the presence of many small gram-negative bacilli that adhere to vaginal epithelial cells.

2. **Urethritis.** Acute urinary frequency, dysuria, and pyuria in the absence of vaginal symptoms favor a diagnosis of urethritis or UTI rather than vaginitis. *Chlamydia trachomatis* is a common cause of the acute urethral syndrome in women, as well as of nonspecific urethritis in men. *Neisseria gonorrhoeae* is also a widespread cause of urethritis and dysuria. The diagnosis and treatment of gonorrhea are now well standardized. Low colony count (100 to 1,000 CFU) infections with coliforms are now a recognized cause of urethritis in symptomatic young women with pyuria. Herpes simplex virus, usually type 2, is another sexually transmitted

agent that can cause severe dysuria through ulcerations in close proximity to the urethral orifice. The diagnosis of herpes progenitalis can be confirmed by finding giant multinucleated transformed cells in epidermal scrapings stained with Wright's stain (Tzanck smear), by isolating the virus in tissue culture, or by direct fluorescent antibody test.

3. **Prostatitis.** Prostatitis is a common affliction in men that causes dysuria and urinary frequency in middle-aged and younger men more frequently than UTIs do. In addition, over 90% of men with febrile UTIs have asymptomatic prostatitis manifested by elevated prostate specific antigens (PSAs) and prostate volume. The PSA may remain elevated for up to 12 months. Prostate syndromes have classically been divided into four clinical entities: (a) acute bacterial prostatitis, (b) chronic bacterial prostatitis, (c) nonbacterial prostatitis, and (d) prostatodynia.

   a. **Acute bacterial prostatitis** is easily distinguished from the other prostatitis syndromes by its acute characteristics. The patient often appears acutely ill, with the sudden onset of chills and fever, urinary frequency and urgency, dysuria, perineal and low back pain, and constitutional symptoms. Rectal examination should not be performed because of the risk of precipitating sepsis, but it may disclose an exquisitely tender, hot, and swollen prostate gland. Microscopical examination of the urine usually displays numerous white blood cells. Urine culture is usually positive for enteric gram-negative bacteria (especially *E. coli*); gram-positive bacteria (staphylococci and enterococci) are less frequently isolated.

   b. **Chronic bacterial prostatitis.** A hallmark of chronic prostatitis is relapsing UTIs. Urinary frequency, dysuria, nocturia, and low back and perineal pain are the usual symptoms, although patients may have a minimum of symptoms between UTIs. The patient is often afebrile, does not appear acutely ill, and may have an unremarkable prostate examination. A proposed mechanism to explain the migration of bacteria into the prostate is by reflux of urine and bacteria into the prostatic ducts from the urethra. This syndrome is distinguished from other forms of chronic prostatitis by displaying an initial negative midstream urine examination and culture; after prostate massage, however, the urine displays a positive microscopical examination for white blood cells, and a uropathogen can be cultured (see section V). Nonbacterial prostatitis is the most common form of chronic prostatitis. It mimics chronic bacterial prostatitis clinically and displays inflammatory cells on post–prostate massage specimens. However, bacteriologic cultures of urine and prostatic secretions are sterile. The etiology is unknown, but some evidence exists for an infectious etiology involving organisms that are difficult to culture.

   c. **Prostatodynia** has also been referred to as chronic noninflammatory prostatitis. Clinically, it presents with symptoms similar to other forms of chronic prostatitis. It is distinguished by the absence of inflammatory cells or uropathogens from all specimens.

B. **UTIs.** Despite the mimicking syndromes, a presumptive diagnosis of infections of the urinary tract can be established economically by analyzing urine in patients with characteristic, albeit nonspecific, signs and symptoms. Acute uncomplicated UTIs occur mainly in women of childbearing age. The presenting features are only suggestive of the site of infection. Patients with bacterial cystourethritis, as distinct from urethritis caused by a sexually transmitted disease (STD) pathogen, will have had prior episodes, experienced symptoms for less than 1 week, and will experience suprapubic pain.

V. **Laboratory diagnosis**

A. **Urine specimens for culture**

1. **Indications.** The diagnosis of UTI, from simple cystitis to complicated pyelonephritis with sepsis, can be established with absolute certainty

only by quantitative cultures of urine. The major indications for urine cultures are:

a. **Patients with symptoms or signs of UTIs**
b. **Follow-up of recently treated UTI**
c. **Removal of indwelling urinary catheter**
d. **Screening for asymptomatic bacteriuria during pregnancy**
e. **Patients with obstructive uropathy and stasis before instrumentation**

2. When universally applied, the first two indications may not be the most cost effective approach to diagnosing UTIs in nonpregnant, young-adult women. These individuals present with dysuria, urgency, and pyuria due to an uncomplicated episode of cystourethritis, with organisms usually susceptible to a variety of antimicrobial agents, or due to an STD pathogen such as gonococcus or chlamydia. Moreover, because the beneficial outcome of therapy is to minimize morbidity rather than prevent life-threatening complications, laboratory costs and use of resources can be minimized if pretreatment cultures are not ordered in this clinical setting. Therefore, women with symptoms consistent with simple uncomplicated lower tract disease and a positive urine dipstick can be treated without obtaining a urine culture. Additionally, if symptoms completely resolve, posttreatment cultures also are unnecessary for patients with uncomplicated infections.

3. **Methods.** Urine specimens must be cultured promptly within 2 hours or be preserved by refrigeration or a suitable chemical additive (e.g., boric acid sodium formate preservative). Acceptable methods of collection are:

a. **Midstream urine voided into a sterile container after careful washing (water or saline) of external genitalia (any soap must be rinsed away)**
b. **Urine obtained by single catheterization or suprapubic needle aspiration of the bladder**
c. **Sterile needle aspiration of urine from the tube of a closed catheter drainage system (do not disconnect tubing to get specimen)**

4. Not acceptable, because of constant contamination and the impossibility of quantitative counts, are tips from indwelling urinary catheters and urine obtained randomly, without adequate patient preparation. The clean-voided, midstream technique of collection is preferred whenever possible to avoid the risk of introducing infection at the time of catheterization, a hazard in elderly patients confined to bed, in men with condom catheters, and in diabetic patients with dysfunctional bladders. Because contamination is exceedingly rare in circumcised men, a clean-catch, midstream specimen is unnecessary in such patients. Occasionally, suprapubic aspiration of the bladder is necessary to verify infection. This technique has been most helpful in obtaining specimens from possibly septic infants and from adults in whom repeated clean-voided specimens have yielded equivocal colony counts on culture.

5. **The usual microbial pathogens** isolated from patients with UTIs are listed in Table 7-1. Results of cultures highly depend, however, on the clinical setting in which bacteriuria occurs. For example, *E. coli* is found in the urine of 80% to 90% of patients with acute uncomplicated cystitis and acute uncomplicated pyelonephritis. Many patients with staghorn calculi of the kidneys harbor urea-splitting *Proteus* organisms in their urine. *Klebsiella*, *Pseudomonas aeruginosa*, and *Enterobacter* infections are commonly acquired in the hospital. The presence of *Staphylococcus aureus* in the urine most often is a clue to concomitant staphylococcal bacteremia, unless an underlying risk factor exists. Microorganisms in young men are similar to the organisms that cause uncomplicated infections in women. Enterococci and coagulase-negative staphylococci are more common in elderly men, most likely representing recent instrumentation or catheterization. *C. albicans* is rarely encountered, except

Table 7-1. Microbial pathogens of kidney and bladder

Organism	Uncomplicated cystitis: young women[a] (%)	Pyelonephritis: outpatient, women[b] (%)	UTI: men[c] (%)	Bacteremic UTIs[d] (%)	Nosocomial UTIs[e] (%)
Gram-negative bacteria					
Escherichia coli	79	86	41	54	29
Klebsiella pneumoniae	3	4	3	9	8
Proteus	2	3	6	8	4
Enterobacter	0	0	1	2	4
Pseudomonas aeruginosa	0	0	NS	3	9
Gram-positive bacteria					
Staphylococcus saprophyticus	11	3	NS	0	0
Staphylococcus aureus	0	1	1	13	
Staphylococcus not *aureus*	0	0	5	1	5
Enterococci	2	0	5	6	13
Other bacteria	0	4	19	4	15
Mixed infections	3	3	18	2	NS
Yeast	0	0	0	3	13

NS, not stated; UTIs, urinary tract infections.

[a]Data from 607 episodes of cystitis; from Stamm WE. Urinary tract infections. In: Root RK, ed. *Clinical infectious diseases: a practical approach*, 1st ed. New York: Oxford University Press, 1999.

[b]Eighty-four episodes from Stamm 1992 and 54 nonhospitalized women; from Pinson AG, Philbrock JT, Lindbeck GH, Schorling JB, eds. Management of acute pyelonephritis in women: a cohort study. *Am J Emerg Med* 1994;12:271–278.

[c]Data from 223 outpatient males with symptoms; from Pead L, Maskell R. Urinary tract infections in adult men. *J Infect* 1981;3:71–78.

[d]185 cases (excluding five cases of *Candida albicans*); from Ackermann RJ, Monroe PW. Bacteremic urinary tract infections in older people. *J Am Geriat Soc* 1996;44:927–933.

[e]90% catheter-associated infections, 1991 experience at the University of Iowa (900-bed hospital); from Bronsema DA, Adams JR, Pallares R, Wenzel RP. Secular trends in rates and etiology of nosocomial urinary tract infections at a university hospital. *J Urol* 1993;150:414–416.

in patients with indwelling catheters, nosocomial UTIs, or relapsing infections after multiple courses of antibiotic therapy. Although the likely microorganism and usual susceptibility patterns are sufficient to guide the initial empiric therapy of uncomplicated cystitis, adequate treatment of acute bacterial pyelonephritis and complicated UTIs necessitates precise therapy based on isolation of the causative bacterium and standardized antimicrobial susceptibility testing using the disc-diffusion or the broth- or agar-dilution methods.

B. Interpretation of urine cultures. Organisms residing in the distal urethra and on pubic hairs contaminate voided, clean-catch specimens. This bacterial contamination must be distinguished from "true infection" or "significant bacteriuria" in urine cultures. Quantitative bacteriology makes this distinction. Because quantitation of bacteriuria is so important clinically, methods for culture of urine must enable the CFU number of a potential pathogen per mL of urine to be assessed. The standard procedure involves the use of calibrated bacteriologic loops that deliver a known volume of urine to the surface of agar plates. Proper plating techniques achieve isolated colonies that can be enumerated accurately. A satisfactory alternative for the diagnosis of uncomplicated UTIs is the dipslide method, which is particularly well suited to quantitative urine cultures in smaller clinics. Rapid methods based on filtration and colorimetry, bioluminescence, growth kinetics, and biochemical reactions are used increasingly to screen urine specimens for the presence of bacteria. The sensitivities of these rapid assays are in the range of 10^4 to 10^5 CFU per mL. The simplest screen is the paper-strip test for detection of leukocyte esterase and nitrite in first morning urine specimens. However, these methods are not a substitute for standard cultures in symptomatic patients with complicated UTIs.

1. Colony counts. Figure 7-2 shows a basic guide to the interpretation of quantitative cultures of urine. Colony counts greater than 10^5 CFU per mL in properly collected and transported specimens usually indicate infection. Colony counts of 10^3 or fewer CFU per mL from untreated patients are uncommon with true UTIs, except in symptomatic young

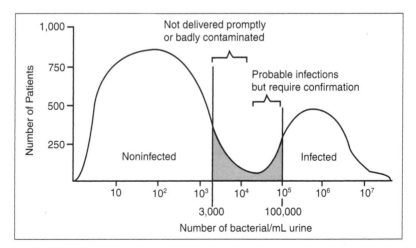

Figure 7-2. Results of quantitative bacterial counts from cultures of urine specimens. (From Brumfitt W, Percival A. Pathogenesis and laboratory diagnosis of nontuberculous urinary tract infection: a review. *J Clin Pathol* 1964;17:482. Reprinted with permission.)

women with pyuria and urethritis, in whom colony counts of *E. coli* as low as 10^3 may be interpretable if the urine was obtained by single catheterization. Intermediate counts, especially with mixed flora, usually imply poor collection or delayed transport and culture. Brisk diuresis may transiently reduce an otherwise high colony count.

2. **Suprapubic needle aspiration.** Any growth from urine obtained by suprapubic needle aspiration may be important. Use of a 0.01-mL quantitative loop for culturing aspirated urine permits the detection of as few as 100 CFU per mL. Two or more colonies (less than or equal to 200 CFU per mL) of the same microorganism ensure the purity of growth from such specimens and permit standardized antimicrobial susceptibility testing. Similar criteria should be used for patients who are receiving antimicrobials at the time of culture. Except in unusual circumstances, the isolation of diphtheroids, alpha-hemolytic streptococci, and lactobacilli indicates contamination of the urine specimen with vaginal or periurethral flora.

3. **Prostatic secretions.** In men, the distinction between a urinary source and a prostatic focus of infection must be made. The procedure for obtaining voided urine and expressed prostatic secretions in partitioned segments that enable proper interpretation is diagrammed in Figure 7-3. Leukocytes (greater than 10 to 15 white blood cells per high-power field) and lipid-laden macrophages are seldom observed in the expressed

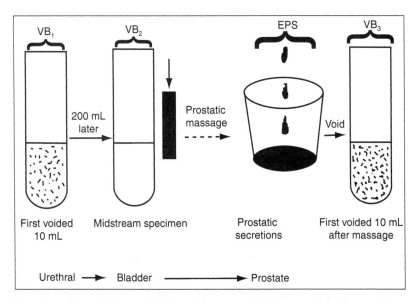

Figure 7-3. Localization of infection with segmented cultures of the lower urinary tract in men. VB_1 is the first 10 mL of voided urine, and VB_2 is the midstream specimen of urine obtained before prostatic massage. Subsequently, the expressed prostatic secretions (EPS) are collected before the final voided urine specimen (VB_3). When the bacterial colony counts in the urethral culture exceed by tenfold or more those of the midstream and prostatic cultures, the urethra is the source of the infection. The diagnosis is bacterial prostatitis if the quantitative counts of the prostatic specimens exceed those of the urethral and midstream samples. (From Meares EM, Stamey TA. Bacteriologic localization patterns in bacterial prostatitis and urethritis. *Invest Urol* 1968;5:492. Reprinted with permission.)

prostatic secretion of healthy men. These agents signify prostatic in-flammation. Therefore, a prostatic focus of infection should be consid-ered when a significant step-up of pyuria or colony counts occurs in the prostate specimens. A UTI of prostatic origin is indicated by colony counts of 10^5 or more CFU per mL of the same microorganism in all four speci-mens. Both urologists and primary care physicians underuse this proce-dure. In one study, a two-step procedure involving microscopical exami-nation and culture of pre– and post–prostate massage urine specimens compared favorably to this four-step procedure. This simplified approach was able to arrive at a similar diagnosis in 91% of patients. Further trials are needed to evaluate this approach, which may improve physician use.

C. **Microscopic examination of urine.** Procedures for the microscopical exam-ination of urine are poorly standardized; nonetheless, visualization of bac-teria leukocytes and epithelial cells in urine can provide some useful infor-mation and enable the clinician to make a presumptive diagnosis of UTI. The advantages of microscopical analysis are immediate availability and low cost. The disadvantages, depending on the method, are lack of sensi-tivity, specificity, or both. Only properly collected and processed specimens for quantitative urine cultures can provide definitive diagnosis. The micro-scopical examination can be done on either unspun urine or the centrifuged sediment. A critical comparison of these two techniques is not available. The presence of squamous epithelial cells and mixed bacterial flora indi-cates contamination and the need for a repeat specimen.

1. **Unspun urine.** When fresh, unspun urine from patients with significant bacteriuria (greater than 10^5 CFU per mL) is examined microscopically (X1,000), 90% of specimens show one or more bacteria, and 75% of spec-imens show one or more white blood cells per oil-immersion field. The best assessment of pyuria is the finding of approximately 10 white blood cells per mm^3 of unspun urine examined in a counting chamber.

2. **Centrifuged sediment.** After 10 mL of urine is centrifuged in a standard 15-mL conical tube for 5 minutes at 2,500 revolutions per minute in a clin-ical centrifuge, three or four drops of the sediment are examined under a coverslip at high power (X400) in diminished light. Patients with signif-icant bacteriuria usually show bacilli in the urinary sediment, whereas only approximately 10% of patients with fewer than 10^5 CFU per mL show bacteria. Approximately 60% to 85% of patients with significant bacteriuria have ten or more white blood cells per high-power field in the sediment of midstream voided urine; however, approximately 25% of pa-tients with negative urine cultures also have pyuria (ten or more white blood cells per high-power field), and only approximately 40% of patients with pyuria have 105 or more bacteria per mL of urine by quantitative culture. The principal pitfall is false-positive pyuria owing to leukocytes from a contaminating vaginal discharge.

3. **Gram's stain.** A simple Gram-stained smear of unspun urine or spun sediment can enhance the specificity of the test, because morphology and stain characteristics aid in identifying the likely pathogen and in targeting empiric therapy.

4. **Pyuria.** Although the presence of pyuria in a midstream specimen has low predictive value for significant bacteriuria, pyuria is a sensitive indica-tor of inflammation. Thus, pyuria may be more accurate than bacteriuria in distinguishing a "true infection" from contamination: 95% of patients with pyuria have a genitourinary tract infection; however, pyuria cannot distinguish a bacterial UTI from acute urethral syndrome. In addition to a UTI, any of the causes of acute urethral syndrome (see section **IV.A**) can result in pyuria. For example, tuberculosis is a cause of pyuria with nega-tive routine urine cultures, although mycobacterial cultures are positive in 90% of instances. Analgesic nephropathy, interstitial nephritis, per-inephric abscess, renal cortical abscess, disseminated fungal infection, and appendicitis may also result in pyuria.

D. **Biochemical tests for bacteriuria.** Two metabolic capabilities shared by most bacterial pathogens of the urinary tract are use of glucose and reduction of nitrate to nitrite; these are properties of all enterobacteriaceae. Because small amounts of glucose and nitrate are normally present in urine, the presence of significant numbers of bacteria in urine results in the absence of glucose and presence of nitrite. Dipstick devices are commercially available for both types of testing. Studies with nitrite-indicator strips show that 85% of women and children with culture-confirmed significant bacteriuria show positive results if three consecutive morning urine specimens are tested. A morning urine specimen is preferred for the nitrite test, because most bacteria take 4 to 6 hours to convert nitrate to nitrite. A negative nitrite test may be observed in patients taking diuretics or with organisms that do not produce nitrate reductase (*Staphylococcus* species, *Enterococcus* species, and *P. aeruginosa*). The sensitivity of the glucose-use test is about 90% to 95% in patients without diabetes mellitus. Both biochemical tests have fewer than 5% false-positive results. Therefore, these biochemical tests can be used by patients or parents, after proper instruction, to determine when quantitative cultures are needed in the management of recurrent episodes of UTI. Spectrum bias in the use of dipsticks must be avoided. Dipsticks should only be used for patients with symptoms suggestive of UTI (i.e., high pretest probability of UTI), and not for asymptomatic screening, as in pregnancy.

E. **Localization of the site of infection.** The site of infection within the urinary tract has great therapeutic and prognostic importance. Upper UTI (pyelonephritis) indicates a much greater likelihood of underlying uropathy (e.g., congenital anomalies, renal stones, ureteral occlusion, vesicoureteral reflux, neurogenic bladder, or prostatic hypertrophy) or previous instrumentation (see section **III.B**). Relapses with the same, often multiple-antibiotic-resistant bacteria are common with pyelonephritis or chronic bacterial prostatitis. Treatment is long (minimum, 10 to 14 days) and may be arduous. On the other hand, cystitis rarely is complicated, and treatment can be short (single-dose or 3-day) and usually is easy. No ready way to distinguish between upper and lower UTIs by simple laboratory tests exists. The difficulty in making this distinction reliably on clinical grounds alone has been discussed (see section **IV.B**). Older, indirect methods (e.g., serum antibodies, urine concentration test, and urinary beta-glucuronidase activity) are neither sensitive nor specific. Direct methods for localization (e.g., ureteral catheterization, renal biopsy, and the bladder washout technique) are hazardous, expensive, or both. Eradication of bacteriuria with single-dose or short-course (3-day) antibiotic therapy in symptomatic patients with uncomplicated disease is a practical method for presumptive localization of infection to the bladder or urethra.

F. **Radiography and other diagnostic procedures: indications.** The principal role of radiographic and urologic studies for patients with UTIs is to detect vesicoureteral reflux, renal calculi, and potentially correctable lesions that obstruct urine flow and cause stasis. Uncomplicated reinfections (cystitis and urethritis) in women who respond to short-course antimicrobial therapy are not an indication for radiographic and cystoscopic investigation of the urinary tract. Radiologic and urologic evaluation should be considered in all children with a first episode of UTIs (except for school-aged girls). Special emphasis should be on the early detection of urologic abnormalities in all young children and boys with a first infection, as well as any child with pyelonephritis or a complicated course. A review of studies evaluating diagnostic imaging in children with UTIs expressed the need for better outcome-based research in this area. Radiologic and urologic evaluation should be considered in adults with UTIs. In the past, all UTIs in males were considered complicated. The conventional recommendation that all males presenting with initial UTIs undergo urologic evaluation to identify predisposing anatomic or functional abnormalities is still followed. However, several studies have indicated that only approximately 20% of men have previously unidentified abnormalities. Some sexually active males are at a higher risk for cystitis (homosexual males, males with a partner who harbors a uropathogen, uncircumcised males). The value of urologic evaluation in this high-risk group, with a single episode of cystitis and an uncomplicated course, is not known. In general, urologic evaluations are recommended in the following situations: (a) males with first episode, (b) all patients with a complicated infection or bacteremia, (c) suspected obstruction or renal stones, (d) hematuria following infection, (e) failure to respond to appropriate antibiotic therapy, and (f) patients with recurrent infections.

Some experts recommend the evaluation of all patients with pyelonephritis. The radiologic evaluation of a subgroup of patients with pyelonephritis (young and otherwise healthy women who respond well to therapy) may have a low diagnostic yield. In one study, only 1 of 25 young women with uncomplicated pyelonephritis had a surgically correctable etiology, and 2 of 25 had focal abnormalities that resolved on a follow-up ultrasound. This has led others to recommend a diagnostic evaluation in young women with uncomplicated pyelonephritis after the second recurrence, or at any time, if a complicating course is present. The ease in obtaining a noninvasive test (ultrasound) has increased radiologic evaluations for most patients admitted with pyelonephritis.

Ultrasound with a plain film of the abdomen has replaced the intravenous pyelogram as the initial radiologic studies for most adults. For a detailed evaluation of the ureterovesical junction, bladder, and urethra, a voiding cystourethrogram and measurement of the residual urine after voiding may be necessary. If vesicoureteral reflux is present after acute infection has been treated, a urologist should be consulted. Cystoscopy may be warranted. Renal calculi can usually be detected on a plain radiograph of the abdomen. An IVP confirms the presence and the location of calculi, detects radiolucent stones (fewer than 10% of renal calculi), and discloses the degree of obstruction and dilation. Ordinarily, radiographic studies should not be performed within 6 weeks of acute infections.

Gram-negative bacilli have the ability to impede ureteral peristalsis, and transient abnormalities of the IVP are common with acute pyelonephritis. These include hydroureter, vesicoureteral reflux, diminished pyelogram, loss of renal outline, and renal enlargement. Acute pyelonephritis with an obstructed ureter is a surgical emergency, and a perinephric abscess also requires surgical drainage. These complications, however, are best detected initially by ultrasound and by computed tomography (CT), respectively. To avoid radiocontrast-induced acute renal failure, excretory urography and other radiocontrast studies should be avoided whenever possible in patients with a serum creatinine above 1.5 mg per dL, diabetes mellitus, dehydration, or advanced age.

VI. Treatment of UTI

A. Principles of underlying therapy and follow-up. To successfully treat a UTI, the clinician must have knowledge of microbial susceptibility and mechanisms of resistance, pharmacokinetics and pharmacodynamics, and status of host defenses. First, most uropathogens are susceptible to a wide range of antibiotics; however, resistant gram-negative bacteria frequently are seen with indwelling catheters, in immunocompromised patients, and in patients with relapsing bacteriuria. Second, the majority of antibiotics are filtered by the kidney and thus achieve a urinary concentration that is many times higher than the minimum inhibitory concentration. Third, although most antibiotics achieve adequate concentration in renal tissue, only tetracyclines, trimethoprim-sulfamethoxazole, and fluoroquinolones achieve any reasonable concentration in the prostate. Finally, patients with systemic or local abnormalities in host defenses usually develop a renal infection that is refractory to therapy. In this case, antibiotics that achieve adequate serum concentrations and are bactericidal are preferable to bacterial static agents. The basic caveats for the effective management of UTIs are outlined here.

1. **Asymptomatic patients** should have colony counts greater than or equal to 100,000 per mL on at least two occasions before treatment is considered.
2. Unless symptoms are present, **no attempt should be made to eradicate bacteriuria** until catheters, stones, or obstructions are removed.
3. **Selected patients with chronic bacteriuria** may benefit from suppressive therapy.
4. A patient who develops **bacteriuria as a result of catheterization** should have treatment to reestablish a sterile urine.
5. **Antimicrobial agents used for treatment** should be the safest and least expensive agents to which the causative microorganisms are susceptible.
6. **Efficacy of treatment** should be evaluated by urine culture 1 week after completion of therapy, except in nonpregnant adult women who respond to therapy for uncomplicated cystitis and uncomplicated pyelonephritis.

B. **Antimicrobial agents**
1. **Beta-lactams.** The increasing antimicrobial resistance observed in *E. coli* makes amoxicillin and ampicillin less attractive choices for empiric therapy in the patient with a complicated UTI, unless enterococcus is strongly considered to be the etiologic agent. Amoxicillin has replaced oral ampicillin due to improved bioavailability and less frequent dosing. Amoxicillin is effective for uncomplicated cystitis, but shortcourse therapy (single-dose and 3-day regimens) has generally been less effective than trimethoprim-sulfamethoxazole or fluoroquinolones given for a similar duration. Cefixime and cefpodoxime are oral thirdgeneration cephalosporins with enhanced activity against enteric gramnegative bacteria, longer serum half-life, and less frequent dosing than first-generation cephalosporins. Parenteral beta-lactams are generally reserved for more complicated infections. Ceftriaxone is a thirdgeneration cephalosporin with good activity against most communityacquired gram-negative enteric bacteria (except *P. aeruginosa*). Ceftazidime and cefepime are examples of cephalosporins with good activity against many gram-negative bacteria, including *P. aeruginosa*.
2. **Nitrofurantoin** is active against many uropathogens, including *E. coli*, *Staphylococcus saprophyticus*, and *Enterococcus faecalis*. Some gramnegative bacteria are resistant to nitrofurantoin (*Klebsiella, Enterobacter*, and *Pseudomonas* species), making it a less than ideal agent for the empiric therapy of complicated UTIs. No clinically significant increase in resistance has been observed. However, this drug is significantly less active than fluoroquinolones and trimethoprim-sulfamethoxazole against non-*E. coli* aerobic gram-negative rods and is inactive against *Proteus* and *Pseudomonas* species. The major role of nitrofurantoin in therapy includes the treatment of uncomplicated cystitis and as an alternative agent for cystitis caused by *E. faecalis*.The oral adult dose for both crystalline and macrocrystalline preparations is 50 to 100 mg every 6 hours for 7 days. Although a 3-day regimen is successful in many patients with uncomplicated cystitis, one clinical trial found nitrofurantoin to be less effective than a 3-day regimen of trimethoprim-sulfamethoxazole. Patients with renal insufficiency (creatinine clearance less than 60 mL per minute) should not receive this agent. Nitrofurantoin has been used in pregnancy [U.S. Food and Drug Administration (FDA) category B], although it is contraindicated in nursing mothers, pregnant women near term, and newborns (in whom it is associated with hemolytic anemia). Suppressive

therapy has been successful in some patients, although concern for less common reactions (e.g., peripheral neuropathy, pneumonitis, and hepatitis) may limit long-term use.

3. **Trimethoprim-sulfamethoxazole and trimethoprim.** Trimethoprim-sulfamethoxazole has a wide spectrum of activity against many uropathogens. However, lack of clinical activity against enterococci and *P. aeruginosa*, as well as increased resistance by some enteric gram-negative bacteria (*Klebsiella* species, *Enterobacter* species), makes trimethoprim-sulfamethoxazole a less than ideal agent for the treatment of complicated UTIs. In addition, resistance patterns tabulated by microbiology laboratories show trimethoprim-sulfamethoxazole resistance variability depending on locale; an 18% incidence of resistance is present in the southeastern and western United States for women with acute cystitis who have had a UTI in the last 6 months. Therefore, some authorities recommend the use of trimethoprim-sulfamethoxazole only if (a) the local resistance pattern is less than 20%, (b) no sulfa allergy exists, and (c) no recent antibiotic use is present. Of interest, despite a 30% resistance prevalence in some locales, at least half of women treated with trimethoprim-sulfamethoxazole have 80% to 85% clinical and microbiologic cures.

Trimethoprim-sulfamethoxazole is well tolerated in most patients. Adverse effects due to sulfonamides are well described and include gastrointestinal symptoms, transient elevation in the serum creatinine, and hematologic and dermatologic reactions. Sulfonamides displace warfarin and hypoglycemic agents from albumin, thus potentiating these drug effects. Trimethoprim-sulfamethoxazole is highly effective for the prophylaxis and therapy of uncomplicated cystitis and for therapy of uncomplicated pyelonephritis. A randomized trial with four different 3-day drug regimens in women with uncomplicated acute cystitis found a 3-day regimen of trimethoprim-sulfamethoxazole was the most cost-effective. Complicated UTIs, especially catheter-associated infections and nosocomial UTIs, should have *in vitro* susceptibility testing performed. Trimethoprim-sulfamethoxazole has been used in pregnancy, but it is not FDA-approved for pregnant women. Other agents, such as amoxicillin, nitrofurantoin, and cephalosporins, are preferred.

Trimethoprim alone is preferred over trimethoprim-sulfamethoxazole by some experts for the prophylaxis and treatment of uncomplicated cystitis, because its efficacy is similar and the side effects fewer (because of the absence of sulfamethoxazole). This agent should not be used alone for the therapy of complicated UTIs.

Trimethoprim monotherapy also achieves good prostate concentrations and is an alternative to fluoroquinolones depending on the susceptibility pattern of the bacteria.

4. Multiple **fluoroquinolones** are now available for clinical use (Tables 7-2 and 7-3). These agents achieve very high concentrations in the urine and renal tissue, easily exceeding the minimal inhibitory concentration of most uropathogens. Fluoroquinolones should not be used as first-line agents for the therapy of uncomplicated cystitis because of concern for the development of resistance and because of the cost. However, their antimicrobial spectrum and generally low side-effect profile make them excellent choices for empiric therapy of complicated UTIs. Among current agents within this antimicrobial class, no particular drug has demonstrated superior clinical efficacy for the therapy of patients with UTIs. An exception is moxifloxacin, which does not achieve adequate urinary concentrations and should be avoided in the treatment of UTIs. Fluoroquinolones should not be used for enterococcal UTIs (only 60% to 70% susceptible), during pregnancy or in children (until further information is available). Aluminum- and magnesium-containing antacids and iron-,

Table 7-2. Oral antimicrobial agents commonly used for treatment of urinary tract infections

	Adult dose	Comment
Miscellaneous agents		
Trimethoprim	100 mg every 12 hr	Prophylaxis, uncomplicated cystitis
Trimethoprim-sulfamethoxazole	160 mg/800 mg every 12 hr	Uncomplicated cystitis; cost-effective
Nitrofurantoin	50–100 mg every 6 hr	Prophylaxis, uncomplicated cystitis
Tetracycline	250–500 mg every 6 hr	Prophylaxis
Beta-lactams[a]		
Amoxicillin	250–500 mg every 8 hr	During pregnancy, enterococcal infections
Cephalexin or cephradine	250 mg every 6 hr	During pregnancy, uncomplicated cystitis
Cefixime	200 mg every 12 h/ 400 mg every 24 hr	Step-down therapy[a]
Cefpodoxime	100–200 mg every 12 hr	Step-down therapy[a]
Fluoroquinolones		
Norfloxacin	400 mg every 12 hr	Low serum drug levels
Ciprofloxacin	250–500 mg every 12 hr	First "systemic" fluoroquinolone
Lomefloxacin	400 mg every 24 hr	Skin photosensitivity reactions
Enoxacin	400 mg every 12 hr	P-450 drug interactions[b]
Ofloxacin	200–400 mg every 12 hr	Generally replaced by levofloxacin
Levofloxacin	250–500 mg every 24 hr	L-isomer of ofloxacin

Note: Comments for miscellaneous agents and beta-lactams relate to role in therapy. The role of fluoroquinolones has been for treatment of complicated UTIs and as an alternative agent for uncomplicated cystitis. Because these agents have not been rigorously compared, comments are related to general spectrum of activity, side-effect profile, and drug interactions.
[a]Short-course therapy for uncomplicated cystitis has generally been less effective than the use of trimethoprim-sulfamethoxazole or fluoroquinolones for a similar duration. The general role of extended-spectrum oral cephalosporins (cefixime, cefpodoxime) has been for the treatment of complicated UTIs (alternative agent) and for intravenous to oral step-down therapy.
[b]Enoxacin is a potent inhibitor of P-450 hepatic isoenzymes. (Inhibition of hepatic isoenzymes causes an elevation of serum levels of theophylline and caffeine.)

calcium-, and zinc-containing preparations should not be administered with oral fluoroquinolones due to a significant decrease in absorption. In general, these agents are well tolerated by most patients. The most common adverse effects are gastrointestinal and on the central nervous system, but these infrequently lead to drug discontinuation. Photosensitivity may limit the use of some of these agents (e.g., lomefloxacin, sparfloxacin). Many of these agents are available for both parenteral and oral administration. Conversion from parenteral to oral therapy (step-down therapy) should be considered for patients who are clinically stable and tolerating oral medications. The excellent bioavailability of these drugs, good clinical success with oral therapy, and the high cost of parenteral therapy due to intravenous catheter–related complications and cost of intravenous preparations are all good reasons for considering oral therapy.

Table 7-3. Intravenous antimicrobial agents commonly used for treatment of urinary tract infections (UTIs)

	Adult dose	Comment
Beta-lactams		
Ampicillin	1–2 g every 4 hr	*Enterococcus faecalis;* usually combined with gentamicin
Ceftriaxone	1 g every 12–24 hr	Pyelonephritis
Ceftazidime	1–2 g every 8–12 hr	Complicated UTI, including *Pseudomonas aeruginosa*
Cefepime	1–2 g every 12 hr	Complicated UTI, including *Pseudomonas aeruginosa*
Aztreonam	1 g every 8-12 hr	Penicillin-allergic patient
Fluoroquinolones[a]		
Ciprofloxacin	200–400 mg every 12 hr	
Ofloxacin	200–400 mg every 12 hr	Generally changed to levofloxacin
Levofloxacin	500 mg every 24 h	
Miscellaneous agents		
Trimethoprim-sulfamethoxazole	160 mg/800 mg every 12 hr	Prophylaxis, uncomplicated cystitis
Vancomycin	1 g every 12 hr	Methicillin-resistant *Staphylococcus aureus;* serious enterococcal infection in the penicillin-allergic patient
Gentamicin	4–7 mg/kg every 24 hr	Serious gram-negative infection
	1.5–2.0 mg/kg every 8 hr	Older dosing schedule; for enterococcus combined with ampicillin

[a]Because oral fluoroquinolones have excellent bioavailability and cost approximately 20% as much as parenteral fluoroquinolones, conversion from intravenous to oral therapy should be done when the patient is clinically stable.

C. Treatment of asymptomatic bacteriuria

  1. Pregnancy increases the risk of UTI complications. The rate of prematurity in children born to women who have bacteriuria during pregnancy is increased, and 20% to 40% of these patients develop pyelonephritis. Successful therapy of these patients with bacteriuria decreases the risk of symptomatic infection by 80% to 90%. Therefore, all women should be screened twice during gestation for asymptomatic bacteriuria. All bacteriuria patients should be treated for 7 days, with follow-up cultures to identify relapses. Long-term prophylaxis offers no advantage over close surveillance. In selecting therapy, the risk to the fetus should be considered. Short-acting sulfonamides or amoxicillin for 7 days usually suffices, because almost all these infections are caused by susceptible *E. coli.* Tetracyclines (FDA category D), trimethoprim (FDA category C), and fluoroquinolones (FDA category C) should be avoided.

  2. Children. Asymptomatic bacteriuria in preschool- and school-aged girls may signify underlying vesicoureteral reflux. Moreover, vesicoureteral reflux, when combined with recurring bacteriuria, can result in progressive renal scarring. Therefore, in this at-risk population, asymptomatic bacteriuria should routinely be detected and treated, with follow-up urologic evaluations after 6 weeks.

3. **General population.** Asymptomatic bacteriuria in men and nonpregnant women, a common condition in the elderly, does not appear to cause renal damage in the absence of obstructive uropathy or vesical ureteral reflux. Prospective randomized studies of therapy for asymptomatic bacteriuria in the elderly have been recently reviewed. Of five clinical trials reviewed, three studies had very small sample sizes, and one non-blinded study displayed a nonstatistical significant decrease in symptomatic infections. The largest randomized trial failed to demonstrate any significant difference in mortality between treated and untreated patients. Therefore, repeated attempts to clear the bacteriuria with antimicrobial agents seem unwarranted; they may only select for more resistant microorganisms and create a need for more toxic and costly antibiotics should the patient subsequently develop symptoms.
4. **Miscellaneous.** Instrumentation of the genitourinary tract should be avoided in patients with asymptomatic bacteriuria or, if necessary, done under the cover of prophylactic antimicrobial therapy. Selected high-risk patients (e.g., with renal transplantation or neutropenia) may benefit from therapy for asymptomatic bacteriuria.
D. **Treatment of uncomplicated cystitis.** Acute cystitis and low-colony-count coliform urethritis are almost exclusively diseases of women, mostly sexually active women between the ages of 15 and 45 years. Although reinfection is common, complications are rare.
   1. **Short-course therapy.** Appreciable evidence exists that infections truly confined to the bladder or urethra respond as well to single-dose or short-course (3-day) therapy as to conventional therapy for 10 to 14 days. Indeed, response to single-dose or short-course therapy implies a lower UTI. Reviews of short-course therapy have concluded that 3-day regimens are more effective than single-dose therapy. One randomized trial evaluated four different 3-day drug regimens in women with uncomplicated acute cystitis. A 3-day regimen of trimethoprim-sulfamethoxazole was more effective than a 3-day regimen of nitrofurantoin. Cure rates for cefadroxil (66%) and amoxicillin (67%) were not statistically different from the cure rate for trimethoprim-sulfamethoxazole (82%). The 3-day regimen of trimethoprim-sulfamethoxazole was the most cost-effective regimen. Further clinical trials are needed to evaluate other patients with uncomplicated cystitis and to measure the impact of newer agents (fluoroquinolones) on outcomes and cost effectiveness. Recommended oral 3-day regimens include trimethoprim-sulfamethoxazole, trimethoprim, and a fluoroquinolone. This variety of treatments is an important breakthrough in the management of uncomplicated cystitis and coliform urethritis, because all patients were treated formerly with the standard 10 to 14 days of therapy. Diabetic women with uncomplicated infections (i.e., with normal urinary tracts) may also be treated with a 3-day course of antibiotic therapy. Post-treatment urine cultures are not required unless symptoms persist. Formal urologic imagings, such as ultrasound, intravenous pyelography, and CT, are not needed in most cases, as correctable abnormalities are rarely found.
   2. **Seven-day regimen.** A longer course of therapy for cystitis should be considered in patients with complicating factors that lead to a lower success rate and a higher risk of relapse. These complicating factors include a history of prolonged symptoms (more than 7 days), recent UTI, diabetic patients with abnormal urinary tracts, age older than 65 years, and use of a diaphragm. Importantly, the elderly frequently have concurrent renal bacteriuria; thus, short-course therapy should not be used.
   3. **Symptomatic pyuria without bacteriuria** in an otherwise healthy young person suggests chlamydial or gonococcal urethritis. The importance of documenting these infections as well as screening for other STDs (e.g., human immunodeficiency virus infection, syphilis), and the necessity of counseling about STD risk reduction cannot be understated.

Recent guidelines suggest that either a single dose of azithromycin or a 7-day course of doxycycline is effective for chlamydial urethritis. Therapy for gonococcal urethritis includes a single dose of ceftriaxone or cefixime, or a fluoroquinolone combined with therapy for chlamydial infection.

E. Management of recurrent cystitis (reinfections). Ten to twenty percent of women develop recurrent UTIs within several months. Some infections are related to inadequate antimicrobial therapy. It is common, however for women whose periurethral and vaginal epithelial cells avidly support attachment of coliform bacteria to suffer from recurrent episodes of cystitis in the absence of recognized structural abnormalities of the urinary tract. A recent prospective study of UTIs in young women identified recent use of a diaphragm and spermicide such as Nonoxynol-9, recent sexual intercourse, and a history of recurrent infection as risk factors for infection.

   1. Antimicrobial strategies. Strategies for managing the disease of women with frequent episodes of cystitis include (a) postcoital prophylaxis, (b) continuous low-dose prophylaxis, (c) patient self-administered therapy, and (d) consideration of contraception or barrier methods against STDs without the use of vaginal spermicides. Postcoital prophylaxis is most helpful for patients who associate recurrent UTIs with sexual intercourse. In these women, a single dose of an antimicrobial after sexual intercourse or thrice weekly at bedtime has been shown to significantly reduce the frequency of episodes of cystitis from an average of three per patient-year to 0.1 per patient-year. Women with frequent recurrent infections (more than three UTIs per year) are offered these prophylactic regimens. Women with fewer than three UTIs per year can be offered self-administered treatment. Multiple antimicrobial agents have demonstrated efficacy in prophylaxis and self-administered therapy. Some of these regimens include nitrofurantoin, 50 or 100 mg; trimethoprim, 100 mg; trimethoprim-sulfamethoxazole, 40 mg per 200 mg; and cephalexin, 250 mg. Fluoroquinolones and cephalosporins are also effective but are more expensive. Although antimicrobial prophylaxis is effective and usually safely tolerated for months to years, single-dose therapy for acute cystitis makes prophylaxis more expensive and possibly more hazardous for most patients because of alterations in fecal and vaginal bacterial flora. Indeed, self-administration of a single-dose regimen at the onset of symptoms has proved to be as cost-effective as prophylaxis.

   2. Nonantimicrobial prophylaxis issues. Encouraging women to practice regular and complete emptying of the bladder may help prevent recurrent cystitis. Postcoital emptying of the bladder has also been widely recommended, although one prospective study failed to demonstrate any relationship with recurrent infections. Moreover, several theoretical preventive measures relate to the use of an alternative contraceptive method: to use a properly fitted diaphragm, to void frequently when wearing a diaphragm, and to limit diaphragm use to the recommended 6 to 8 hours after intercourse. In postmenopausal women, intravaginal administration of estriol can reduce recurrent UTIs by modifying the milieu for vaginal flora. Cranberry juice (300 mL per day) was effective in decreasing asymptomatic bacteriuria with pyuria in postmenopausal women. The small difference in symptomatic UTIs was not statistically significant.

F. Treatment of acute bacterial pyelonephritis. The occurrence of flank pain, chills and fever, and nausea and vomiting with or without dysuria suggests acute bacterial pyelonephritis. In this clinical setting, blood cultures and quantitative cultures of urine should be obtained. Whether ambulatory patients should be admitted to the hospital for treatment depends in part on a subjective assessment of toxicity, likely compliance with therapy, and the home situation. When the assessment is doubtful, the patient should be treated in the hospital, at least until a clear response to therapy has occurred. This policy also applies to patients with known underlying uropathies, because complications are more common in these patients.

1. **Outpatient therapy.** Recommendations for therapy of uncomplicated pyelonephritis are outlined in Table 7-4. Fluoroquinolone or trimethoprim-sulfamethoxazole is the drug of choice for initial therapy of pyelonephritis in outpatients. Local susceptibility patterns will influence

Table 7-4. Recommendations for therapy for urinary tract infections

Infection	Group	Medication	Duration
Uncomplicated cystitis	Young women	Trimethoprim-sulfamethoxazole, trimethoprim, fluoroquinolone[a]	3 d
Cystitis	Women with risk factors including recent UTI, symptoms >7 d, diaphragm use, age >65 yr, diabetics with abnormal GU structures	Trimethoprim-sulfamethoxazole, trimethoprim, fluoroquinolone, nitrofurantoin, cephalosporins	7 d
	Pregnant women	Amoxicillin, cephalosporins[b], nitro-furantoin, sulfonamides, trimethoprim-sulfamethoxazole[c]	7 d
Acute uncomplicated pyelo-nephritis	Women (outpatient)	Fluoroquinolone, trimethoprim-sulfamethoxazole, oral cephalosporin[d]	10–14 d
	Women (inpatient)	Fluoroquinolone[e], ceftriaxone, ampicillin plus gentamicin[f], trimethoprim-sulfamethoxazole	14 d
Complicated infection	Outpatient	Fluoroquinolone	10–14 d
	Inpatient	Fluoroquinolone[e], cephalosporins[g], ampicillin plus gentamicin[f]	14 d

UTI, urinary tract infection.

[a] Oral fluoroquinolones are listed in Table 7-2; they offer no significant advantage over trimethoprim-sulfamethoxazole in women with uncomplicated cystitis.

[b] Oral cephalosporins: cephradine, cephalexin.

[c] Trimethoprim-sulfamethoxazole has been used in pregnancy, but it has not been approved by the U.S. Food and Drug Administration for pregnant patients.

[d] Oral cephalosporins with an extended spectrum: cefpodoxime, loracarbef.

[e] Fluoroquinolones available for intravenous administration are listed in Table 7-3.

[f] Increasing ampicillin resistance among many enteric bacteria, including *Escherichia coli*, limits ampicillin as a single agent for complicated UTIs. If enterococcus is not likely, then a fluoroquinolone or a parenteral third- or fourth-generation cephalosporin is recommended.

[g] Some examples of parenteral cephalosporins are listed in Table 7-3.

Adapted from Falagas ME. Practice guidelines: urinary tract infections. *Infect Dis Clin Pract* 1995;4: 241–257; Kunin CM. *Detection, prevention, and management of urinary tract infections*, 5th ed. Philadelphia: Lea & Febiger, 1997; Stamm WE. Urinary tract infections. In: Root RK, ed. *Clinical infectious diseases: a practical approach*, 1st ed. New York: Oxford University Press, 1999.

the choice for initial therapy. After culture results and susceptibility tests are available, a full 10- to 14-day course of antimicrobial therapy may be completed with the least expensive drug to which the patient's microorganism is susceptible.

2. **Inpatient therapy.** Patients who require admission to the hospital should be treated initially with a third-generation cephalosporin or a fluoroquinolone (intramuscular or intravenous), or gentamicin or tobramycin (1.5 to 2.0 mg per kg every 8 hours or 4.0 to 7.0 mg per kg every 24 hours, with appropriate alteration of the dose interval if the serum creatinine exceeds 1 mg per dL) if the urine shows gram-negative bacilli on microscopical examination. If gram-positive cocci are seen in the urine, intravenous ampicillin (1 g every 4 hours) should be given in addition to the aminoglycoside, to cover the possibility of enterococcal infection while the results of urine and blood cultures and antimicrobial susceptibility tests are pending. If no complications ensue and the patient becomes afebrile, the remaining days of a 10- to 14-day course can be completed with oral therapy. However, persistent fever, persistent bacteriuria in 48 to 72 hours, or continual signs of toxicity beyond 3 days of therapy suggest the need for an evaluation to exclude obstruction, metastatic focus, or the formation of a perinephric abscess. The urinary tract is a common source of sepsis and bacteremic shock in patients with underlying uropathies. As with other patients in septic shock, intravenous fluids must be given to maintain adequate arterial perfusion, which usually results in a urinary output in excess of 50 mL per hour. Failure to respond to seemingly appropriate therapy suggests the possibility of undrained pus. Examination by ultrasound or CT may disclose an obstructed ureter or perinephric abscess, both of which require surgical drainage.

G. **Management of recurrent renal infections (relapses).** Chronic bacterial pyelonephritis is one of the most refractory problems in clinical medicine; relapse rates are as high as 90%. The entity is a heterogeneous one with multiple underlying factors.

1. **Risk factors.** To improve the success rate, it is of utmost importance that any correctable lesion be repaired, that obstructions to urine flow be relieved, and that foreign bodies (e.g., indwelling urinary catheters or renal staghorn calculi) be removed if possible. If the risk factors cannot be corrected, long-term eradication of bacteriuria is almost impossible. To attempt eradication in such instances leads only to the emergence of more resistant strains of bacteria or fungi; consequently, the physician must be resigned to treating symptomatic episodes of infection and suppressing bacteriuria in selected patients.

2. **Acute symptomatic infection.** The treatment of the acute symptoms and signs of UTI in a patient with chronic renal bacteriuria is the same as for patients with acute bacterial pyelonephritis. Urine cultures to detect a possible change in antimicrobial susceptibility of the infecting microorganism are important. Toxic patients also should have blood cultures.

3. **Prolonged treatment.** Some patients with relapsing bacteriuria after 2 weeks of therapy respond to 6 weeks of antimicrobial therapy. This is especially true of patients with no underlying structural abnormalities. Men may require 6 to 12 weeks of antibiotic therapy for febrile UTIs, since over 90% have associated asymptomatic prostatitis. Patients who fail the longer therapy, who have repeated episodes of symptomatic infection, or who have progressive renal disease despite corrective measures are candidates for suppressive chemotherapy.

4. **Suppressive therapy.** To reduce the colony counts in their urine, patients selected for suppressive therapy should have 2 to 3 days of specific high-dose antimicrobial therapy, to which their infecting bacteria are susceptible. The preferred agent for long-term suppression is methenamine mandelate, 1 g four times daily in adults. To be most effective, the pH of the urine should be maintained below 5.5; this can be accomplished

with ascorbic acid, 500 mg two to four times daily. Alternatively, the dosage of methenamine mandelate alone can be increased to 8 g or even 12 g per day. The dosage should be adjusted to the minimum amount required to keep the urine free of bacteria. To avoid metabolic acidosis, the dosage of methenamine mandelate must be reduced in patients with renal insufficiency, in whom 2 g per day may suffice. In these patients, methenamine mandelate should not be used at all unless the creatinine clearance exceeds 10 mL per minute. Alternative therapy is trimethoprim-sulfamethoxazole (160 mg/800 mg tablets twice daily) or nitrofurantoin (50 to 100 mg once or twice daily).

5. **Prognosis.** Although a common cause of appreciable morbidity, UTIs do not play a major role in the pathogenesis of end-stage renal disease. Patients who come to renal dialysis or transplantation because of chronic bacterial pyelonephritis almost always have an underlying structural defect. Most often, the lesion is chronic atrophic pyelonephritis associated with vesicoureteral reflux that started in infancy. The role of surgical correction of vesicoureteral reflux is not clear despite years of debate; what is certain, however, is the importance of meticulous control of infection in children to prevent progressive renal scarring and renal failure by early adulthood.

H. **Treatment of prostatitis**
1. **Acute bacterial prostatitis** is commonly accompanied by acute cystitis, which enables the recovery of its causative pathogen by culture of voided urine. Massage of an acutely inflamed prostate gland often results in bacteremia; therefore, this procedure should be avoided unless the patient is already receiving effective antibiotic therapy. Antimicrobial selection depends on (a) the susceptibility pattern of the causative bacteria and (b) the ability of the drug to achieve concentrations in the prostate that exceed the minimum inhibitory concentrations of the bacteria. The drug of choice most commonly is either the combination of trimethoprim-sulfamethoxazole (cotrimoxazole) or a fluoroquinolone; treatment, however, must be based ultimately on an accurate microbiological diagnosis. Beta-lactam antibiotics should be avoided because of the low concentrations achieved in prostatic tissue and lower cure rates. Treatment should be given for 30 days to prevent chronic bacterial prostatitis. After acute symptoms subside, a suitable oral antibiotic can be given in full dose for at least 30 days. Urethral catheterization should be avoided. If acute urinary retention develops, drainage should be by suprapubic needle aspiration or, if prolonged bladder drainage is required, by a suprapubic cystostomy tube, placed while the patient is under local anesthesia.

2. **Chronic bacterial prostatitis.** The hallmark of chronic bacterial prostatitis is relapsing UTI. It is most refractory to treatment. Although erythromycin with alkalinization of the urine has been effective against susceptible gram-positive pathogens, most instances of chronic bacterial prostatitis are caused by gram-negative enteric bacilli. Cotrimoxazole or a fluoroquinolone is the drug of choice. Approximately 75% of patients improve, and 33% are cured with 12 weeks of cotrimoxazole therapy (160 mg/800 mg twice daily). For patients who cannot tolerate cotrimoxazole or a fluoroquinolone, nitrofurantoin, 50 or 100 mg once or twice daily, can be used for long-term (6 to 12 months) suppressive therapy.

3. The therapy for **nonbacterial chronic prostatitis** is difficult because an exact etiology has not been identified. Due to a concern for *C. trachomatis*, *Ureaplasma urealyticum*, and other fastidious and difficult to culture organisms, many experts recommend a 6-week trial of a tetracycline or erythromycin. Symptomatic therapy with nonsteroidal anti-inflammatory drugs (NSAIDs) and alpha-receptor blockers has also been used.

I. **Recommendations for the care of urinary catheters.** Urinary catheters are valuable devices for enabling drainage of the bladder, but their use is

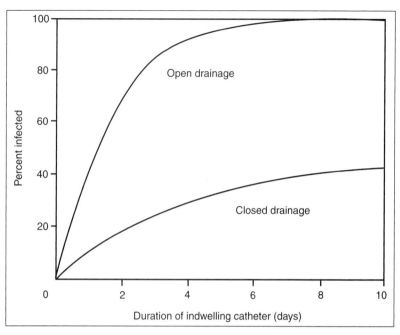

Figure 7-4. Prevalence of bacteriuria in catheterized patients according to duration of catheterization and type of drainage system. (From Fass RJ, Klainer AS, Perkins RL. Urinary tract infection: practical aspects of diagnosis and treatment. *JAMA* 1973;225:1509. Reprinted with permission.)

associated with an appreciable risk of infection in the urinary tract. For a single (in-and-out) catheterization, the risk is small (12%), though this prevalence is much higher in diabetic and elderly women. However, bacteriuria occurs in virtually all patients with indwelling urinary catheters within 3 to 4 days unless placement is done under sterile conditions and a sterile, closed drainage system is maintained (Fig. 7-4). The use of a neomycin-polymyxin irrigant does not prevent catheter-associated infections. Urinary catheters are the single most common cause of nosocomial infections and are responsible for more than 5,000 deaths from gram-negative sepsis each year in the United States. Explicit recommendations for the prevention of catheter-associated UTIs, formulated by the Centers for Disease Control and Prevention, are as follows:

1. **Indwelling urinary catheters should be used only when absolutely necessary.** They should never be used solely for nurse or physician convenience, and they should be removed as soon as possible.
2. **Catheters should be inserted only by adequately trained personnel.** If practical, a team of individuals should be given responsibility for catheter insertion and maintenance.
3. **Urinary catheters should be aseptically inserted using proper sterile technique and the following sterile equipment:** gloves, a fenestrated drape, sterile sponges and an iodophor solution for periurethral cleansing, a lubricant jelly, and an appropriately sized urinary catheter. After insertion, catheters should be properly secured to prevent movement and urethral traction.

4. **Once- or twice-daily perineal care for catheterized patients** should include cleansing of the meatal-catheter junction with an antiseptic soap; subsequently, an antimicrobial ointment may be applied.

5. **A sterile closed drainage system should always be used.** The urinary catheter and the proximal portion of the drainage tube should not be disconnected (thus opening the closed system) unless it is required for irrigation of an obstructed catheter. Sterile technique must be observed whenever the collecting system is opened and catheter irrigation is done. A large-volume sterile syringe and sterile irrigant fluid should be used and then discarded. If frequent irrigations are necessary to ensure catheter patency, a triple-lumen catheter that permits continuous irrigation within a closed system is preferable.

6. **Small volumes of urine for culture can** be aspirated from the distal end of the catheter with a sterile syringe and 21-gauge needle. The catheter must first be prepared with tincture of iodine or alcohol. Urine for chemical analyses can be obtained from the drainage bag in a sterile manner.

7. **Nonobstructed gravity flow must be maintained at all times.** This requires emptying the collecting bag regularly, replacing poorly functioning or obstructed catheters, and ensuring that collection bags always remain below the level of the bladder.

8. **All closed collecting systems contaminated by inappropriate technique, accidental disconnection, leaks, or other means should be immediately replaced.**

9. **Routine catheter change is not necessary** in patients with urinary catheterization of less than 2 weeks' duration, except when obstruction, contamination, or other malfunction occurs. In patients with chronic indwelling catheters, replacement is necessary when concretions can be palpated in the catheter or when malfunction or obstruction occurs.

10. **Catheterized patients should be separated from each other whenever possible** and should not share the same room or adjacent beds if other arrangements are available. Separation of bacteriuric and nonbacteriuric patients is particularly important.

   These guidelines should be adhered to meticulously, and the use of indwelling urinary catheters should be kept to a responsible minimum.

J. **Catheter-associated infections.** Catheter-associated bacteriuria should only be treated in the symptomatic patient. When the decision to treat a patient with a catheter-associated infection is made, removal of the catheter is an important aspect of therapy. If an infected catheter remains in place, relapsing infection is very common. The interaction between the organisms and catheter (foreign body) cause the organism to form a biofilm or area in which antibiotics are unable to completely eradicate these organisms. Recommendations for empiric therapy are similar to recommendations for complicated UTIs (see Table 7-4). The choice of empiric therapy is based on an initial Gram's stain of the urine, local susceptibility patterns, host factors, and the patient's recent antibiotic use. The final choice of an antibiotic and duration of therapy should be based on the identification and susceptibility of the etiologic agent and the host's response to therapy. Patients who respond rapidly to therapy may be treated for 7 days, although making firm conclusions about duration of therapy is very difficult.

   Patients with candiduria may fall into several different clinical categories. Otherwise healthy patients with asymptomatic candiduria often require only a urinary catheter change and may not require antifungal therapy. On the other end of the spectrum is the immunocompromised host, in whom candiduria may represent disseminated infection. The patient with disseminated candidiasis requires systemic therapy with either fluconazole or amphotericin B or a liposomal preparation of amphotericin. General recommendations for treating patients with candiduria and without evidence of disseminated infection include the removal of the urinary catheter

and discontinuation of antibiotics. Antifungal options include either fluconazole (200 mg the first day, then 100 mg for 4 days), continuous bladder
irrigation with amphotericin B (50 mg per 1,000 mL of sterile water via a
three-way catheter for 5 days), or low-dose intravenous therapy with amphotericin (0.3 mg per kg in a single dose). Occasionally, longer systemic
therapy with oral 5-fluorocytosine, intravenous amphotericin B, or both is
required.

REFERENCES

1. Stamm WE, Hooton TM. Management of urinary tract infections in adults. *N Engl J Med* 1993;329:1328–1334.
2. Hooton TM, Scholes D, Hughes JP, et al. A prospective study of risk factors for symptomatic urinary tract infection in young women. *N Engl J Med* 1996;335: 468–474.

Suggested readings

Ang BSP, Telenti A, King B, Steckelberg JM, Wilson WR. Candidemia from a urinary source: microbiological aspects and clinical significance. *Clin Infect Dis* 1993;17:662–666.
Domingue GJ, Hellstrom WJG. Prostatitis. *Clin Microbiol Rev* 1998;11:604–613.
Edelstein H, McCabe RE. Perinephric abscess: modern diagnosis and treatment in 47 cases. *Medicine (Baltimore)* 1988;67:118–131.
Fihn SD. Acute uncomplicated urinary tract infection in women. *N Engl J Med* 2003;349:259–266.
Fisher JF, Newman CL, Sobel JD. Yeast in the urine: solutions for a budding problem. *Clin Infect Diseases* 1995;20:183–189.
Fowler JE Jr., Pulaski ET. Excretory urography, cystography, and cystoscopy in the evaluation of women with urinary-tract infection. *N Engl J Med* 1981;304:462–465.
Godfrey KM, Harding MD, Zhanel GG, et al. Antimicrobial treatment in diabetic women with asymptomatic bacteriuria. *N Engl J Med* 2002;347:1576–1583.
Hooton TM, Fihn SD, Johnson C, Roberts PL, Stamm WE. Association between bac-
terial vaginosis and acute cystitis in women using diaphragms. *Arch Intern Med* 1989;149:1932–1936.
Hooton TM, Stamm WE. Diagnosis and treatment of uncomplicated urinary tract infections. *Infect Dis Clin North Am* 1997;11:551–582.
Hooton TM, Winter C, Tiu F, Stamm WE. Randomized comparative trial and cost analysis of 3-day antimicrobial regimens for treatment of acute cystitis in women. *JAMA* 1995;273:41–45.
Kincaid-Smith P, Becker G. Reflux nephropathy and chronic atrophic pyelonephritis: a review. *J Infect Dis* 1978;138:774–780.
Krieger JN. Complications and treatment of urinary tract infections during pregnancy. *Urol Clin North Am* 1986;13:685–693.
Kunin CM. *Detection, prevention, and management of urinary tract infections,* 5th ed. Philadelphia: Lea & Febiger, 1997.
Kunin CM, Chin QF, Chambers S. Indwelling urinary catheters in the elderly: relation of "catheter life" to formation of encrustations in patients with and without blocked catheters. *Am J Med* 1987;82:405–411.
Kunin CM, Van Arsdale White L, Hua TH. A reassessment of the importance of "low-count" bacteriuria in young women with acute urinary symptoms. *Ann Intern Med* 1993;119:454–460.
Lachs MS, Nachamkin I, Edelstein PH, Goldman J, Feinstein AR, Schwartz JS. Spec-
trum bias in the evaluation of diagnostic tests: lessons from the rapid dipstick test for urinary tract infection. *Ann Intern Med* 1992;117:135–140.
Lipsky BA, Baker CA. Fluoroquinolone toxicity profiles: a review focusing on new agents. *Clin Infect Dis* 1999;28:352–364.
Nickel JC. The Pre and Post Massage Test (PPMT): a simple screen for prostatitis. *Tech Urol* 1997;3:38–43.

Nicolle LE. Asymptomatic bacteriuria in the elderly. *Infect Dis Clin North Am* 1997;11:647–662.

Nicolle LE, Bjornson J, Harding GK, MacDonell JA. Bacteriuria in elderly institutionalized men. *N Engl J Med* 1983;309:1420–1425.

Nicolle LE, Harding GK, Preiksaitis J, Ronald AR. The association of urinary tract infection with sexual intercourse. *J Infect Dis* 1982;146:579–583.

Silverman DE, Stamey TA. Management of infection stones: the Stanford experience. *Medicine (Baltimore)* 1983;62:44–51.

Stamm WE. Guidelines for prevention of catheter-associated urinary tract infections. *Ann Intern Med* 1975;82:386–390.

Stamm WE, Counts GW, Wagner KF, et al. Antimicrobial prophylaxis of recurrent urinary tract infections: a double-blind, placebo-controlled trial. *Ann Intern Med* 1980;92:770–775.

Stapleton A, Latham R, Johnson C, Stamm WE. Postcoital antimicrobial prophylaxis for recurrent urinary tract infection: a randomized, double-blind, placebo-controlled trial. *JAMA* 1990;264:703–706.

Stapleton A, Stamm WE. Prevention of urinary tract infection. *Infect Dis Clin North Am* 1997;11:719–733.

Strom BL, Collins M, West SL, Kreisberg J, Weller S. Sexual activity, contraceptive use and other risk factors for symptomatic and asymptomatic bacteriuria: a case-control study. *Ann Intern Med* 1987;107:816–823.

Talan DA, Klimberg IW, Nicolle LE, Song J, Kowalsky SF, Church DA. Once daily, extended release ciprofloxacin for complicated urinary tract infections and acute uncomplicated pyelonephritis. *J Urol* 2004 Feb;171(2):734–739.

Ulleryd P. Febrile urinary tract infection in men. *Intnl J Antimicrobial Agents* 2003; 22:S89–S93.

Velasco M, Martinez JA, Moreno-Martinez A, et al. Blood cultures for women with uncomplicated acute pyelonephritis: are they necessary? *Clin Infect Dis* 2003;37:1127–1130.

Warren JW. Catheter-associated urinary tract infections. *Infect Dis Clin North Am* 1997;11(3):609–622.

The Patient with Hematuria, Proteinuria, or Both, and Abnormal Findings on Urinary Microscopy

Sharon G. Adler and
Kenneth Fairley

I. **Urine analysis.** A urine sample is usually easy to obtain, and it can be studied by very simple techniques on the ward or in the physician's office. Examination of the urine is one of the most rewarding steps in clinical medicine. Not only does it uncover renal parenchymal and urinary tract disease that eludes detection by other methods of investigation, but it frequently points to a specific diagnosis. Almost every patient with parenchymal renal disease shows abnormal findings on urine microscopy, an increase in urine protein, or both. Urine microscopy reveals abnormalities in many patients with renal disease who have no significant proteinuria. Many renal diseases that require treatment are first suspected on the basis of urinary findings—in particular, infections, glomerulonephritis, and interstitial nephritis.

A. **Method of collection of urine specimens.** The method of collecting a urine sample is of critical importance when the specimen is to be examined microscopically. For dipstick testing, the sample should be examined promptly for accurate results. Urine pH may change with time after collection, and contaminating bacteria multiply and convert nitrate to nitrite, causing a false-positive test for bacteriuria. At low specific gravity (less than 1.010), cells lyse and casts form less readily. Casts also dissolve in alkaline urine.

1. **Midstream urine collection.** In collecting urine for microscopical examination, avoiding contamination with bacteria, squamous cells, and leukocytes is important. Contamination is very common in women, in whom contaminating cells and bacteria arise in the vagina and vulval area. The important points in collecting a good midstream urine sample are shown in Table 8-1. Although bacteria are often detected on microscopy, infection is best proved by culture, which also allows the antibiotic sensitivity of infecting organisms to be determined. Special media are required for the culture of some organisms, such as the tubercle bacillus, *Mycoplasmas*, anaerobic organisms, and yeasts. Culture results are reported as colony-forming units (CFU) per mL of urine; the significance of a count depends on the method of collection (Table 8-2).

2. A catheter specimen in women is best collected as a **midcatheter specimen** using a short open-ended catheter. At least 200 mL must pass through the catheter to flush out contaminating urethral contents before the specimen is collected. Conventional "side hole" catheters push urethral contents into the bladder before urine can run out, and critical bacterial counts are 30-fold higher using a conventional catheter than those obtained on urine collected with an open-ended catheter.

3. **Suprapubic aspiration.** A fine lumbar puncture needle with stylet in place is passed through sterilized suprapubic skin directly into a full bladder. Uncontaminated urine can then be aspirated.

B. **Dipstick testing.** Dipstick testing of urine provides a rapid determination of urine pH, specific gravity, and the presence of protein, blood (hemoglobin), leukocytes, nitrites, glucose, and bile. Dipsticks are less sensitive in detecting pyuria and bacteriuria.

The method of screening for proteinuria is the examination of a randomly excreted urine sample by dipstick. Tetrabromophenol is buffered to a pH of 3, and this results in a yellow-to-blue color that changes with increasing protein concentration. False-positive dipstick results for proteinuria are

Table 8-1. Guidelines for collecting midstream urine sample

Women

When possible use a vaginal tampon.

Hold labia well separated during collection of the specimen.

Gently cleanse the periurethral area from anterior to posterior with several moistened gauze squares.

Men

Hold the retracted foreskin back throughout the collection.

Clean the urethral meatus with moist gauze.

If urethral or prostatic infection is suspected:

The first 10 mL of voided urine reflects urethral infection (it also includes bladder contents).

The midstream urine collected, as above, reflects the bladder contents.

Prostatic fluid, if available, reflects prostatic infection most accurately.

The first 10 mL of urine voided after prostatic massage provides information on infection in prostatic secretions (it also includes bladder contents).

Note: In both sexes, at least 200 mL should be passed before a midstream urine specimen is collected without interruption of the flow of urine.

seen when urine pH is greater than or equal to 8 and when the patient is excreting metabolites of penicillins, aspirin, or oral hypoglycemic agents in the urine. Standard dipsticks for protein fail to detect very small quantities of abnormal albuminuria (e.g., microalbuminuria) and are relatively insensitive to even large amounts of nonalbumin protein. To alleviate the first of these shortcomings, dipsticks capable of detecting microalbuminuria are currently available and are useful, when used properly, as a screening test to identify patients with diabetes mellitus and incipient nephropathy or to detect patients with a high risk of coronary artery and/or cerebrovascular disease. Dipsticks that are more sensitive to nonalbumin proteins are under development. Currently, a 24-hour urine collection is required to detect such proteins.

Urine color varies with its concentration and with the presence of drugs such as phenazopyridine (Pyridium), phenindione, and multivitamin tablets, and of blood, bile, porphyrin, melanin, and homogentisic acid. Some of these color changes may be mistaken for hematuria. Dipstick examination of the urine accurately determines the presence of hemoglobin, which depends on the oxidation of orthotolidine by cumene hydroperoxide, although cross-reactivity with myoglobin does occur. Although the microscopic examination of urine for erythrocytes provides far more information about the underlying renal lesion, a dipstick is quick, simple, and provides quantitative information. The Ames N Multistix and Boehringer nephron tests provide sensitive and specific methods of detecting microscopical

Table 8-2. Influence of collection technique on accuracy of detection of urine abnormalities

Collection technique	Hematuria	Pyuria	Significant bacteriuria (CFU/mL)	Fastidious microorganisms
Midstream urine	Excellent	Fair[a]	>100,000	Poor
Open-ended catheter	Good	Very good	>1,000	Good
Suprapubic aspiration	Poor	Excellent	>1	Excellent

CFU, colony-forming units.

[a]Depends on collection technique.

hematuria. Ascorbic acid, a strong reducing agent, prevents the chemical reaction in dipsticks that detects hemoglobin and is the cause of many false-negative tests. In the case of a low-specific-gravity urine (below 1.010), lysis of erythrocytes leads to false-negative microscopy, but the dipsticks provide a positive test.

C. **Microscopic analysis.** In the United States, urine is characteristically examined using a standard light microscope to make a semiquantitative estimate of the frequency of the formed elements in the urine by counting their number per high-power field. More quantitative measures can be obtained by examining the urine on a coverslipped counting chamber rather than on a plain glass slide. The counting-chamber method is more accurate, largely because it eliminates the error introduced by the variability of the depth of the layer of urine on the slide, which occurs as a function of viscosity. The accuracy of the microscopic examination can also be enhanced by using phase-contrast microscopy, which allows for more sensitivity in the observation of morphologic detail. If a phase-contrast microscope is unavailable, staining the urine sediment with Sternheimer-Malbin stain may also enhance visualization of cellular elements using a standard light microscope.

1. **Hematuria.** A large amount of blood present in the urine is obvious to the naked eye. The red blood cell count in such cases is always well above 10^6 cells per mL. The morphology and quantitation of the urinary erythrocytes are two of the most important investigations in clinical nephrology. They not only provide information about the underlying cause, but also assist in determining the nature of investigations required. Because the recognition that glomerular bleeding can be determined by the appearance of erythrocytes on phase-contrast microscopy, prompt assessment of the number and morphology of urinary erythrocytes in the urine has assumed new significance. In the case of crescentic glomerulonephritis, which can be suspected when red blood cell casts and large numbers of dysmorphic erythrocytes are seen on urine microscopy, the physician is alerted to the urgent need for biopsy confirmation and appropriate treatment.

A high count of glomerular erythrocytes (more than 10^6 red blood cells per mL) has both prognostic and therapeutic implications, because it suggests the presence of crescents on renal biopsy. If 4+ dipstick testing for heme is present, immediate urine microscopy is indicated to determine the nature and hence the source of erythrocytes, and, if possible, the count per mL. The source of erythrocytes can be determined by measuring their size and by examining their morphology. After centrifuging the urine specimen, if a red pellet results, adequate numbers of erythrocytes are present to measure their volume in an automated counter of the type customarily used for complete blood cell counts (CBCs). If the urinary erythrocyte mean corpuscular volume is less than 72 fL, a glomerular bleeding source is likely.

The best method for assessing erythrocyte morphology is phase-contrast microscopy. If bright-field illumination is used, many erythrocytes will not be correctly identified. In particular, those that have lost their hemoglobin staining are not seen, a common occurrence in an acid urine. The small and distorted erythrocytes characteristic of glomerular bleeding may also be missed. Characteristic dysmorphic erythrocytes, which indicate that hematuria is arising in glomeruli, are illustrated in Fig. 8-1. These vary considerably in size, shape, and hemoglobin content, and many bizarre forms are present. Normal urine contains up to 8,000 glomerular erythrocytes per mL in a centrifuged specimen and 13,000 per mL in uncentrifuged urine. Erythrocytes arising from a nonglomerular source are uniform in size and shape but may show some "ghost cells," cells that are losing their hemoglobin (Fig. 8-2). The latter change occurs particularly in an acid urine.

Figure 8-1. Erythrocytes, showing the wide variation in size, shape, and hemoglobin content, in the urine of a patient with glomerulonephritis (phase-contrast microscopy). (From Fairley KF. Urinalysis. In: Schrier RW, Gottschalk CW, eds. *Diseases of the kidney*, 4th ed. Boston: Little, Brown, 1988. Reprinted with permission.)

2. **Urinary casts.** Casts are formed from Tamm-Horsfall glycoprotein, which is synthesized and secreted in the ascending limb of the loop of Henle and distal convoluted tubules.
   a. **Physiologic casts.** Hyaline casts are transparent and cylindrical and are seen in the urine of normal subjects. Their presence does not indicate renal disease. Granular casts are semitransparent cylinders with refractile granules of uncertain origin. These, too, are present in individuals without renal disease. The number of hyaline and granular casts in urine may be increased by fever, exercise, and volume depletion.
   b. **Pathologic casts.** Casts may contain cellular material (erythrocytes, leukocytes, tubular cells, bacteria, or fungi), fibrin, lipids, bile, and crystals.

      The most important cellular cast is that composed of erythrocytes (Fig. 8-3). This indicates glomerular bleeding, as do erythrophagocytic cells. Large numbers of erythrocyte casts also increase the likelihood of crescents in glomeruli. Casts composed of polymorphonuclear leukocytes usually indicate renal parenchymal infection. These may also be seen in acute interstitial nephritis and occasionally in glomerular lesions, where numerous polymorphonuclear leukocytes are in glomeruli. Casts may also contain all varieties of mononuclear

Figure 8-2. Nonglomerular bleeding, showing two populations of cells (phase-contrast microscopy). (From Fairley KF. Urinalysis. In: Schrier RW, Gottschalk CW, eds. *Diseases of the kidney*, 4th ed. Boston: Little, Brown, 1988. Reprinted with permission.)

Figure 8-3. An erythrocyte cast in an acid urine, composed of red cells from which much of the hemoglobin has disappeared. (From Fairley KF. Urinalysis. In: Schrier RW, Gottschalk CW, eds. *Diseases of the kidney*, 4th ed. Boston: Little, Brown, 1988. Reprinted with permission.)

Figure 8-4. A cholesterol ester spherulite approximately the same size as an erythrocyte. (From Fairley KF. Urinalysis. In: Schrier RW, Gottschalk CW, eds. *Diseases of the kidney*, 4th ed. Boston: Little, Brown, 1988. Reprinted with permission.)

leukocytes and may include tubular epithelial cells from all segments of the nephron. In nephrotic syndrome, all casts usually contain fat particles and some contain oval fat bodies. Because the fat bodies consist of cholesterol esters, they can be easily identified by their "Maltese cross" birefringence (Figs. 8-4 and 8-5). Many fat bodies, however, are composed of fat particles too small to show crosses, and these appear as a faint glow in polarized light.

Crystals in casts are commonly present in patients who are taking triamterene. The crystals disappear when the urine is alkalinized or the drug is discontinued. Crystals may also occasionally be present in casts in patients with hypercalcemia or hyperuricosuria, or as an isolated finding.

Figure 8-5. The particle in Figure 8-4, when viewed with polarized light, shows the classic "Maltese cross." (From Fairley KF. Urinalysis. In: Schrier RW, Gottschalk CW, eds. *Diseases of the kidney*, 4th ed. Boston: Little, Brown, 1988. Reprinted with permission.)

Broad waxy casts signify chronic renal disease. These typically have a very sharp border and are easily seen with bright-field illumination. They do not dissolve in alkaline urine.

3. **Leukocytes and nucleated cells in the urine.** Normal midstream urine contains up to 2,000 nucleated cells per mL, and most of these are leukocytes. Normal bladder urine obtained by needle aspiration contains very low counts of leukocytes (mean, 283 per mL, with only 2 of 25 urines containing more than 1,000 per mL). In one author's (KF) laboratory, the mean count in a midstream specimen in the same subjects performed at the same time was 2,018 leukocytes per mL, even when meticulous care was taken to avoid contamination. The additional cells in the midstream sample presumably arise in the urethra.

An increase in the leukocyte count in the urine most commonly implies infection. Infected urines show an increase in leukocytes in more than 90% of cases. When pyuria is present without bacteriuria, three-fourths of patients show an underlying urinary tract abnormality.

Sterile pyuria may be seen in tuberculosis, renal papillary necrosis, acute interstitial nephritis, urate nephropathy, glomerulonephritis, and polycystic disease of the kidney. It may also be present in patients with calculi and in a variety of other urinary tract abnormalities. Before a diagnosis of sterile pyuria is made, fastidious organisms such as ureaplasmas, anaerobic bacteria such as *Gardnerella vaginalis*, and chlamydia should be sought in an appropriate specimen using special cultural techniques.

When it is difficult to distinguish leukocytes from renal tubular epithelial cells, a drop of acetic acid makes it easier to recognize the lobed nuclei of polymorphonuclear leukocytes. Staining the cells also distinguishes them.

4. **Renal tubular cells.** Large numbers of renal tubular cells are found in the urine in acute tubular necrosis and acute interstitial nephritis. Acute interstitial nephritis can be distinguished by a much higher count of leukocytes (more than 15,000 per mL) and a higher total nucleated cell count (more than 75,000 per mL) than are seen in acute tubular necrosis. Eosinophils are present in the urine in most cases of interstitial nephritis, in counts above 5,000 per mL; these are rare in acute tubular necrosis. Eosinophils in the urine are best seen with Hansel's stain, which, unlike Wright's stain, is not pH dependent.

Nucleated cells are also present in the urine in glomerulonephritis, particularly crescentic glomerulonephritis, in which total cell counts, leukocytes, and renal tubular cells are present in higher numbers than in noncrescentic glomerulonephritis. Glomerular epithelial cells identified by monoclonal antibody staining are also present in a much higher percentage of urines from patients with crescentic glomerulonephritis than from those with noncrescentic glomerulonephritis.

5. **Crystals.** Although crystals of calcium oxalate and uric acid may be seen in normal urine samples, large, bizarre crystals of any type, including calcium oxalate and uric acid, usually indicate increased urinary excretion and may indicate calculous disease. Cystine crystals are always abnormal and indicate cystinuria.

II. **Hematuria**

A. **Localization and differential diagnosis.** An abnormal quantity of erythrocytes in the urine can either be due to a glomerular disorder or to nonglomerular bleeding. Glomerular bleeding should be suspected if any of the following are present: dysmorphic urinary erythrocytes, erythrocytes with mean corpuscular volume less than 72 fL, red blood cell casts, and concomitant proteinuria, especially higher than 1 g per day. In Table 8-3, an asterisk denotes those glomerular disorders that frequently manifest hematuria. Nonglomerular hematuria is characterized by the presence of isomorphic urinary erythrocytes with a mean corpuscular volume of more than 72 fL in the absence of red blood cell casts or significant proteinuria. The further

Table 8-3. Causes of glomerular proteinuria

"Primary" glomerular disorders
  Minimal change, mesangial proliferative (IgA, IgM*), focal and segmental
    glomerulosclerosis*, membranous, membranoproliferative*, crescentic*
Hereditary
  Alport syndrome*, Fabry disease*, nail-patella syndrome*
Infectious
  Bacterial*, viral*, fungal*, protozoal*, and helminthic* causes, including bacterial
    endocarditis*, poststreptococcal glomerulonephritis*, visceral abscesses*,
    secondary syphilis*, hepatitis B and C*, human immunodeficiency virus*,
    malaria*
Metabolic
  Diabetes mellitus
Immunologic
  Systemic lupus erythematosus*, mixed connective tissue disease, Sjögren
    syndrome, Henoch-Schönlein purpura*, Wegener granulomatosis*, microscopic
    polyarteritis nodosa*, Goodpasture syndrome*, cryoglobulinemia*
Medications
  Penicillamine, gold- or mercury-containing compounds, lithium, nonsteroidal
    anti-inflammatory drugs, angiotensin-converting enzyme inhibitors, heroin*
Neoplasms
  Multiple myeloma*; colon, lung, or breast carcinoma; lymphoma; leukemia
Miscellaneous
  Sickle cell disease*, allergies*, immunizations*, cirrhosis*, immunotactoid
    glomerulopathy*, amyloidosis*, reflux nephropathy*, congenital nephrotic
    syndrome

IgA, immunoglobulin A; IgM, immunoglobulin M.
*Denotes glomerular disorders that frequently present with hematuria.

localization of nonglomerular bleeding can be suggested by the three-glass
test. In this procedure, patients with macroscopic hematuria urinate 10- to
15-mL aliquots of urine each into three containers. A urethral site of bleeding is suggested if the hematuria predominates in the first 10 mL, whereas
a bladder origin is implied if the majority of blood is in the final aliquot.
Upper-tract bleeding is characterized by hematuria in all three collection
vessels. The differential diagnosis of nonglomerular proteinuria is outlined

Table 8-4. Causes of tubular proteinuria

Hereditary
  Polycystic kidney disease, medullary cystic disease
Infectious
  Pyelonephritis, tuberculosis
Metabolic
  Diabetes mellitus, hyperuricemia, uricosuria, hypercalcemia, hypercalciuria,
    hypokalemia, oxalosis, cystinosis
Immunologic
  Sjögren syndrome, renal transplant rejection, drug hypersensitivity, sarcoidosis
Toxic
  Analgesic abuse, radiation nephritis, lithium, heavy metals (lead, cadmium,
    mercury), Balkan nephritis, cyclosporine, cisplatinum, aminoglycosides
Anatomic
  Obstruction, ureterovesical reflux, medullary sponge kidney
Miscellaneous
  Multiple myeloma, amyloidosis, sickle cell disease, medullary sponge kidney

in Table 8-4. Many of these disorders are either characterized by or occasionally present with hematuria.

B. Clinical evaluation and treatment. Patients with hematuria may present with quantities of blood visible to the naked eye (macroscopic or gross hematuria) or visible only by microscopic examination (microscopic hematuria). The initial evaluation of the patient with gross or microscopic hematuria should include those steps outlined above to distinguish glomerular from nonglomerular causes. If a glomerular cause is suspected, patients should be further evaluated as described in section **III.C.**

For patients who have been determined to have nonglomerular hematuria, the differential diagnosis outlined in Table 8-4 may be narrowed by obtaining a relevant history and physical examination. The history and review of systems should include questions regarding passage in the urine of stones, tissue, or blood clots; frequent urinary tract infections (UTIs); episodic gross hematuria; fever; weight loss; medication or drug use, particularly oral contraceptives or analgesics; dysuria; tuberculosis; diabetes mellitus; trauma; coagulation disorders; and family history of renal disease. Pertinent aspects of the physical examination should include auscultation for renal bruits, palpation of the prostate for nodules or prostatitis, and palpation of the abdomen for enlarged kidneys indicative of polycystic kidney disease.

Table 8-5 outlines a suggested diagnostic approach to the patient with nonglomerular hematuria. Initial laboratory studies should include a complete blood count (CBC), prothrombin time, and partial thromboplastin time to rule out coagulopathy and hemoglobinopathy. A serum chemistry

Table 8-5. A diagnostic approach in the patient with nonglomerular hematuria

Urinary findings
No erythrocyte casts
Urinary RBC of normal morphology
Proteinuria <1 g/d/1.73 m^2
Urinary RBC >72 fL
↓

Urine culture and sensitivity, acid-fast bacteria × 3	Diagnostic → → →	Urinary tract infection
Prostate examination		Tuberculosis
Cytology		Tumors
↓		
Nondiagnostic		
↓		
Intravenous urography (or ultrasound)	Diagnostic → → →	Cystic disorders
		Intrarenal tumors
		Calculi
↓		Papillary necrosis
Nondiagnostic		Trauma/fracture
		Medullary sponge kidney
↓		Horseshoe kidney
Cystoscopy/retrogrades	Diagnostic → → →	Urethral lesions
		Cystitis
↓		Collecting system/bladder tumors
Nondiagnostic		
↓		
Angiography	Diagnostic → → →	Ureteral varices
		Aneurysm
		Arteriovenous malformation

RBC, red blood cells.

panel is useful to determine the level of renal function and to rule out the presence of hypercalcemia, hyperuricemia, and hyperglycemia. Urine should be cultured for bacterial and mycobacterial infection and, if clinically suspected, mycoplasma or other more fastidious organisms. Once a UTI has been excluded, an examination of the urinary tract anatomy should be undertaken to define the bleeding site. In the presence of normal or near-normal glomerular filtration rate (GFR), intravenous urography is the most useful diagnostic radiologic procedure available for defining renal anatomy. It should disclose the presence of renal cysts (hereditary and acquired); calculi; papillary necrosis; medullary sponge kidney; renal, pelvic, and ureteral tumors; and ureteral strictures. In the event of a nondiagnostic intravenous urographic study, cystoscopy can be performed to more definitively examine the bladder for the presence of tumors or infectious (inflammatory/interstitial) cystitis and the urethra for the presence of urethritis, strictures, or both. A nondiagnostic cystoscopic examination can be followed, if clinically indicated, by arteriography to pursue the possibility that hematuria is secondary to ureteral varices or aneurysms, arteriovenous malformations, or the loin-pain hematuria syndrome.

The treatment of hematuric states is entirely dependent on the underlying cause of erythrocyturia. The reader is therefore referred to textbooks of internal medicine, nephrology, and urology for detailed coverage of these topics. In this section, however, UTIs are discussed briefly, because they are commonly encountered by the general practitioner as well as by the specialist.

The most common presentation with UTI is dysuria and frequency in a woman of childbearing years. The urine may show macroscopic or heavy nonglomerular microscopic hematuria, as well as pyuria and bacteriuria. Some have recently advocated that even in patients with diabetes, pyuria without clinical signs or symptoms of infection should not be treated with antibiotics. In those in whom treatment is indicated, a single dose of an appropriate antibiotic (e.g., 2 g of amoxicillin or ampicillin) cures the infection in 80% of cases. Antibiotic resistance may be responsible for some treatment failure (e.g., ampicillin-resistant *Escherichia coli*). However, unresponsiveness to treatment may be an indication for further investigation, because a high percentage of those who do not respond to a single dose show abnormalities on further investigation by imaging techniques, such as intravenous urography. Failure to respond to treatment may also suggest an upper rather than lower UTI.

Urinary tract infection in a child or a man should always be investigated, because of the high incidence of underlying abnormalities. Infection in the presence of an underlying urinary tract abnormality usually requires longer courses of treatment. Eradicating the infection without removing the abnormality may be impossible in some cases, notably with infected stones or staghorn calculi.

III. Proteinuria

A. Biochemical evaluation.
Although not specific for glomerular disease, an abnormal amount of protein excreted in the urine is a cardinal manifestation of disease in virtually all patients with glomerulonephritis. Fever, exercise, hyperglycemia, and severe hypertension can transiently increase proteinuria.

To precisely quantitate and qualitatively analyze the amount and composition of urinary proteins, an examination of a 24-hour collection of urine is usually required. The collection method involves emptying the bladder and discarding the first urine on the morning of collection, and scrupulously collecting all subsequent urine for the next 24 hours. The final urine at the end of the 24-hour period is also kept as part of the collection. If the urine is refrigerated during the 24-hour period, no preservative is required. If refrigeration is unavailable, a preservative such as acetic acid (or a cup of vinegar) can be added to the collection vessel.

Quantification of the 24-hour urine creatinine should be performed to ensure that a complete collection was submitted. In female patients under steady-state conditions of renal function, the 24-hour urinary excretion of creatinine should equal approximately 15 to 20 mg per kg of ideal body weight; in male patients, the excretion should be 18 to 25 mg per kg. Accurate quantitative methods of protein excretion by precipitation include the sulfosalicylic acid precipitation test, the micro-Kjeldahl method, Esbach's picric acid–citric acid reagent, and the biuret method. Results are expressed either as grams excreted in 24 hours or as a ratio of protein to creatinine excretion.

In following a patient with heavy proteinuria (e.g., when assessing responsiveness to therapy), a urinary protein–creatinine concentration ratio is useful as a substitute for repeated full 24-hour urine collections. The normal 24-hour urine protein excretion in the adult ranges from 30 to 130 mg. Children and adolescents may excrete as much as twice this amount. Normal spot urinary protein–creatinine ratios on random samples generally fall below 0.2. Values higher than 3 suggest the presence of nephrotic-range proteinuria.

Qualitative assessments of urinary protein composition are often a valuable addition to the quantitative examination. Urine protein electrophoresis (UPEP) separates urinary proteins on the basis of molecular weights into five peaks: albumin and α_1, α_2, β, and γ globulins. Normally, urinary proteins are composed of filtered proteins from plasma (50%) and proteins that are secreted into the urine from urinary tract cells (50%). Of the filtered proteins, albumin is the most abundant, representing approximately 15% of the total urinary protein. This is followed by immunoglobulins (5%), light chains (5%), β_2 microglobulin (<0.2%), and other plasma proteins (25%). Of the secreted proteins, Tamm-Horsfall protein enters the urine after synthesis in the tubular cells of the ascending limb of the loop of Henle. It is the single most abundant protein in normal urine, accounting for 50% of the total urinary protein.

UPEP and immunoelectrophoresis (IEP) can be helpful in identifying the nature of proteins present in the urine. Immunofixation may be more sensitive than either of the two latter methods. Examining the urine for Bence-Jones proteinuria by seeking urinary precipitates at 45° to 55°C that redissolve at a higher temperature is a less sensitive method than are UPEP and IEP for identifying overflow proteinuria.

B. Pathophysiologic classification of proteinuria. Given the diverse sources of urinary proteins and the implication of source for the site of pathology, proteinuria is classified into three major categories reflecting pathogenesis.

1. Overflow proteinuria is due to the filtration by the normal glomerulus of an abnormally large amount of small-molecular-weight protein present in serum whose filtration exceeds the capacity of normal tubules for reabsorption. This occurs in monoclonal gammopathies (such as multiple myeloma), in intravascular hemolysis (hemoglobinuria), and in rhabdomyolysis (myoglobinuria). Overflow proteinuria can be identified by an abnormal peak or "spike" on the UPEP. For example, a "spike" occurring in the γ region (or, less commonly, in the α_2 or β region) suggests the presence of a monoclonal gammopathy. Further identification of the protein can be accomplished by performing IEP.

2. Tubular proteinuria is found in both acute and chronic injuries involving the renal tubulointerstitial region. Usually quantitatively less than 2 g per day, tubular proteinuria is derived from three sources. First, injured tubules fail to completely reabsorb small-molecular-weight proteins filtered by the glomerulus, such as β_2 microglobulin and amylase. Second, injured tubules secrete brush border components and cellular enzymes, such as n-acetylglucosamine and lysozyme, into the urine. Finally, with tubulointerstitial injury, Tamm-Horsfall protein may be secreted into the urine in greater amounts by the tubular cells of the ascending limb of the loop of Henle and the distal nephron. UPEP and IEP may also aid in distinguishing glomerular from tubular proteinuria. The overwhelming predominance of albumin rather than globulins on a UPEP suggests the presence of glomerular proteinuria. A quantitative comparison of the urinary albumin and β_2 microglobulin levels performed by IEP or other immunologic techniques (including immunoprecipitation, immunodiffusion, or radioimmunoassay) may also be helpful in this regard. A urinary albumin to β_2 microglobulin ratio of 10 to 1 suggests the presence of tubular proteinuria, whereas in glomerular proteinuria, this ratio usually exceeds 1,000 to 1. In normal urine, the albumin to β_2 microglobulin ratio ranges from 50 to 1 to 200 to 1.

3. **Glomerular proteinuria** occurs when injury to the glomerulus results in an ultrafiltrate characterized by a fractional increase in the clearance of serum proteins. In some forms of glomerulonephritis, this is due to changes in the size-selective properties of the glomerular capillary wall that allow the passage of larger-molecular-weight proteins or even of cells (e.g., in crescentic glomerulonephritis). In other forms, this is due to changes in the charge-selective properties of the glomerular capillary wall that enhance the ultrafiltration of negatively charged albumin (e.g., minimal change nephropathy). Some glomerular disorders are characterized by changes in both size and charge selectivity (e.g., diabetic nephropathy). Mesangial injury may also induce proteinuria, perhaps by interfering with normal mesangial clearance functions.

   Glomerular proteinuria is composed predominantly of albumin and, when quantitatively large (i.e., more than 3.0 to 3.5 g per day, or more than 2 g per day per m^2), it is said to be in the nephrotic range. The nephrotic syndrome consists of a pentad of nephrotic-range proteinuria, hypoalbuminemia, hyperlipidemia, lipiduria, and edema. With the exception of minimal-change glomerulopathy, the occurrence of heavy proteinuria in glomerular disorders is associated with a higher risk for progressive renal insufficiency.

4. **Other types of proteinuria.** Two forms of proteinuria do not fit easily into the classification described above. Benign orthostatic proteinuria is typically found in tall adolescents and occurs in the lordotic position. Protein is found in the urine collected on retiring and in the morning after the patient has been ambulant, but not in the overnight specimen collected immediately on rising. No abnormality should be present in the urine sediment, and proteinuria should not exceed 1 g per day. In one-half of these patients, proteinuria disappears within 10 years; however, in a small proportion, overt renal disease develops in later life. Finally, functional, transient proteinuria may be associated with such diverse causes as cardiac failure, fever, or heavy exercise. It disappears within hours after cessation of exercise and with resolution of the disease process. Proteinuria after marathon running may be as heavy as 5 g per L of urine.

C. **Clinical evaluation and treatment.** The most important first step in the development of an appropriate differential diagnosis and subsequent treatment plan for patients with proteinuria is classification of the urinary protein.

1. **Classification of proteinuria**
    a. **Overflow proteinuria.** The presence of overflow is suggested by a disparity characterized by a small amount of proteinuria demonstrated by dipstick and a disproportionately larger amount measured on a 24-hour collected specimen. This is most often due to excretion of monoclonal light chains, which can be confirmed by IEP. Identification of a monoclonal immunoglobulin in the urine should stimulate diagnostic testing for multiple myeloma, amyloidosis, or a lymphoproliferative disorder. Hemoglobinuria and myoglobinuria can also cause overflow

proteinuria. However, these are readily identifiable, because in these conditions the dipstick for blood is strongly positive, whereas the microscopical examination of urine demonstrates few or no red blood cells. This finding should stimulate an evaluation for hemolysis and for rhabdomyolysis.

b. Tubular proteinuria. A wide range of conditions can cause tubulointerstitial injury (see Table 8-4). An investigation of tubular proteinuria should begin with a detailed history regarding other affected family members (to rule out polycystic kidney disease); prescribed or over-the-counter medication use (analgesic nephropathy); frequent UTIs (reflux); flank pain; passage of renal stones; skin rash, arthralgias, arthritis (drug hypersensitivity, collagen-vascular disease); dry mouth or eyes (Sjögren's syndrome); occupational or recreational exposure to potential toxins; and manifestations of systemic disease. Physical findings confirmatory of disorders in the differential diagnosis listed in Table 8-4 should be sought. These might include palpably enlarged kidneys (polycystic kidney disease), band keratopathy (hypercalcemia, hyperparathyroidism), skin rash (systemic lupus, drug hypersensitivity), arthritis (gout, lupus), or oral mucosal lead line (lead toxicity). Laboratory tests including CBC with examination of the peripheral smear; measurements of serum creatinine, urea nitrogen, glucose, calcium, phosphorus, uric acid, and potassium; and urine culture are adjunctive information to the history, physical examination, urinalysis, and quantitative urine studies in focusing the differential diagnosis. Positive or negative results in these areas may suggest the need for further tests, which may include renal ultrasound (polycystic kidney disease, renal stones, obstruction); urine, serum, or hemoglobin electrophoresis (monoclonal gammopathy, sickle cell disease or trait); urine culture and sensitivity (pyelonephritis, renal tuberculosis); serum angiotensin-converting enzyme level (sarcoidosis); intravenous urography (medullary sponge kidney); or serum lead levels (lead toxicity). Although some tubulointerstitial disorders have characteristic histomorphologic features (medullary cystic disease, amyloidosis, myeloma kidney, hypokalemia), the microscopic appearance of most tubulointerstitial disorders lacks uniquely distinguishing characteristics. Renal biopsy is therefore used infrequently in the diagnosis of patients with tubulointerstitial disease. Therapy for the tubulointerstitial disorders is dependent on the underlying cause.

c. Glomerular proteinuria. When proteinuria is characterized by a disproportionate amount of albumin, a glomerular origin is implied. Mild transient proteinuria, especially associated with acute and reversible disease, is usually of little long-term significance. However, heavy and sustained proteinuria suggests a more serious disorder. Because the differential diagnosis is large, and many of the implicated disorders are uncommon, consultation with a nephrologist is recommended during the initial evaluation and treatment.

Patients with constant heavy proteinuria require close diagnostic scrutiny. Glomerular proteinuria in this group is often categorized either as non-nephrotic (less than 3.5 g per day per 1.73 m^2 body surface area) or nephrotic (more than 3.5 g per day per 1.73 m^2 body surface area). This somewhat arbitrary division of patients into those with lesser and greater amounts of urinary protein is justified by two major observations. First, patients with non-nephrotic proteinuria tend to have a better prognosis with regard to renal function than do patients with heavier proteinuria. As a result, an aggressive diagnostic or therapeutic approach may not be immediately indicated. Thus, after a search for underlying causes discernible by history, physical examination, and serologic assessment (see section **III.D.**), therapy including the use of antiproteinuric agents such as angiotensin converting enzyme inhibitors (ACEi) with or without angiotensin receptor blockers (ARB), and follow-up to observe the course of the renal function and degree of proteinuria may be indicated in individual patients before a consideration of renal biopsy and the use of potentially risky immunosuppressive therapeutic regimens. Second, the morbidity and prognosis of patients with heavier proteinuria is conferred not only by the patient's renal functional outcome, but also by the pathophysiologic consequences of heavy proteinuria (e.g., the nephrotic syndrome).

The nephrotic syndrome is defined by the presence of more than 3.5 g of proteinuria per 1.73 m^2 of body surface area per day, hypoalbuminemia, hyperlipidemia, lipiduria, and edema. Heavy proteinuria induces enhanced tubular reabsorption and catabolism of proteins leaked into the glomerular ultrafiltrate, thus contributing to hypoproteinemia. Sodium and water retention, with resultant edema, occurs secondary to hypoproteinemia in some patients and as a direct result of glomerular injury in others. Hypoproteinemia and an associated decrement in plasma oncotic pressure may stimulate apolipoprotein synthesis in the liver, causing hyperlipidemia and lipiduria. It is postulated that in nephrotic disorders that persist for many years (e.g., membranous nephropathy), hyperlipidemia may contribute to accelerated atherosclerosis. Heavy proteinuria also predisposes to hypercoagulability; variable losses of antithrombin III, protein S, and protein C have been described in some but not all nephrotic patients. Other urinary losses may variably induce subtle abnormalities of function in some patients with nephrotic syndrome, including losses of immunoglobulin and complement (predisposition to infection), thyroid-binding globulin (low total thyroxine, normal thyroid-stimulating hormone), and vitamin D (hypovitaminosis, hypocalcemia, and secondary hyperparathyroidism). Individuals with heavy proteinuria express the complications of nephrotic syndrome variably, further reflecting differences in urinary protein losses, dietary intake, and genetic predisposition.

D. **The differential diagnosis of heavy proteinuria.** Once proteinuria is determined to result from glomerular injury, an underlying disorder should be sought. The very large number of differential diagnoses outlined in Table 8-3 can be narrowed substantially by obtaining a detailed history, physical examination, and appropriate serologic testing. The history should cover the following important details: the presence of diabetes; deafness; similarly affected family members (suggestive of Alport nephropathy or other familial nephritis); ethnicity [immunoglobulin A (IgA) nephropathy is frequent in Asians and infrequent in African Americans]; presence of fever; travel; medication use; transfusions, drug abuse, sexual orientation and partners [human immunodeficiency virus (HIV), hepatitis, syphilis]; arthritis, arthralgias, malar or skin rash, oral ulcers, alopecia [systemic lupus erythematosus (SLE) and other immune or hypersensitivity disorders]; hemoptysis (Goodpasture disease, Wegener granulomatosis); sinusitis, sterile otitis (Wegener granulomatosis); paresthesias, angiokeratomas, dyshidrosis, focal neurologic deficits (Fabry disease); weight loss, cough, breast mass (malignancy and secondary membranous nephropathy); allergies; childhood or adolescent UTI's (focal sclerosis secondary to reflux nephropathy); and episodes of gross or persistent microhematuria (IgA nephropathy, thin basement membrane nephropathy). The physical examination should be directed at establishing whether systemic disease is present and whether the nephrotic syndrome or its complications are present. All adult patients with abnormal proteinuria should also have, at a minimum, a chest x-ray; CBC; serum and urine protein electrophoresis; serum chemistry panel, including tests of renal and hepatic function; and a measurement of serum albumin, total protein, total and high-density lipoprotein cholesterol, triglycerides, glucose, and calcium levels. For patients older than the age of 40, stool guaiac examination in men and women and mammography in women should also be performed. For those over the age of 50, a screening colonoscopy should be performed if it has not already been done. Additional serologic testing may be warranted, depending on the presence or absence of hematuria and the results of the aforementioned studies. Such additional tests include, but are not limited to, antinuclear and anti-double stranded DNA antibodies (lupus); antineutrophil cytoplasmic antibody (ANCA), anti-proteinase 3 and anti-myeloperoxidase antibodies (Wegener granulomatosis and other vasculitic syndromes); C3, C4 (may be low in endocarditis, poststreptococcal glomerulonephritis, lupus, membranoproliferative glomerulonephritis, cryoglobulinemia); antihyaluronidase, anti-DNase B, antistreptolysin O (poststreptococcal glomerulonephritis); anti-glomerular basement membrane antibody (Goodpasture disease); rheumatoid factor (endocarditis, cryoglobulinemia, rheumatoid arthritis); serum cryoglobulins; angiotensin-converting enzyme (sarcoidosis); glycosylated hemoglobin; serologic testing for syphilis; hepatitis B antigens and antibody; recombinant immunoblot testing and viral load for hepatitis C; and enzyme-linked immunoabsorbent assay/Western blot for human immunodeficiency virus. In the spirit of cost-consciousness, these tests should not be routinely ordered in all patients with glomerular proteinuria. Rather, a thoughtful synthesis of the history and physical examination should guide the selection of appropriate tests among those listed (and potentially others not mentioned).

A renal biopsy should be considered if no underlying disorder emerges as a cause for glomerular proteinuria after a thorough evaluation. In addition, renal biopsy is indicated when a secondary cause has been identified and a histologic examination of the renal tissue would help guide therapy, as is the case for SLE.

IV. **Therapy.** The treatment of glomerular disorders falls into three categories: treatment of the underlying systemic disease, general management of the nephrotic syndrome, and therapies for specific glomerular diseases.

A. **Treatment of underlying systemic disease.** Due to the large number of entities that potentially cause glomerulonephritis, the reader is referred to a textbook of internal medicine or nephrology for their treatment. However, special mention should be made of diabetes mellitus. Data suggest that tight glycemic control and ACEi and/or ARBs are useful in preventing or forestalling the development of overt diabetic nephropathy in patients with diabetes mellitus. These also have been shown to have a favorable impact on serum creatinine levels, progression to end-stage renal disease, and overall mortality in patients with diabetic nephropathy.

1. **General management of the nephrotic syndrome.** The treatment of edema due to the nephrotic syndrome begins with sodium restriction and diuretics. Care should be taken to avoid inducing a state of marked prerenal azotemia.

Many strategies have been advocated to decrease heavy proteinuria. Nonsteroidal anti-inflammatory drugs (NSAIDs) reportedly produce a decrease in proteinuria in some patients, along with a smaller decrement in GFR. Despite their utility in a few patients, however, the overall impact of NSAIDs in substantially diminishing proteinuria for the majority of patients with nephrosis is disappointingly small. ACEi and ARBs are also useful to decrease proteinuria, and their efficacy has been tested both in patients with diabetic nephropathy and in patients with the idiopathic nephrotic syndrome. Combinations of these agents appear to be additive in limiting proteinuria. Many months may elapse between ACEi and/or ARB initiation and the achievement of the maximal decrement in proteinuria from that dose, a phenomenon that suggests more than hemodynamic change as its mechanism of action. Proteinuria may also be reduced by lowering patients' mean arterial pressure to levels below 92 mm Hg, independent of the class of antihypertensive agents used to achieve this target. Finally, dietary protein restriction in the range of 0.6 to 0.8 g per kg per day has been suggested, both to slow the rate of loss of renal function and as a further means of diminishing proteinuria. The efficacy of angiotensin blockade, the conflicting supporting data for the effcicacy of low-protein diets, and concerns regarding nutritional safety in patients with heavy proteinuria (i.e., more than 10 g per day) has made stringent dietary protein restriction less frequently prescribed in recent years. Nevertheless, patients with heavy proteinuria should be advised to eat a diet close to the recommended daily allowance of protein, which is 0.8 gm protein/kg body weight.

The hyperlipidemia of the nephrotic syndrome may contribute to accelerated atherosclerosis. Use of the HMG-CoA (3-hydroxy-3-methylglutaryl–coenzyme A) reductase inhibitors or agents such as gemfibrozil often lower serum low-density lipoprotein cholesterol and triglyceride levels substantially in patients with nephrosis. However, they should not be used together because of the increased risk of rhabdomyolysis. For the patient with venous or, less commonly, arterial thrombosis or pulmonary emboli, long-term anticoagulation for the duration of the nephrotic syndrome is recommended.

2. **Therapies for specific glomerular diseases.** The so-called primary glomerular disorders fall into essentially seven histologic categories: minimal-change glomerulopathy, IgM mesangial proliferative glomerulonephritis, focal and segmental glomerulosclerosis, IgA nephropathy, membranous nephropathy, membranoproliferative glomerulonephritis (MPGN), and crescentic glomerulonephritis. From a therapeutic standpoint, the first three are often considered as a group, and the latter four are considered separately. Because these disorders are relatively uncommon and therapies often involve the use of potentially toxic drugs, referral to a nephrologist is advised.

a. **Minimal-change glomerulopathy—IgM mesangial proliferation glomerulonephritis—focal and segmental glomerulosclerosis.** If the nephrotic syndrome is present, conservative general care as described in section **IV.A.1** may be appropriate as an adjunct to specific therapy. These glomerular disorders are variably responsive to high-dose prednisone (1 mg per kg, maximum, 80 mg). More than 90% of children with minimal-change glomerulopathy have a complete remission of proteinuria within 2 months of starting steroid therapy. In adults, this figure is approximately 80% to 90%. Response rates for the latter two disorders are not as high (approximately 40% to 50% and 20% to 30%, respectively). Extending the duration of high-dose prednisone to 4 to 6 months may accrue as many as 10% to 15% additional complete remissions. Prednisone should then be slowly tapered over approximately 4 months. Relapse, steroid dependence, or both can be treated with the addition of cytotoxic agents (e.g., cyclophosphamide or chlorambucil), cyclosporine A, or possibly mycophenolate mofetil, depending on the severity of the nephrotic syndrome and the level of renal function. Treatment of prednisone-resistant patients is controversial. Genetically inherited forms of focal and segmental glomerulosclerosis have been identified and involve mutations of podocyte proteins. These inherited forms may or may not be steroid-responsive.

b. **IgA nephropathy (Berger's disease).** This is the most common form of primary glomerular disease in the world. It is particularly prevalent in Asia and Australia, and rare in African-Americans. Originally thought to be benign, it is now apparent that the condition progresses to end-stage renal disease in 20% to 40% of patients affected. Occasionally, reversible acute renal failure has been noted, particularly in association with gross hematuria. It may, rarely, be complicated by the presence of crescents. Clinically, it may be confused with a benign familial disorder, thin basement membrane nephropathy, because the presenting manifestation of each is predominantly glomerular hematuria. These two entities may be distinguished by a family history of hematuria (occasional in IgA nephropathy, frequent in thin basement membrane nephropathy), the presence of abnormal proteinuria (frequent in IgA nephropathy, uncommon in thin basement membrane nephropathy), and renal biopsy (no glomerular immunoglobulins present in thin basement membrane nephropathy, mesangial IgA in Berger's disease). No therapeutic regimen is agreed upon to clearly affect outcome in IgA nephropathy, although there is support in different geographic locations for warfarin and dipyridamole with or without cyclophosphamide, omega-3 fatty acids, ACEi with or without ARBs, long-term steroids, and steroids with cytotoxic agents, the latter particularly for those with progressive renal insufficiency.

c. **Membranous nephropathy.** Two-thirds of patients with this disorder either have a spontaneous remission or have stable or very slowly progressive renal insufficiency. Thus, the majority do well with conservative therapy (including ACEi and ARBs) directed at minimizing complications from the nephrotic syndrome. For patients at high risk for progression (e.g., those with heavy proteinuria, more than 10 g per day; hypertension; diminished GFR; male gender; or tubulointerstitial fibrosis on renal biopsy), specific therapy may be indicated. In this setting, steroids with a cytotoxic agent (either chlorambucil or cyclophosphamide) appears to be preferable to steroids alone in inducing a timely complete or partial remission. Cyclosporine A has been shown to be of benefit in a randomized trial; the benefit of mycophenolate mofetil remains anecdotal.

d. **MPGN.** Hepatitis C is the most common cause of MPGN type 1. Definitive therapy is uncertain, but a combination of interferon-alpha and ribavirin (or pegylated interferon alpha with ribavirin) may be indicated. Side effects due to ribavirin increase when the GFR falls below 50 mL per min. Steroids and cytotoxics may increase viral load, and should be used only for the cryoglobulinemic vasculitis complications of hepatitis C. Some investigators controversially suggest that children with MPGN type I (mesangial and subendothelial deposits) benefit from steroid therapy. Initial enthusiasm for the use of aspirin and dipyridamole has waned. No therapy is effective for type II (dense-deposit disease).

e. **Crescentic glomerulonephritis.** When glomerulonephritis is accompanied by crescents, a nephrologic emergency is present, due to the propensity for rapid progression to end-stage renal disease. Early diagnosis and implementation of therapy are essential to preserve renal function. After excluding poststreptococcal glomerulonephritis, three forms of crescentic glomerulonephritis are recognized. The reader is referred to a textbook of nephrology for the treatment of type I (antiglomerular basement membrane nephritis, or Goodpasture syndrome) and type III (pauci-immune glomerulonephritis, Wegener granulomatosis). Type II (immune complex–mediated glomerulonephritis) is treated initially with intravenous methylprednisolone sodium succinate (Solu-Medrol®), followed by high-dose oral prednisone with or without cytotoxics. Because of the relative rarity of the syndrome, no randomized controlled trials have proved that additional benefits accrue from the use of cytotoxic agents. However, largely due to the clearcut benefits of cyclophosphamide in types I and III and plasmapheresis in type I, some investigators have recommended their use in type II.

Suggested readings

Addis T. The number of formed elements in the urinary sediment of normal individuals. *J Clin Invest* 1926;2:409.

Birch DF, Fairley KF, Whitworth JA, et al. Urinary erythrocyte morphology in the diagnosis of glomerular hematuria. *Clin Nephrol* 1983;20:78.

Fairley KF, Birch DF. Haematuria: a simple method for identifying glomerular bleeding. *Kidney Int* 1982;21:105.

Gadehold H. Quantitative estimation of cells in the urine. *Acta Med Scand* 1968; 183:309.

Godfrey K, Harding M, Zhanel GG, Nicolle LE, Cheang M, for the Manitoba Diabetes Urinary Tract Infection Study Group. Antimicrobial treatment in diabetic women with asymptomatic bacteriuria. *N Engl J Med* 2002;347:1576–1583.

Haver MH. *Urinary sediment: a textbook atlas.* Chicago: American Society of Pathologists, 1983.

Kincaid-Smith P, Whitworth JA, eds. *The kidney,* 2nd ed. Oxford, UK: Blackwell, 1987.

Murphy BM, Fairley KF, Birch DF, et al. Culture of mid catheter urine collected via an open-ended catheter: a reliable guide to bladder bacteriuria. *J Urol* 1984;131:19.

Kim M, Corwin H. Urinalysis. In: Schrier RW ed. *Diseases of the kidney and urinary tract,* 7th ed. Philadelphia: Lippincott Williams & Wilkins: 317–332.

Nakao N, Yoshimura A, Morita H, Takada M, Kayano T, Ideura T. Combination of treatment of angiotensin II receptor blocker and angiotensin-converting enzyme inhibitor in nondiabetic renal disease (COOPERATE): a randomised controlled trial. *Lancet* 2003;361:117–124.

Ruggenenti P, Gaspari F, Perna A, Remuzzi G. Cross-sectional longitudinal study of spot morning urine protein: creatinine ratio, 24-hour urine protein excretion rate, glomerular filtration rate, and end-stage renal failure in chronic renal disease in patients without diabetes. *BMJ (Clinical Research Edition)* 1998;316(7130):504.

Scherberich JE. Urinary proteins of tubular origin: basic immunochemical and clinical aspects. *Am J Nephrol* 1990;10[Suppl 1]:43.

Waller KV, Ward KM, Mahan JD, Wismatt DK. Current concepts in proteinuria. *Clin Chem* 1989;35:755.

The Patient with Glomerulonephritis or Vasculitis

Alexander Wiseman

I. **Overview** Glomerular diseases are most simply defined as either a primary process, in which the disease process is confined to the kidney, or a secondary process, in which a systemic disease impacts the kidney. A wide variety of incompletely understood disease processes may lead to histologic abnormalities in the mesangial region, the subepithelial space (the urinary side of the glomerular capillary basement membrane), the subendothelial space (the vascular side of the glomerular basement membrane), or any combination of the above within the glomerulus. These distinct patterns of injury seen on renal biopsy form the basis for classification of these diseases and guide therapy. Because a number of systemic vasculitides can cause small vessel inflammation, often the small vessels of the kidney and the glomerular capillaries are targets of vascular inflammation and can be recognized on renal biopsy.

Clinically, the presence of a glomerular disease should be considered when proteinuria is present; glomerulonephritis and vasculitis should be considered when hematuria and/or proteinuria are present. Thus, the approach to the patient with possible glomerular disease should begin with an assessment of the protein excretion in the urine and a microscopical analysis of the urine for dysmorphic red blood cells and/or red blood cell casts.

II. **Proteinuria** Although a number of conditions, such as interstitial nephritis, can cause proteinuria, typically the quantity of nonglomerular proteinuria is less than 1 g on a 24-hour urine collection, whereas clinically and therapeutically relevant glomerular diseases are associated with proteinuria of greater than 1.5 to 3 g per day. The clinician must assess the presence and degree of proteinuria in order to screen for possible glomerular disease.

A. **Evaluation of proteinuria.** A number of methods are utilized to assess the presence and degree of proteinuria:

1. **24-hour urine collection.** When done properly, the 24-hour urine collection provides the most accurate measure of urinary protein excretion. This method involves emptying the bladder and discarding the first morning urine, then collecting all urine for the subsequent 24 hours, including the first morning void the following day. The urine should be refrigerated during the collection period. If this is not possible, one cup of vinegar can be added to the collection container to act as a preservative. To ensure adequate collection, a 24-hour total creatinine excretion should be obtained on the same sample. In females under steady-state conditions of renal function, the 24-hour urinary excretion of creatinine should equal approximately 15 to 20 mg per kg of ideal body weight; in males, the excretion should be 18 to 25 mg per kg of ideal body weight.

2. **Urine dipstick test.** As a rapid screen for the presence of albuminuria, commercially available dipsticks can provide the clinician a gross estimate of the presence and degree of proteinuria. Quantification of proteinuria, however, must be performed using a 24-hour urine collection or alternatively, multiple early morning spot urine collections for the calculation of the protein to creatinine ratio.

3. **Urine sulfosalicylic acid test.** The urine dipstick detects albuminuria, but not smaller molecular weight proteins such as immunoglobulin light

chains. The urine sulfosalicylic acid (SSA) test detects the presence of all proteins in the urine, including light chains. This test is particularly helpful in patients with chronic renal insufficiency of unknown etiology, no abnormalities on urinalysis, and little or no protein detected on dipstick screening. A positive SSA test with a normal dipstick indicates the presence of nonalbumin proteins in the urine, leading to further investigation of light chain deposition disease, most frequently associated with multiple myeloma.

4. **Urine protein–creatinine ratio.** A urinary protein–creatinine concentration ratio on the first voided morning urine sample can be used as a quick assessment of proteinuria, and it can be useful as a substitute for repeated full 24-hour urine collections to assess responsiveness to therapy. The normal 24-hour urine protein excretion in the adult can range from 30 to 130 mg, whereas children and adolescents may excrete as much as twice this amount. With the assumption taken that the average individual excretes approximately 1 g of creatinine per day, normal spot urinary protein–creatinine ratios on random samples generally fall below 0.2 (mg protein per mg creatinine), whereas values greater than 3 suggest the presence of nephrotic-range proteinuria. This ratio should not be used as a substitute for an initial 24-hour collection in cases in which glomerulonephritis is considered or in cases in which the creatinine generation is likely greater than 1 g per day (for example, in individuals with large muscle mass).

B. **Classification of proteinuria.** As mentioned above, a number of nonglomerular diseases can lead to proteinuria. When proteinuria is identified, it is important to identify whether it is glomerular or nonglomerular in origin, because the treatments for these conditions are dramatically different. In general, proteinuria can be classified into three major categories:

1. **Overflow proteinuria.** Overflow proteinuria is caused by the filtration of an abnormally large amount of small-molecular-weight proteins from the serum (by normal glomeruli) that exceeds the capacity of normal tubules for reabsorption. Diseases associated with overflow proteinuria include rhabdomyolysis (myoglobinuria), intravascular hemolysis (hemoglobinuria), and monoclonal gammopathies (such as the light chain deposition disease seen in multiple myeloma). Evaluation of overflow proteinuria may be aided by urine protein electrophoresis (UPEP), which separates urinary proteins into five peaks based on the molecular weights of the proteins. The five peaks include albumin and α_1, α_2, β, and γ globulins. For example, an abnormal peak or "spike" occurring in the γ region (or, less commonly, in the α_2 or β region) suggests the presence of a monoclonal gammopathy.

2. **Tubular proteinuria.** In contrast to overflow proteinuria, in which normal tubular reabsorption is overwhelmed by an abnormally large amount of filtered proteins, tubular proteinuria is caused by damage to the renal tubulointerstitial region, which leads to a failure to reabsorb small-molecular-weight proteins. Under normal conditions, the small amount of urinary protein is composed of filtered proteins from plasma (50%) and proteins that are secreted into the urine from urinary tract cells (50%). Filtered proteins include small amounts of albumin (approximately 15% of the total urinary protein), immunoglobulins (5%), light chains (5%), β_2 microglobulin (<0.2%), and other plasma proteins (25%). The most prevalent tubular protein (and the most abundant protein in normal urine) is Tamm-Horsfall protein, which enters the urine after synthesis in the tubular cells of the ascending limb of the loop of Henle and is secreted into the urine. Under conditions of tubulointerstitial injury, both filtered and secreted proteins are found in increased amounts in the urine, up to 1 to 2 g per day. Increases in tubular proteinuria may occur by three mechanisms. First, injured tubules are unable to reabsorb the small-molecular-weight proteins normally filtered by the glomerulus, such as

β_2 microglobulin. Second, brush border components and cellular enzymes such as N-acetylglucosamine and lysozyme are secreted into the urine under conditions of tubular injury. Lastly, increased amounts of Tamm-Horsfall protein may be secreted into the urine by injured tubular cells of the ascending limb of the loop of Henle and the distal nephron. When the source of proteinuria is unclear, urine electrophoresis (UPEP) and immunoelectrophoresis (IEP) can be utilized to aid in diagnosis. In glomerular proteinuria, a UPEP demonstrates primarily albumin rather than globulins, whereas tubular proteinuria demonstrates a predominance of small-molecular-weight proteins. IEP can quantify this distinction further if a definitive spike is not present on UPEP. A urinary albumin to β_2 microglobulin ratio of 10 to 1 is indicative of tubular proteinuria, in contrast to glomerular proteinuria, in which this ratio usually exceeds 1,000 to 1. In comparison, in normal urine, the albumin to β_2 microglobulin ratio ranges from 50 to 1 to 200 to 1.

3. **Glomerular proteinuria.** Glomerular proteinuria results from injury to the glomerulus, leading to an increase in filtered proteins. This injury may result in changes in the *size*-selective properties of the glomerular basement membrane, allowing the passage of larger-molecular-weight proteins or even of cells (as in crescentic glomerulonephritis), or may result in changes in the *charge*-selective properties of the glomerular basement membrane, permitting the ultrafiltration of negatively charged albumin (as in minimal change nephropathy). Glomerular injury may lead to a combination of defects in both size and charge selectivity (as in diabetic nephropathy). Finally, mesangial injury may also induce proteinuria via mechanisms that are not clear, perhaps by interfering with normal mesangial clearance functions.

   As described, glomerular proteinuria is identified by the preponderance of albumin compared to smaller molecular weight proteins. Generally, the greater the degree of proteinuria, the worse the renal prognosis. In this regard, nephrotic-range proteinuria, defined by significant proteinuria greater than 3.0 to 3.5 g per day, often requires specific therapeutic intervention based upon the underlying disease.

4. **Other proteinuria.** Although most forms of proteinuria may be classified into overflow, tubular, or glomerular sources, two additional causes of proteinuria exist that do not fall into these categories. Benign orthostatic proteinuria is proteinuria of less than 1 gram per day without other urinary abnormalities; this is typically found in tall adolescents. When split urine collections are performed (a 12-hour overnight collection and 12-hour daytime collection), protein is found only in the daytime collection. The condition is considered to be benign and often disappears in adulthood; however, in a very small proportion, overt renal disease develops in adulthood. Proteinuria can occur with cardiac failure, fever, or heavy exercise. It is transient and disappears within hours after cessation of exercise or with recovery from the disease process. Table 9.1 lists the most common causes of nonglomerular proteinuria.

C. **Clinical assessment of proteinuria.** The clinical approach to a patient with proteinuria identified on a screening test (such as a urine dipstick or spot urine protein measurement) should be tailored to assess the presence of concurrent renal injury and the potential for future renal damage. A 24-hour urine protein measurement and a serum creatinine measurement should first be obtained, and the urine should be evaluated for the presence of red blood cells and casts (described in **III.A**). If renal function is normal, no red cells are present, and proteinuria is less than 200 mg per day, the renal injury sustained from a potential low-grade glomerular disease is minimal, and the risk of future renal injury is low if diabetes and/or hypertension are not present. Proteinuria in the range of 200 mg per day to 2 g per day with no hematuria and normal renal function can be caused by

Table 9-1. Common causes of nonglomerular proteinuria

Overflow	Tubular	Other
Rhabdomyolysis	Polycystic kidney disease	Benign orthostatic proteinuria
Hemoglobinuria	Pyelonephritis	Transient protein-uria (cardiac failure, fever, heavy exercise)
Monoclonal gammo-pathy (light chain deposition disease)	Obstruction	
	Vesicoureteral reflux	
	Medications (chronic lithium exposure, analgesic nephro-pathy, aminoglycosides)	
	Metabolic defects (oxalosis, cystinosis, hypercalcemia, hypercalciuria, hyperuricemia)	
	Trace metals (lead, mercury, cadmium)	

glomerular lesions, but is more likely to be related to tubular abnormalities; investigation should be directed accordingly, because a glomerular disease in this clinical scenario carries a good prognosis if blood pressure is adequately controlled. Proteinuria greater than 2 to 3 grams per day needs further evaluation for the presence of glomerular injury regardless of renal function. This evaluation is outlined in section **IV**. Any presentation in which red blood cell casts or dysmorphic red blood cells are present, regardless of the degree of renal function or proteinuria, must be further evaluated for the presence of a glomerulonephritis or vasculitis.

III. **Hematuria.** The pathognomonic finding of glomerular injury is the presence of dysmorphic red blood cells or red blood cell casts in the urine. This finding is a hallmark of glomerular capillary injury and limits the differential diagnosis significantly. However, care must be taken to rule out other causes of hematuria that produce red blood cells in the urine that are of normal morphology and do not form casts (typical of lower urinary tract abnormalities) and positive dipstick hematuria due to myoglobinuria or hemoglobinuria.

A. **Evaluation and classification of hematuria.** The initial evaluation is typically provoked either by macroscopic hematuria (visible discoloration of the urine) or by incidental findings on dipstick. Similar to the evaluation of proteinuria, hematuria can either be due to a glomerular disorder or to a nonglomerular source. Glomerular bleeding should be suspected if dysmorphic urinary red blood cells, red blood cell casts, and proteinuria are present. Nonglomerular hematuria is characterized by the presence of isomorphic urinary erythrocytes without red blood cell casts or significant proteinuria. Hematuria secondary to nonglomerular causes can be differentiated by the three-glass test. In this procedure, an initial stream, mid-stream, and end-stream sample of urine (10 to 15 mL each) is collected in three separate containers. A urethral site of bleeding is likely if the hematuria predominates in the inital sample, whereas a bladder origin is suggested if hematuria is predominately identified in the final sample. Ureteral and renal sources are suspected if hematuria is present in all three collection samples.

B. **Clinical assessment of hematuria.** The initial evaluation of the patient with gross or microscopic hematuria should be focused upon differentiating

Table 9-2. Systemic diseases that cause glomerular injury and a nephritic clinical presentation

Disease	Specific examples	Laboratory findings
Infections	Hepatitis C (B less commonly)	Low C3, Hep C Ab, Hep C viral PCR, cryoglobulins
	Post-streptococcal GN	Low C3, Anti-streptolysin Ab
	Bacterial endocarditis	Low C3, positive blood cultures
	MRSA infection	Low C3, positive blood cultures
Vasculidities	SLE	Low C3, ANA, anti-DNA
	Wegener's granulomatosis	c-ANCA
	Goodpasture's syndrome	Anti-GBM Ab
	Churg-Strauss syndrome	p-ANCA
	Henoch-Shönlein purpura	IgA in skin biopsy
	Polyarteritis nodosa	ANCA in 20% (c- or p-ANCA)
	Mixed cryoglobulinemia	Rheumatoid factor, low C4
Thrombotic microangiopathy	Scleroderma renal crisis	Anti-Scl-70
	Thrombotic thrombocytopenic purpura	Low platelets, hemolysis
	Hemolytic uremic syndrome	Low platelets, hemolysis, *E. coli* enteritis
	Malignant hypertension	

glomerular from nonglomerular causes. If microscopy suggests a glomerular cause, with dysmorphic red blood cells and red blood cell casts, patients should be further evaluated for renal dysfunction and glomerulonephritis as described in section **IV.C.** Nonglomerular hematuria typically entails an evaluation for the possibility of a urogenital malignancy, infection, stone, or cystic disease. In this regard, the history and review of systems should focus upon the frequency and nature of hematuria (gross or microscopic), pain, burning with urination, increased frequency of urination, fever, weight loss, and passage of stones. Medications that may lead to hematuria should be reviewed, including oral contraceptives and analgesics, particularly in patients with diabetes. Other causes of hematuria, including trauma, coagulation disorders, and family history of renal disease should be considered. The physical examination can identify certain causes of hematuria, such as renal bruits suggestive of arteriovenous fistulae; an enlarged prostate or nodules suggestive of hypertrophy, prostatitis, or malignancy; or enlarged kidneys on abdominal palpation, suggestive of polycystic kidney disease.

The diagnostic evaluation of nonglomerular hematuria should include urine culture for bacterial infection, and if suspected, mycobacterial and mycoplasma infection. Once a UTI has been excluded, the urinary tract anatomy should be evaluated via radiologic imaging or direct visualization to rule out malignancy, stone disease, and hereditary renal disease. The upper tract (the kidneys and ureters) can be evaluated by either a renal ultrasound, computed tomography (CT) scan, or intravenous pyelography (IVP), whereas the lower tract (bladder and urethra) is best evaluated by cystoscopy. Urine cytology can serve as an additional test to screen for the abnormal cellularity suggestive of urogenital malignancy. At the discretion of a urologist, a combination of the above tests should be performed in the patient with unexplained hematuria.

In the presence of a normal or near-normal glomerular filtration rate (GFR), intravenous urography is the most useful diagnostic radiologic procedure available for defining renal anatomy. It should disclose the presence of renal cysts (hereditary and acquired); calculi; papillary necrosis; medullary sponge kidney; renal, pelvic, and ureteral tumors; and ureteral strictures. In the event of a nondiagnostic intravenous urographic study, cystoscopy can be performed to more definitively examine the bladder for the presence of tumors or infectious (inflammatory/interstitial) cystitis and the urethra for the presence of urethritis, strictures, or both. A nondiagnostic cystoscopic examination can be followed, if clinically indicated, by arteriography to pursue the possibility that hematuria is secondary to ureteral varices or aneurysms, arteriovenous malformations, or the loin-pain hematuria syndrome.

IV. **Glomerular hematuria and/or proteinuria.** Once the evaluation of hematuria and/or proteinuria lead the clinician to consider a glomerular disease as the most likely etiology, further clinical information can assist in the classification of the renal disorder prior to invasive testing. Although it is often difficult to predict the histologic pattern of injury in a patient with glomerular disease, one can first consider if a pattern of injury exists that may be segregated based upon two general clinical presentations—the nephritic syndrome and the nephrotic syndrome—to assist in serologic testing.

   A. **The nephritic syndrome.** This clinical syndrome typically presents with clinical findings of hematuria, proteinuria, and dysmorphic red blood cells and/or red blood cell casts. The proteinuria can range from 200 mg per day to heavy proteinuria (greater than 10 grams per day). Clinically, it is accompanied by hypertension and edema. Renal insufficiency is common and typically progressive. The term "rapidly progressive glomerulonephritis" refers to diseases with a nephritic syndrome that lead to a rapid deterioration in renal function, defined as a doubling of serum creatinine or a 50% decrease in glomerular filtration rate over 3 months or less.

   B. **The nephrotic syndrome.** This clinical syndrome also presents with proteinuria and edema, but unlike the nephritic syndrome, proteinuria is the most prominent feature (greater than 3.5 g per 1.73 m^2 per day). Dysmorphic red blood cells and casts are typically absent [exceptions do exist: focal segmented glomerulosclerosis (FSGS) and IgA nephropathy, conditions that usually present with nephrotic proteinuria, also can present with hematuria]. Additional features of the nephrotic syndrome include hypercholesterolemia and hypoalbuminemia (serum albumin less than 3.0 mg per dL). The diseases that cause the nephrotic syndrome can lead to chronic, progressive renal injury, but typically are more indolent than diseases that lead to a nephritic syndrome.

   Once the clinical pattern has been identified, the clinician must consider if there is a systemic process that may be causing the proteinuria. Tables 9-2 and 9-3 list systemic diseases that present with a nephritic and nephrotic syndrome, respectively, and also highlight key laboratory findings that may aid in an initial diagnosis.

   In the absence of evidence of systemic disease, the clinician must consider primary (or islolated) glomerular diseases in the differential diagnosis. Histologically, these primary diseases are not distinct from the injury pattern seen in systemic diseases. The primary glomerulopathies are recognized by the histologic pattern defined by light microscopy, immunofluorescent staining for immunogloulins, and the characteristics and location of immune deposits on electron microscopy. The primary glomerular diseases are listed in Table 9-4, with the prominent histologic findings on biopsy that define the disorder.

   C. **Clinical assessment of glomerular disease**

   1. **The nephritic syndrome.** In cases in which the nephritic syndrome is the predominant clinical presentation, a search for systemic diseases is warranted. The history and physical exam should particularly focus on the assessment of rashes, lung disease, neurologic abnormalities, evidence of viral or bacterial infections, and musculoskeletal and hematologic abnormalities. Laboratory assessment should be tailored to the clinical

Table 9-3. Systemic diseases that cause glomerular injury and a nephrotic clinical presentation

Disease state	Common stiologies	Laboratory findings
Infections	Hepatitis B (C less common)	Hep B SAg, Hep B eAg
	HIV	HIV Ab
	Syphilis	RPR
Chronic diseases	Diabetes	Elevated HgbA1c, blood glucose
	Amyloidosis	UPEP/IEP (when associated with light chains)
	Sickle cell disease	Hemoglobin electrophoresis
	Obesity	
Malignancies	Multiple myeloma	SPEP, UPEP
	Adenocarcinoma (lung, breast, colon most common)	Abnormal cancer screening studies (usually clinically evident tumor burden)
	Lymphoma	
Rheumatologic	Systemic lupus erythematosus	ANA, anti-dsDNA Ab
	Rheumatoid arthritis	Rheumatoid factor
	Mixed connective tissue disease	Anti-RNP Ab
Medications	NSAIDs	
	Bucillamine	
	Penicillamine	
	Lithium	
	Ampicillin	
	Captopril	
	Probenecid	
	Gold	

findings in the history and physical examination. A complete blood count (CBC), electrolyte panel, 24-hour urine collection for protein and creatinine clearance, and liver function tests should be obtained initially. Serum complement (C3) levels are often clinically helpful to assist in the diagnosis of a specific renal disease (Table 9-5). Further laboratory assessment may be performed based on these findings, and may include an anti-streptolysin (ASO) titer, antinuclear antibody (ANA), antineutrophil cytoplasmic antibodies (ANCA), cryoglobulins, and/or an anti-GBM antibody. These early assessments may provide a presumptive diagnosis and should lead the clinician to an appropriate therapeutic intervention while awaiting renal biopsy results. These laboratory assessments should not substitute for the renal biopsy; only with a tissue diagnosis that confirms the clinical findings and provides information regarding the acuity and chronicity of the disease process can a glomerular disease can be properly managed.

2. **The nephrotic syndrome.** With the identification of significant proteinuria, with or without other features of the nephrotic syndrome, secondary causes of proteinuria should be assessed. History and physical examination should evaluate for the presence of viral and bacterial infections, malignancies (particularly lung, breast, and lymph node), chronic diseases (such as diabetes), and medications should be reviewed for their potential to cause glomerular proteinuria. Laboratory assessment initially includes CBC, electrolyte panel, 24-hour urine collection for protein and creatinine clearance, liver function tests, and a cholesterol panel. Further assessment may include hepatitis and human immunodeficiency

Table 9-4. Primary glomerular diseases, defined by histology

Nephritic	Histologic findings	Nephrotic	Histologic findings
Renal-limited vasculitis/ microscopic polyangiitis	Necrotizing capillary lesions, crescents; negative IF, EM	Minimal-change disease	Normal light microscopy, effaced foot processes on EM
Anti-glomerular basement membrane disease	Linear IgG staining along glomerular basement membrane	Membranous nephropathy	Subepithelial "spikes" on light, IF, EM
Essential cryoglobulinemia	Fibrils on electron microscopy	Membranoproliferative glomerulonephritis	Thickened mesangial matrix, splitting ("double contour") of the glomerular basement membrane, C3 granular staining on IF
		Focal segmental glomerulosclerosis	Sclerosis in portions of glomeruli, C3 in areas of sclerosis on IF
		IgA nephropathy	IgA in mesangium on IF
		Fibrillary glomerulonephritis	Fibrillar deposits in mesangium, negative congo red staining on IF

Table 9-5. Clinical approach to glomerulonephritis based upon serum complement level

Low serum complement level		Normal serum complement level	
Systemic diseases	*Primary renal diseases*	*Systemic diseases*	*Primary renal diseases*
SLE	Post-streptococcal glomerulonephritis	Polyarteritis nodosa	IgA nephropathy
Subacute bacterial endocarditis	Membranoproliferative glomerulonephritis (MPGN) Type 1 Type 2	Hypersensitivity vasculitis	Idiopathic rapidly progressive glomerulonephritis (anti-glomerular basement membrane disease, pauci-immune glomerulonephritis, immune complex disease)
"Shunt" nephritis Cryoglobulinemia		Wegener's granulomatosis Henoch-Schönlein purpura Goodpasture's syndrome Visceral abcess	

(Adapted from Madaio MP, Harrington JT. Current concepts. The diagnosis of acute glomerulonephritis. *N Eng J M* 1983;309:1299, with permission.)

virus (HIV) serologies, ANA, rapid plasma reagin (RPR), and serum and urine electropheresis. Renal biopsy should be performed in all cases in which no cause is evident, or to determine the extent of renal disease to guide therapy or prognosis.

V. Therapy for glomerulonephritis. The management of systemic diseases that cause secondary glomerular injury is rapidly changing (for example, new antiviral therapies for HIV and Hepatitis B and C, and clinical trials using chemotherapeutic regimens for malignancies and vasculidities), thus the reader is encouraged to refer to recent disease-specific reviews of the literature for current management strategies for these systemic diseases. This chapter reviews the treatment of the most frequent systemic diseases that cause glomerular injury. The treatment of glomerular disorders can be approached by general management of the nephrotic syndrome and proteinuria, and immunomodulating therapies for specific glomerular diseases and vasculidities.

A. General management of the nephrotic syndrome and proteinuria. Four general treatment strategies should be considered in the patient with nephrotic syndrome: managment of edema, management of proteinuria, mangagement of hyperlipidemia, and management of hypercoagulability. Management of edema should initially focus on sodium restriction and diuretics. Thiazides are a reasonable treatment choice for patients with mild edema and normal renal function; however, the majority of patients will require a loop diuretic such as furosemide for adequate sodium balance. The cornerstone to management of proteinuria is the inhibition of the renin-angiotensin system using either angiotensin converting enzyme inhibitors (ACEi) or angiotensin receptor blockers (ARB). Using these medications, intraglomerular pressure is reduced due to efferent arteriolar vasodilation, thus resulting in a reduced amount of protein filtrated. In diabetes, ACEi have been shown to be critical in slowing the development of overt diabetic nephropathy in patients with type 1 diabetes and microalbuminuria (30 to 300 mg per day), and reducing the incidence of end-stage renal disease (ESRD) and overall mortality in patients with type 1 diabetes and overt diabetic nephropathy (urine protein excretion greater than 300 mg per day). ARBs have shown similar benefits in patients with type 2 diabetes with either microalbuminuria or overt nephropathy. In nondiabetic proteinuric renal disease, ACEi also significantly reduces the risk of developing ESRD. The maximal therapeutic dose of single agent, and the role a combination of ACE and ARB for treatment of significant proteinuria and progression of renal disease remains unknown. Proteinuria may also be reduced by lowering patients' mean arterial pressure to levels lower than 92 mm Hg, independent of the class of antihypertensive agents used to achieve this target. Finally, dietary protein restriction in the range of 0.6 to 0.8 g per kg per day has been suggested, both to slow the rate of loss of renal function and as a further means of diminishing proteinuria. Long-term studies regarding nutritional safety are still necessary before this strategy should be advocated in patients, particularly those with heavy proteinuria (i.e., more than 10 g per day).

Control of hyperlipidemia often can be accomplished with use of the HMG-CoA reductase inhibitors or agents such as gemfibrozil. The issue of anticoagulation arises due to a hypercoagulable state induced by nephrotic proteinuria. Protein losses include the loss of antithrombotic factors such as antithrombin III, leading to an increased frequency of renal vein thrombosis and, less commonly, arterial thrombosis or pulmonary emboli. Long-term anticoagulation for the duration of the nephrotic syndrome is recommended for patients with documented thrombotic episodes. Debate still exists regarding prophylactic anticoagulation for all patients with nephrotic syndrome.

B. Therapies for specific glomerular diseases. The specific management of glomerular diseases may be initiated following renal biopsy. Histologically, glomerular disorders associated with the nephrotic syndrome fall into five

Table 9-6. Histologic classification of crescentic (or rapidly progressive) glomerulonephritis

Linear immunofluorescence	Granular immunofluroescence	Absent (pauci-immune) immunofluorescence
Goodpasture's disease	SLE	ANCA-associated vasculitis: Wegener's granulomatosis, Churg-Strauss syndrome, microscopic polyangiitis
Anti-GBM disease	Henoch-Schonlein purpura, IgA nephropathy Cryoglobulinemia	

general categories: minimal-change glomerulopathy, membranous nephropathy, mesangial proliferative glomerulonephritis (MPGN), focal and segmental glomerulosclerosis, and IgA nephropathy. Glomerular disorders with a nephritic clinical presentation typically show disruption of the glomerular basement membrane with cellular crescent formation in Bowman's space on renal biopsy (crescentic glomerulonephritis). These disorders generally fall into three histologic categories defined by the immunofluorescence patterns of immune deposits within the glomerulus (Table 9-6): linear immunofluorescence, granular immunofluorescence, and absent immunofluoresence. This categorization is a generalization, since aggressive forms of IgA nephropathy and MPGN may clinically appear nephritic and may be associated with glomerular crescents.

1. **Minimal-change glomerulopathy.** Approximately 15% of cases of idiopathic nephrotic syndrome in adults, and 85% in children, are due to minimal-change disease (MCD). Light microscopy is normal, and in combination with findings of effacement of foot processes on electron microscopy, is diagnostic of MCD on renal biopsy. IgM deposits may be seen in the mesangium on immunofluorescence, which may protend a poorer prognosis. In addition to the conservative managment of nephrotic syndrome, high-dose prednisone (1 mg per kg, maximum, 80 mg) is used as primary therapy for at least 12 weeks. Whereas greater than 90% of children with MCD will have a complete remission of proteinuria within 2 months of starting steroid therapy, in adults this figure is approximately 50% to 60%. Extending the duration of high-dose prednisone to 5 to 6 months increases the rate of complete remission to 80%. Prednisone should then be slowly tapered over approximately 4 months. For relapsing cases and cases in which steroids cannot be tapered (steroid dependence), recycling of steroids with or without the addition of cytotoxic agents (e.g., cyclophosphamide or chlorambucil), cyclosporine A, or possibly mycophenolate mofetil, may be effective.

2. **Membranous nephropathy.** Approximately 30% to 40% of cases of idiopathic nephrotic syndrome in adults are due to membranous nephropathy. Typically, this disease is slowly progressive and frequently patients may have spontaneous remissions, particularly female patients. However, certain patients are at high risk for progressive renal injury. Clinical risk factors associated with progression include heavy proteinuria greater than 8 g per day; hypertension; diminished GFR (creatinine greater than 1.2 for women, greater than 1.4 for men), male gender, and a greater than 20% tubulointerstitial fibrosis on renal biopsy. For these patients, steroids combined with a cytotoxic agent (either chlorambucil or cyclophosphamide) alternating monthly for 6 months appears to be more effective than steroids alone in inducing a complete or partial

remission. Preliminary data suggest that mycophenolate therapy also may be effective in the management of low- to moderate-risk patients.

3. **MPGN.** Idiopathic MPGN can be subcategorized to two types, type 1 (immune complex-mediated) and type II (thought to be complement-mediated). Both types, however, appear similar on light microscopy with expansion of the mesangial matrix. On electron microscopy, type II MPGN shows dense longitudinal deposits within the GBM versus the dense subepithelial deposits seen in type 1 MPGN. Together, these entities make up 5% of idiopathic nephrotic syndrome in adults, and they tend to carry a poor renal prognosis. Of patients with type 1 MPGN and nephrotic proteinuria, 60% will progress to ESRD in 10 years. Unfortunately, no established therapy exists for MPGN. Despite conflicting data regarding its efficacy, long-term alternate-day prednisone is the current therapy of choice, particularly for children and teenagers. In any case of MPGN, secondary causes must be fully evaluated, because diseases such as chronic bacterial infection, Hepatitis C infection, and cryoglobuline-mia, as well as leukemias and lymphomas all have therapies that may lead to remission of the renal disease.

4. **Focal and segmental glomerulosclerosis.** Approximately 20% of cases of idiopathic nephrotic syndrome in adults is due to focal segmental glomerulosclerosis (FSGS). FSGS may represent a more severe form of minimal-change disease, because glomerular epthelial cell foot process effacment is present on electron microscopy. Unlike MCD, however, focal areas within the kidney demonstrate sclerosis in segments of individual glomeruli. Previously considered an untreatable renal lesion, recent evidence suggests that with prolonged courses (at least 6 months) of high-dose corticosteroid therapy approximately 30% of patients will acheive remission of the nephrotic syndrome. The remaining 70% who fail to respond to steroids may occasionally experience remission on cytotoxic agents such as cyclosporin, cyclophosphamide, or chlorambucil.

5. **IgA nephropathy (Berger's disease).** IgA nephropathy is the most common form of primary glomerular disease in the world. It is particularly prevalent in Asia and Australia (perhaps due to sampling bias resulting from a more frequent biopsy rate in these regions), and rare in African-Americans. Although generally considered to be a slowly progressive renal disease, with ESRD occuring in 20% to 40% of patients by 20 years, a minority of patients may experience a rapidly progressive glomerulonephritis with crescent formation on biopsy. Occasionally, reversible acute renal failure occurs, particularly in association with gross hematuria. Treatment of IgA nephropathy remains controversial, because no therapeutic regimen has been shown to clearly affect outcome. Some studies advocate the use of fish oil in slowing the progression of renal insufficiency. For crescentic disease, short-term, high-dose prednisone may be of benefit. The use of cytotoxic agents such as cytoxan remains investigational at this time.

6. **Crescentic glomerulonephritis, linear immunofluorescence.** When glomerulonephritis is accompanied by crescents, and immunofluorescent staining for IgG demonstrates a linear pattern along glomerular capillaries on biopsy, the presence of an anti-glomerular basement membrane autoantibody (anti-GBM) is the most likely etiology. Clinically, this may present either as isolated renal dysfunction (anti-GBM disease) or as renal disease in conjunction with pulmonary involvement (Goodpasture's syndrome) with IgG staining of the pulmonary capillary basement membrane. Treatment of this disorder involves the combination of high-dose steroids, cytoxan therapy, and plasmapheresis to remove the anti-GBM antibody. Patients who present with oliguria have a poor renal prognosis, but occasionally may avoid chronic dialysis with aggressive and early therapy.

7. **Crescentic glomerulonephritis, granular immunofluorescence.** In this form of glomerulonephritis, immune complexes deposit within the glomeruli in a nonlinear fashion, giving the appearance of "lumps and bumps" when stained by immunofluorescent markers. Diseases within this histologic category include postinfectious GN (in which C3 and IgG stains in the subepithelial space), Henoch-Schönlein purpura, and occasionally IgA nephropathy (in which IgA predominantly stains in the mesangial space), cryoglobulinemia (in which IgM rheumatoid factor or light chains are identified in the subendothelial space) and systemic lupus erythematosus (SLE; in which C3, IgG, IgM, IgA, and C1q all are present on immunofluorescence). In general, therapy for immune complex–mediated glomerulonephritis includes high-dose corticosteroids and cytoxan, particularly for the treatment of diffuse proliferative lupus nephritis. Plasmapheresis has not been demonstrated to be of benefit in this class of renal diseases, with the exception of cryoglubinemia.

8. **Crescentic glomerulonephritis, absent immunofluorescence.** When crescentic glomerulonephritis is accompanied by necrotizing capillary lesions, but no immunofluorescent staining of immune deposits are present on renal biopsy, the differential diagnosis of "pauci-immune" diseases are considered. These diseases are generally considered to be secondary to antibodies to lysosomal enzymes of neutrophils (ANCA). Two ANCAs have been identified. Antibody to myeloperoxidase (MPO) results in perinuclear staining of neutrophils (p-ANCA), whereas antibody to proteinase-3 results in cytoplasmic staining of neutrophils (c-ANCA). Both systemic diseases (such as Wegener's granulomatosis, associated primarily with c-ANCA; Churg-Strauss syndrome, associated with either c- or p-ANCA; and polyarteritis nodosa) and primary renal disease (microscopic polyangiitis) can cause a pauci-immune necrotizing glomerulonephritis. Whether systemic or primary, these diseases are managed with high-dose steroids and cyclophosphamide as the therapy of choice. Oral cytoxan seems to be more effective than i.v. pulse cytoxan therapy. Eighty percent of patients respond to therapy, and unlike anti-GBM disease, patients may ultimately cease dialysis requirements, although patients with a serum creatinine of greater than 6 mg per dL at presentation are less likely to respond than patients with lower serum creatinine at the time of presentation.

VI. **The thrombotic microangiopathies: glomerular injury that masquerades clinically as glomerulonephritis.** Systemic disorders that may produce a nephritic clinical presentation include a number of diseases that are not classical inflammatory diseases or vasculidities. Systemic diseases such as scleroderma, thrombotic thrombocytopenic purpura (TTP), hemolytic uremic syndrome (HUS), malignant hypertension, and antiphospholipid syndrome (APS) can present with hematuria, hypertension, and proteinuria (although usually less than 1 to 1.5 g per day), but all have renal histologic findings distinct from glomerulonephritis. Common histologic findings on renal biopsy in HUS, TTP, and APS include glomerular capillary thrombi and afferent arterioles, with fibrinoid necrosis from endothelial injury. Immunofluorescence is typically negative, with the exception of the presence of fibrinogen. Electron microscopy is also usually unremarkable, with no deposits noted. Additionally, malignant hypertension and scleroderma can cause subintimal proliferation within blood vessels, leading to an "onion-skin" appearance of arterioles. Microthrombi may be present as well.

The specific management of the thrombotic microangiopathies differs significantly from other disorders that lead to a nephritic clinical presentation, thus a correct diagnosis rather than empiric therapy is critical under circumstances of a nephritic presentation. For treatment of malignant hypertension and scleroderma renal crisis, blood pressure control is paramount. ACE inhibitor therapy is the first-line therapy in the setting of scleroderma, since data demonstrate improved patient survival and renal outcomes using this form of therapy. In HUS, the clinical picture is predominantly one of acute renal failure, thrombocytopenia, and hemolysis resulting either from verotoxin (from *E. coli* 0157:H7 gastrointestinal infection) or from secondary causes such as idiosyncratic reactions to medications such as cyclosporin and mitomycin, or postpartum HUS. Therapy is supportive, with dialysis and correction of electrolytes and treatment of anemia providing reasonable short-term outcomes. Ninety percent of cases of diarrhea-associated HUS will completely recover, whereas 5% die within the acute phase and 5% remain with severe renal and extrarenal complications. Long-term follow-up demonstrates a diminished GFR in 40% of these patients at 10 years. For TTP, the clinical picture is a pentad of neurologic signs, purpura, fever, thrombocytopenia, hemolysis, and renal failure that usually do not coexist but rather wax and wane. Secondary forms of TTP exist, and include pregnancy-associated, malignancy-associated, and HIV-associated causes. However, the most common cause of primary TTP is secondary to endothelial injury and the release of abnormally large von Willebrand factor (vWF) multimers into the microcirculation. This leads to platelet aggregation and thrombi formation. For this syndrome, fresh frozen plasma exchange or infusion is the most effective therapeutic intervention, although the mechanism for its beneficial effect remains under investigation. Plasma exchange should be continued until the platelet count has normalized and the serum lactate dehydrogenase (LDH) enzyme level returns to normal range. This typically takes 7 to 16 exchanges to induce remission, followed by a slow taper of therapy. Additional therapies that have been described include high dose prednisone therapy, vincristine, and other chemotherapeutic agents. The benefit of these therapies is not clear. In some patients in whom plasma exchange is only transiently effective, splenectomy may be necessary.

Suggested readings

Contreras G, Roth D, Pardo V, Striker LG, Schultz DR. Lupus nephritis: a clinical review for practicing nephrologists. *Clin Nephrol* 2002;57(2):95–107.

Falk RJ, Nachman, PH, Hogan SL, Jennette JC. ANCA glomerulonephritis and vasculitis: a Chapel Hill perspective. *Semin Nephrol* 2000;20(3):244–255.

Jennette JC, Falk RJ. Diagnosis and management of glomerular diseases. *Med Clin North Am* 1997;81(3):653–677.

Kuhn K, Haas-Wohrle A, Lutz-Vorderburgge A, Felten H. Treatment of severe nephrotic syndrome. *Kidney Int* 1998;64(S):S50–53.

Madaio MP, Harrington JT. The diagnosis of glomerular diseases, acute glomerulonephritis and the nephrotic syndrome. *Arch Intern Med* 2001;161(1):25–34.

Schnaper HW. Idiopathic focal segmental glomerulosclerosis. *Semin Nephrology* 2003; 23(2):183–193.

Tsai HM. Advances in the pathogenesis, diagnosis, and treatment of thrombotic thrombocytopenic purpura. *J Am Soc Nephrol* 2003;14(4):1072–1081.

The Patient with Acute Renal Failure

Sarah Faubel, Charles L. Edelstein, and Robert E. Cronin

I. **Definition and recognition of acute renal failure.** Acute renal failure (ARF) is a sudden decrease in the glomerular filtration rate (GFR) occurring over a period of hours to days and resulting in the failure of the kidney to excrete nitrogenous waste products and maintain fluid and electrolyte homeostasis. Clinically, it is recognized by an increase in serum creatinine and blood urea nitrogen (BUN). ARF may occur in patients with previously normal renal function or patients with chronic kidney disease (CKD); in either case, the clinical approach to find and treat the cause remains similar.

A. **Serum creatinine as a marker for ARF and GFR.** Normal serum creatinine is 0.6 to 1.2 mg per dL and is the most commonly used parameter to assess renal function. Practically, and in clinical trials of ARF, an increase in creatinine of 50% above baseline or an increase of 0.5 mg per dL are commonly used definitions of ARF. Unfortunately, the correlation between serum creatinine concentration and GFR may be confounded by several factors.

1. **Creatinine excretion is dependent on glomerular filtration and proximal tubular secretion.** Certain medications such as trimethoprim interfere with proximal tubular creatinine secretion and may cause a rise in serum creatinine without a fall in GFR (see Table 10-1). Once filtered, creatinine cannot be reabsorbed.

2. **Creatinine production is dependent on muscle mass.** Muscle mass declines with age and illness. Therefore, a serum creatinine of 1.2 mg per dL in an elderly, 40-kg patient with cancer and wasted muscles may represent a severely impaired GFR, whereas a serum creatinine of 1.2 mg per dL in a 100-kg weightlifter with large muscle mass may represent a normal GFR.

3. **Creatinine production and excretion must be in a steady state before creatinine may be used in any formula for the estimate of GFR.** The most commonly used formulae to estimate GFR are the Cockcroft-Gault, Modification of Diet in Renal Disease (MDRD), and the modified MDRD. In a steady state, the modified MDRD is as good as the MDRD for estimating renal function; both equations are superior to the Cockcroft-Gault formula. After an acute insult, it may take several days for creatinine excretion and production to reassume a steady state. For example, if a 60 kg, 30-year-old woman with a serum creatinine of 1.0 mg per dL suddenly loses all renal function, her serum creatinine may only rise to 2.0 mg per dL after one day. By the modified MDRD her GFR is 31 mL per minute; by Cockgroft-Gault it is 39 mL per minute, but it is actually zero.

a. **Cockcroft-Gault formula:**

$$GFR = \{[(140 - \text{Age [years]}) \times \text{Lean body weight in kg}] / [\text{serum Cr} \times 72]\} \times (0.85 \text{ if female})$$

b. **MDRD formula:**

$$GFR, \text{ in mL/min per } 1.73 \text{ m}^2 =$$
$$(170 \times (\text{Serum Cr}^{-0.999}) \times (\text{Age}^{-0.176}) \times (\text{BUN}^{-0.170})$$
$$\times (\text{Serum albumin}^{+0.318}) \times (0.762 \text{ if female}) \times (1.180 \text{ if black})$$

Table 10-1. Medications that affect serum creatinine without actually affecting renal function

Mechanism and medication
Increased serum creatinine by the inhibition of creatinine secretion
Trimethoprim
Cimetidine
Probenecid
Triamterene
Amiloride
Spironolactone
Increased serum creatinine due to interference with creatinine measurement
Ascorbic acid
Cephalosporins

Where serum Cr (creatinine) and BUN are in mg per dL; serum albumin is in g per dL

  c. Modified MDRD formula:

$$\text{GFR, in mL/min per } 1.73\,\text{m}^2 = 186.3 \times (\text{serum Cr}^{-1.154})$$
$$\times (\text{Age}^{-0.203}) \times (0.742 \text{ if female}) \times (1.21 \text{ if black})$$

  d. Creatinine clearance (CCr) gives a better estimate of GFR than the formulae listed above in the acute setting. This requires a 24-hour urine collection. Normal ranges for CCr are 120 ± 25 mL per minute for men and 95 ± 20 mL per min for women.

$$\text{CCr} = [\text{Urine creatinine (mg/dL)} \times \text{Urine volume (mL/24 hr)}] /$$
$$[\text{Serum Cr (mg/dL)} \times 1{,}440 \text{ min}]$$

B. BUN as a marker for ARF and GFR. Normal BUN is 8 to 18 mg per dL. An increase in BUN typically accompanies a rise in serum creatinine in the setting of ARF. Urea is filtered, but not secreted. Increased reabsorption of urea by the proximal tubule and AVP-sensitive urea transporters in the collecting duct occurs in states of volume depletion. In this setting, BUN can rise without a rise in creatinine, resulting in a BUN to serum creatinine ratio that is greater than 20 (see section IV.H.3).

BUN levels are affected by multiple factors not related to GFR. Because BUN production is related to protein metabolism, an increase in BUN without a decline in GFR may occur with hypercatabolic states, protein loading, and steroid administration. Conversely, a low BUN may be present in the setting of reduced GFR in patients who are on a low-protein diet, are severely malnourished, or have severe liver disease.

C. Distinguishing acute from chronic renal failure. Distinguishing acute from chronic renal failure (CRF) may be challenging. Laboratory findings such as hyperphosphatemia, hypoalbuminemia, and hyperkalemia are unreliable factors to distinguish acute from chronic renal failure and may be present in either case. Symptoms such as nausea, vomiting, and malaise may also occur in acute or chronic renal failure. Potential methods to distinguish between the two include:

  1. Old records. The most reliable way to distinguish acute from chronic renal failure is an evaluation of old records. Increased BUN or serum creatinine documented months earlier and/or a history of kidney disease suggest that the renal failure is chronic.

2. **Small kidneys (less than 10 cm) on renal ultrasound.** Normal-sized kidneys may be present in some patients with chronic kidney disease, such as diabetic nephropathy, amyloidosis, autosomal dominant polycystic kidney disease, rapidly progressive glomerulonephritis, or malignant hypertension.

3. **Anemia.** Normochromic normocytic anemia is common in patients with CKD and a GFR less than 30 mL per min; in patients with a GFR of 30 to 44 mL per minute, only about 20% of patients have anemia. Therefore, with a GFR of 30 mL or below, the absence of anemia suggests that renal failure is acute. In some etiologies of CKD (e.g., autosomal dominant polycystic kidney disease), anemia may be absent.

D. **Urine output in ARF.** ARF is typically described as either oliguric or non-oliguric. **Oliguria** is defined as a urine output of less than 400 mL per day; 400 mL is the minimum amount of urine that a person in a normal metabolic state must excrete to get rid of the daily solute production. For example, a person with a daily solute production of 500 mOsm who concentrates urine to a maximum of 1,200 mOsm per L, would need to pass 400 mL of urine per day to excrete the daily solute production.

Anuria is defined as a lack of urine obtained from a bladder catheter; it has a short list of potential causes. It is most often caused by complete bilateral urinary tract obstruction and shock. Less common causes are the hemolytic-uremic syndrome and rapidly progressive glomerulonephritis, particularly anti-GBM antibody disease; bilateral renal arterial or venous occlusion can also cause anuria.

II. **Classifications of ARF: definitions and causes.** ARF is classified as prerenal, intrinsic renal, and postrenal.

A. **Prerenal ARF (Fig. 10-1).** Prerenal ARF is a fall in the GFR due to reduced renal perfusion in which no structural or cellular damage to the kidney has occurred. Urine sediment is typically bland. Essential to this diagnosis is

Figure 10-1. Causes of Prerenal ARF. Prerenal ARF may be secondary to true intravascular volume depletion or arterial underfilling from a decrease in cardiac output or arterial vasodilatation. The extracellular fluid volume (ECF) comprises the intravascular and the interstitial body water compartments.

that renal function returns to normal within 24 to 72 hours of correction of the hypoperfused state. Prerenal ARF occurs in the following situations:

1. **Total intravascular volume depletion.** This condition can occur in a number of settings where intravascular volume is reduced and may be secondary to
   a. Hemorrhage
   b. Renal fluid loss
      Excessive diuresis (e.g., diuretics)
      Osmotic diuresis (e.g., glucosuria)
      Primary adrenal insufficiency (i.e, hypoaldosteronism)
      Salt-wasting nephritis
      Diabetes insipidus
   c. Gastrointestinal fluid loss
      Vomiting
      Diarrhea
      Nasogastric tube drainage
   d. Skin fluid loss
      Burns
      Excessive sweating
      Hyperthermia
   e. Third-space fluid loss
      Peritonitis
      Pancreatitis
      Systemic inflammatory response syndrome (SIRS)
      Profound hypoalbuminemia

2. **Effective volume depletion from arterial underfilling.** Arterial underfilling is a state in which intravascular volume is actually normal (or even increased) but circulatory factors are inadequate to maintain renal perfusion pressure. Underfilling may be due to either a decrease in cardiac output or arterial vasodilatation and may occur in a number of clinical settings:
   a. Reduced cardiac output
      Congestive heart failure
      Cardiogenic shock (e.g., acute myocardial infarction)
      Pericardial effusion with tamponade
      Massive pulmonary embolism
   b. Peripheral vasodilation
      Sepsis
      Antihypertensive medications
      Anaphylaxis
      Anesthesia
      Cirrhosis and other liver diseases

3. **Intrarenal hemodynamic changes**
   a. Glomerular afferent arteriole vasoconstriction (preglomerular effect)
      Nonsteroidal anti-inflammatory drugs (NSAIDs) (prostaglandin inhibition)
      Cyclo-oxygenase 2 inhibitors (Cox 2 inhibitors) (prostaglandin inhibition)
      Cyclosporine
      Tacrolimus
      Radiocontrast dye
      Hypercalcemia
   b. Glomerular efferent arteriole vasodilitation (postglomerular effect)
      Angiotensin converting enzyme (ACE) inhibitors
      Angiotensin II receptor blockers (ARBs)

B. **Postrenal ARF.** Postrenal ARF is caused by the acute obstruction of the flow of urine. Urinary obstruction of both ureters, the bladder, or the urethra may cause postrenal ARF. Patients most at risk for postrenal ARF are elderly men, in whom prostatic hypertrophy or prostatic cancer may lead to complete or partial obstruction of urine flow. In women, complete urinary tract obstruction is relatively uncommon in the absence of pelvic surgery, pelvic malignancy, or previous pelvic irradiation. The causes of postrenal ARF include:

1. **Bilateral ureteral obstruction or unilateral obstruction in a solitary kidney (upper urinary tract obstruction)**
   a. Intraureteral
      Stones
      Blood clots
      Pyogenic debris or sloughed papillae
      Edema following retrograde pyelography
      Transitional cell carcinoma
   b. Extraureteral
      Pelvic or abdominal malignancy
      Retroperitoneal fibrosis
      Accidental ureteral ligation or trauma during pelvic surgery
   c. Bladder neck/urethral obstruction (lower urinary tract obstruction)
      Prostatic hypertrophy
      Prostatic and bladder carcinoma
      Autonomic neuropathy or anticholinergic agents causing urinary retention
      Urethral stricture
      Bladder stones
      Fungal infection (e.g., fungus balls)
      Blood clots
C. **Intrarenal or intrinsic ARF.** In contrast to prerenal and postrenal ARF, the disorders listed here represent problems within the kidney itself. These problems may be vascular, glomerular, interstitial, or tubular. The diseases may be primary renal or part of a systemic disease. The course of ARF in these situations cannot be changed by manipulating factors outside the kidney (e.g., performing volume repletion, improving cardiac function, correcting hypotension, or removing obstruction).
   1. **Vascular.** Vascular disorders causing ARF are classified based on the size of the vessels involved.
      a. Large- and medium-sized vessels
         Renal artery thrombosis or embolism
         Operative arterial cross-clamping
         Bilateral renal vein thrombosis
         Polyarteritis nodosa
      b. Small vessels
         Atheroembolic disease
         Thrombotic microangiopathies
            Hemolytic-uremic syndrome (HUS)
            Thrombotic thrombocytopenic purpura (TTP)
            Scleroderma renal crisis
            Malignant hypertension
         Thrombotic microangiopathies of pregnancy
            Hemolysis, elevated liver enzymes, and low platelets (HELLP) syndrome
         Postpartum ARF
   2. **Glomerular.** Glomerular diseases are typically categorized based on urine findings as either nephrotic or nephritic.
      a. **Nephrotic** glomerular disorders are characterized by large proteinuria (greater than 3 grams in 24 hours) and minimal hematuria. Nephrotic glomerular disorders are uncommonly associated with ARF, but may occur in minimal-change disease or focal segmental glomerulosclerosis (FSGS), particularly collapsing FSGS.
      b. **Nephritic** glomerular disorders (glomerulonephritis) are characterized by hematuria and proteinuria (typically 1 to 2 grams in 24 hours).

Patients with known glomerulonephritis may develop ARF; alternatively, glomerulonephritis may commonly present as ARF. Rapidly progressive (crescentic) glomerulonephritis (RPGN) should be suspected in a patient with glomerulonephritis who has a doubling of serum creatinine within a 3-month period. RPGN is caused by injury to the glomerular capillary wall, which results in subsequent inflammation, fibrosis, and crescent formation. Urgency is required to make the diagnosis of RPGN, because crescent formation can rapidly destroy the glomeruli; response to therapy is directly correlated with the percent of glomeruli having crescents. Because the diagnosis is typically made by renal biopsy, the causes of glomerulonephritis and RPGN are classified according to immunofluorescence staining on renal biopsy.

(1) **Diseases with linear (antiglomerular basement membrane) immune complex deposition**

Goodpasture's syndrome (renal and pulmonary complications are present)

Renal-limited Goodpasture's syndrome

(2) **Diseases with granular immune complex deposition**

Acute postinfectious glomerulonephritis

Lupus nephritis

Infective endocarditis

Immunoglobulin A (IgA) glomerulonephritis

Henoch-Schönlein purpura

Membranoproliferative glomerulonephritis

Cryoglobulinemia

(3) **Diseases with no immune deposits (pauci-immune)**

Wegener's granulomatosis

Microscopic polyangiitis

Churg-Strauss syndrome (CSS)

Idiopathic crescentic glomerulonephritis

3. **Interstitium.** ARF from an interstitial cause is known as **acute interstitial nephritis (AIN).** The primary histologic lesion of AIN is marked edema of the interstitial space with a focal or diffuse infiltration of the renal interstitium with inflammatory cells. AIN (also called acute tubulointerstitial nephritis) is most commonly due to drug hypersensitivity, but may also be a consequence of infections or systemic disease [e.g., systemic lupus erythematosus (SLE)].

a. **Drug-induced AIN.** Over 100 drugs have been implicated in drug-induced AIN. Some of the drugs which are most commonly associated with acute interstitial nephritis are:

Antibiotics (e.g., methicillin, cephalosporins, rifampicin, sulfonamides, erythromycin, and ciprofloxacin)

Diuretics (e.g., furosemide, thiazides, chlorthalidone)

NSAIDs

Anticonvulsant drugs (e.g., phenytoin, carbamazepine)

Allopurinol

b. **Infection-associated AIN**

Bacterial (e.g., staphococcus, streptococcus)

Viral (e.g., cytomegalovirus, Epstein-Barr virus)

Tuberculosis

4. **Tubular.** Acute tubular necrosis (ATN) is characterized by an abrupt decrease in the GFR due to proximal tubular dysfunction caused by ischemia (50% of cases) and nephrotoxins (35% of cases). Although this type of renal injury has long been designated ATN, in many cases little true necrosis of tubular cells is present on histologic examination. Rather, the tubules demonstrate morphologic changes of sublethal injury (e.g., swelling, vacuolization, loss of brush border, apical blebbing, and loss of basolateral infoldings). Loss of viable tubular epithelial cells

into the urine also occurs. The presence of tubular dysfunction, rather than necrosis, may explain the abrupt recovery of renal function that is seen in some patients with ATN.

Ischemic ATN is a consequence of reduced blood flow to the kidneys, which results from a decreased total blood volume or arterial underfilling with a redistribution of blood away from the kidney. Ischemic ATN is seen most commonly after septic or hemorrhagic shock. **Nephrotoxic ATN** is most commonly caused by aminoglycoside antibiotics and radiocontrast dye.

Causes of ATN include:

a. Renal ischemia

Shock
Hemorrhage
Trauma
Gram-negative sepsis
Pancreatitis

b. Nephrotoxic drugs

Aminoglycoside antibiotics
Amphotericin B
Pentamidine
Foscarnet
Acyclovir
Indinavir
Antineoplastics (e.g., cisplatin)
Hypotension from any cause
Radiocontrast dye
Organic solvents (e.g., carbon tetrachloride)
Ethylene glycol (antifreeze)
Anesthetics (enflurane)

c. Endogenous toxins

Myoglobin (e.g., rhabdomyolysis)
Hemoglobin (e.g., incompatible blood transfusion, acute falciparum malaria)
Uric acid (e.g., acute uric acid nephropathy)

III. Epidemiology of ARF. See Table 10-2.

A. Community-acquired ARF. ARF is present on admission in about 1% of hospitalized patients. Half of cases are in patients with CKD. The most common causes of community-acquired ARF include prerenal (70%) and postrenal (17%). The overall mortality of patients presenting with ARF is 15%.

B. Hospital-acquired acute renal failure. The development of ARF in hospitalized patients is common and carries with it a significant independent risk of mortality. In patients with normal renal function, the incidence of hospital-acquired ARF is approximately 5%; in patients with CKD, it is approximately 16%. Overall, approximately 40% of ARF in hospitalized patients is due to ATN; medications account for about 15%; radiocontrast dye, 10%, and AIDS-associated, 5%.

In ARF developing outside the intensive care unit (ICU), prerenal accounts for 28% of ARF, whereas ATN accounts for 38% of ARF. If ARF develops in the ICU, prerenal accounts for 18% of ARF and ATN accounts for 76%. ATN in the ICU is typically multifactorial and is frequently part of multisystem organ failure syndrome.

C. Prevention of ARF. Numerous factors predispose hospitalized patients to the development of ARF: volume depletion, drugs which affect renal blood flow (e.g., NSAIDs and Cox-2 inhibitors), and the use of nephrotoxic medications and contrast dye.

Although data are limited on treatments to prevent ARF, it is prudent to carefully follow volume status and maintain adequate hydration, discontinue (when possible) medications that affect renal blood flow; choose

Table 10-2. Characteristics of ARF in regard to the location of its development

Community acquired acute renal failure

History/symptoms	Predisposing factor(s)	Type of ARF
Acute systemic illness (e.g., viral influenza, gastroenteritis)	Volume depletion	Prerenal or ATN
Streptococcal pharyngitis or pyoderma (vesicular skin lesions, typically located on the extremities, which become pustular and then crust)	Immune complex deposition in the glomeruli	Acute poststreptococcal glomerulonephritis
Trauma, crush injury, prolonged immobilization, "found down"	Extensive muscle damage and tissue breakdown	Rhabdomyolysis
Urinary tract symptoms such as difficulty voiding, incontinence, dribbling	Obstruction to urine flow or neurogenic bladder	Postrenal
Fever and/or rash in a patient recently prescribed a new medication	NSAIDS, antibiotics, and diuretics are frequently prescribed on an outpatient basis	Allergic interstitial nephritis
Accidental or intentional overdose of a nephrotoxin (altered mental status may be a frequent accompaniment)	Heavy metal compounds, solvents, ethylene glycol, salicylates, and acetaminophen	ATN

Acute renal failure occurring inside the hospital

History/symptoms	Predisposing factor(s)	Type of ARF
Excessive fluid loss from aggressive diuresis, nasogastric suction, surgical drains, diarrhea, etc.	Volume depletion	Prerenal or ATN
Surgery with or without concomitant volume depletion	Anesthesia causes renal vasoconstriction, which reduces renal blood flow	Prerenal or ATN
Radiologic (contrast CT) or other procedures (e.g., coronary angiography)	Intravenous contrast dye	ATN
Sepsis	Infection, volume depletion, hypotension, nephrotoxic antibiotics (e.g., aminoglycosides)	ATN

alternate nonradiocontrast imaging techniques [e.g, magnetic resonance imaging (MRI) with gadolinium]; and use non-nephrotoxic antibiotics.

D. Morbidity and mortality associated with ARF. It is commonly thought that ARF from ATN is a completely reversible disorder. Recent data suggest that of patients who develop ARF in the ICU and require dialysis, up to 30% will require maintenance dialysis after discharge from the hospital.

Table 10-3. Mortality of ARF

Type of ARF	Mortality
ARF in the ICU associated with respiratory failure and the requirement of dialysis	>90%
ARF in the ICU	72%
ARF in hospitalized patients, not in the ICU	32%
ARF following i.v. contrast	34% (compared to 7% in controls) Adjusted odds ratio of death: 5.5
ARF following cardiac surgery	64% (compared to 4.3% in controls) Adjusted odds ratio of death: 7.9
ARF following administration of amphotericin B	Adjusted odds ratio of death: 6.6

Another widely held belief is that patients die with ARF, not from ARF. Numerous well-controlled studies have challenged this notion and found that after adjusting for comorbidities, the development of ARF in hospitalized patients is an independent and significant predictor of in-hospital mortality (Table 10-3).

IV. **Evaluation of the patient with ARF.** A stepwise evaluation approach to the patient with ARF is recommended. A comprehensive **history** and thorough **physical examination** suggest the diagnosis in the majority of patients.

Whether the patient is seen for the first time in the office, emergency room, hospital, or ICU, careful tabulation and recording of data are the first steps in determining the diagnosis. Vital signs, daily weights, records of intake and output, past and current laboratory data, and the fluid and medication list should be recorded on a flow sheet and included in the patient's chart. When the patient has been hospitalized for several days or weeks with a complicated course before developing ARF, a carefully prepared flow sheet may often be the only way to comprehend the problem and guide the selection of proper therapy.

Urinalysis by dipstick and the evaluation of **urine sediment** by microscopy should always be performed in patients with ARF. **Urine chemistries** that may be helpful in the diagnosis of ARF include sodium, creatinine, osmolality, and protein content.

Clinical features of the common causes of ARF are described in the following sections.

A. **Prerenal ARF.** Prerenal ARF may occur in patients who are clinically hypovolemic (total intravascular volume depletion) or hypervolemic (arterial underfilling).

1. **History.** The following history is suggestive of prerenal ARF from true volume depletion or hypovolemia: thirst, decreased fluid intake, fever, nausea, vomiting, diarrhea, burns, peritonitis, and pancreatitis. Prerenal ARF from arterial underfilling occurs most commonly in patients with congestive heart failure (CHF) or liver disease. Features of the history that are suggestive of CHF include: recent myocardial infarction, orthopnea, paroxysmal nocturnal dyspnea, or dyspnea on exertion. Features suggesting liver disease and cirrhosis include a history of alcohol abuse or hepatitis. A complete documentation of medications (prescribed and over-the-counter) is important in the evaluation of prerenal ARF. Medications that affect intrarenal hemodynamics include cyclosporine, tacrolimus, NSAIDs, Cox-2 inhibitors, ACE inhibitors, and ARBs.

2. **Physical examination.** Assessment of volume status and the adequacy of the extracellular fluid volume (ECF) are critical to the diagnosis of prerenal ARF.

   a. **Physical findings that suggest a reduction in intravascular volume** include:

Absence of axillary sweat

A recent reduction in body weight

Orthostatic hypotension. Defined as a fall in systolic blood pressure of more than 20 mm Hg or a rise in pulse rate of more than 10 beats per minute after standing

Tachycardia

Dry mucus membranes

"Tenting" of upper thorax skin when pinched between the fingers

Jugular venous pressure not visible

  b. **Physical examination findings generally found in arterial underfilling states with an excess of ECF** include:

Elevated jugular venous pressure

Ascites

Lower extremity pitting edema

Anasarca

CHF in particular may be identified by:

Pulmonary crackles

S3 gallop

Liver failure may be identified by:

Jaundice

Decreased liver size

Palmar erythema

Spider angiomas

3. **Urinary findings.** Regardless of the cause of prerenal ARF (hypovolemic, arterial underfilling, or medication-induced) the urine dipstick, sediment, and chemistries will be the same. (See Table 10-4 for a comparison of urinary findings in various types of ARF.)

  a. The urine **dipstick** should be normal with negative protein, heme, leukocyte esterase, and nitrate. The specific gravity is increased (greater than 1.020).

  b. The **urine sediment** is bland (no cells or casts).

  c. **Urine chemistry and indices.** Frequently it is difficult to distinguish between prerenal ARF and other forms of renal disease, particularly ATN. Laboratory tests and indices characteristic of prerenal ARF versus other causes of ARF are summarized in Table 10-5. A discussion of the pathophysiologic basis of these tests is in section **IV-G.3.**

4. **Specific disorders of prerenal ARF**

  a. **Hepatorenal syndrome (HRS)** occurs in patients with severe liver failure. It is characterized by peripheral vasodilatation (low systemic vascular resistance) accompanied by intense renal vasoconstriction that causes renal insufficiency. Two forms of HRS are recognized. **Type 1 HRS** is the more severe form and is characterized by an abrupt (within 2 weeks) decline of renal function, defined as a doubling of serum creatinine to greater than 2.5 or a 50% reduction in creatinine clearance to less than 20 mL per minute. Without liver transplantation, the mortality of this condition is greater than 90% at 3 months. **Type II HRS** is characterized by slowly progressing renal insufficiency in a patient with refractory ascites; it has a much better prognosis. Patients with type II HRS may convert to type I in the setting of certain insults such as the development of infections (e.g., spontaneous bacterial peritonitis) or the use of NSAIDs. HRS is typical of other forms of prerenal azotemia, and the kidney functions normally if transplanted into a person with a normal liver. The only permanent cure for HRS is liver transplantation.

  As agreed upon by the International Ascites Club, the **diagnostic criteria for HRS** are divided into major and additional criteria. To diagnose HRS, each of the major criteria must be present. The additional criteria provide supporting evidence for the diagnosis, but are not required to make the diagnosis.

Table 10-4. Urinary findings in various causes of ARF

Dipstick	Prerenal[a]	Post renal[b]	Small vessel vascular	Nephrotic glomerular	Nephritic glomerular	AIN	ATN[c]
Leukocyte esterase	(−)	(−)	(−)	(−)	(−)	(+)	(−)
Heme	(−)	(−)	(+)	(−) or trace	(+)	(+)	(−)
Protein	(−)	(−)	(+)	(+)	(+)	(+)	(−) or trace
Specific gravity	>1.020	1.010	variable	variable	variable	1.010	1.010
Microscopy							
RBCs	(−)	(−)	(+)	(−) or few	(+)	(+)	(−)
WBCs	(−)	(−)	(−)	(−)	(−)	(+)	(−)
RBC casts	(−)	(−)	(+)	(−)	(+)	(−)	(−)
WBC casts	(−)	(−)	(−)	(−)	(−)	(+)	(−)
Granular casts	(−)	(−)	(−)	(−)	(−)	(−)	(+)
Renal tubular epithelial cells	(−)	(−)	(−)	(−)	(−)	(−)	(+)
Tests							
Osmolality (mOsm/L)	>500	≤350	variable	variable	variable	≤350	≤350
Protein (g/day)	(−)	(−)	1–2	>3	1–2	1–2	≤1

[a] Although classically associated with a bland urinary sediment, a few granular casts may occasionally be present.
[b] If a superimposed infection is present due to urine stasis, the leukocyte esterase, heme, protein, RBCs, and WBCs may be positive.
[c] If ATN is secondary to rhabdomyolysis, heme will be positive on dipstick and RBCs will be absent on microscopy.

Table 10-5. Urinary diagnostic indices

Index	Prerenal ARF	Acute tubular necrosis
Urine sodium (UNa), mEq/L	<20	>40
Urine osmolality, mOsm/kg H_2O	>500	<350
Urine creatinine (UCr) to plasma creatinine (PCr)	>40	<20
Serum BUN/serum creatinine	>20	≤10
Fractional excretion of sodium (FENa): FENa = [(Una/Pna)/(Ucr/Pcr)] × 100	<1	>1
Fractional excretion of urea (FeUN): FeUn = [(Uun/Pun)/(Ucr/Pcr)] × 100	<35	>50

UNa, urine sodium (mEq/L); PNa, plasma sodium (mEq/L); Ucr, urine creatinine (mg/dL); Pcr, plasma creatinine (mg/dL); Uun, urine urea (mg/dL); Pun, BUN (mg/dL).

Major criteria

Severe liver failure (acute or chronic)

Serum creatinine greater than 1.5 mg per dL or 24 hour creatinine clearance less than 40 mL per minute

Absence of another cause of renal failure (e.g., proteinuria less than 500 mg per dL; no obstruction on renal ultrasound)

Absence of ongoing infection or fluid loss

Absence of a sustained improvement in renal function following diuretic withdrawal and administration of 1.5 liters of isotonic saline

Additional criteria

Oliguria

Urine sodium less than 10 mEq per L

Urine osmolality greater than plasma osmolality

Urine RBCs less than 50 per high powered field

Serum sodium less than 130 mEq per L

b. **Vasomotor ARF due to NSAIDs.** A history of NSAID use in all patients with ARF should be aggressively sought. Under euvolemic conditions with normal kidney, liver, and cardiac function, the administration of NSAIDs does not cause an increase in serum creatinine. In the presence of clinical conditions with increased renal vasoconstrictor activity (e.g., CHF, cirrhosis, nephrotic syndrome, hypertension, sepsis, volume depletion, anesthesia), NSAIDs can cause ARF. Patients with chronic renal insufficiency (e.g., diabetic nephropathy) are also at risk of acute vasomotor decline in renal function with NSAIDs. Typical clinical features include the presence of risk factors, decreased urinary output, bland urine sediment, low (less than 1%) fractional excretion of sodium, and prompt improvement in renal function after discontinuation of NSAIDs. NSAIDs may also cause AIN and ATN.

c. **Cyclosporine and tacrolimus** may cause a dose-dependent, hemodynamically mediated ARF in solid-organ and bone marrow transplant patients. A large increase in renal vascular resistance occurs. The loss of renal function is reversible when the dosage of the drug is reduced. The urine sediment is bland, and ATN is not typically present.

d. **ACE inhibitors** and ARBs are widely used for the treatment of hypertension, CHF, and diabetic nephropathy. ARF may occur in conditions where angiotensin plays a crucial protective role in maintaining GFR by constricting the glomerular efferent arteriole, such as volume depletion, bilateral renal artery stenosis, autosomal dominant polycystic kidney disease, cardiac failure, cirrhosis, and diabetic nephropathy. Diuretic-induced sodium depletion and underlying chronic renal insufficiency are other major predisposing factors. ARF is usually asymptomatic, nonoliguric, and associated with hyperkalemia. ARF is reversible in most cases after discontinuation of the ACE inhibitor or ARB. ARF can usually be managed in the outpatient setting by discontinuation of the ACE inhibitor and discontinuation of diuretics if present. An increase in BUN and serum creatinine in a patient on an ACE inhibitor or ARB should raise the possibility of renal artery stenosis.

B. Postrenal ARF

1. **History.** Symptoms that suggest urinary tract obstruction are anuria or intermittent anuria and polyuria, prostatic symptoms (urinary frequency and urgency, dysuria, straining upon urination), pelvic malignancy on previous radiotherapy, and recurrent renal stones. Patients may complain of pain over a distended bladder; severe pain (renal colic) may be present if obstruction is due to renal calculi. Patients with diabetes mellitus, sickle cell anemia, and analgesic nephropathy are predisposed to papillary necrosis that causes obstruction.

2. **Physical examination.** The physical examination is important in diagnosing postrenal ARF, especially in the unconscious patient or in the confused patient in whom otherwise unexplained agitation may be the only clue to acute urinary retention. Careful abdominal examination may uncover a distended, tender bladder or bilaterally hydronephrotic kidneys. A digital examination of the prostate should be performed routinely in any male patient with ARF, and pelvic masses should be sought in female patients through a bimanual pelvic examination. In any patient in whom lower tract obstruction is suspected as the cause of acute ARF, a sterile in-and-out diagnostic postvoid bladder catheterization should be performed as a routine part of the physical examination. The postvoid residual urine volume should be less than 50 mL. The urine volume should be recorded and the specimen saved for studies.

3. **Urine findings.** The typical urinalysis and sediment finding in postrenal ARF compared to other causes of ARF is presented in Table 10-4.

   a. **Urinalysis.** The urine dipstick should be normal with negative protein, heme, leukocyte esterase, and nitrate. The specific gravity is typically isosmotic (1.010). Heme test for red blood cells (RBCs) may be positive if obstruction is due to renal calculi. A secondary infection may be present due to urine stasis; in this setting the dipstick may be positive for leukocyte esterase, nitrate, heme, and trace protein.

   b. **Urine sediment** is typically bland without cells or casts. As noted, hematuria may be present if obstruction is due to renal calculi. Prostatitis and some cases of benign prostatic hypertrophy may also be associated with hematuria. In the setting of a secondary urinary tract infection (UTI), the sediment may contain white blood cells, red blood cells, and/or bacteria.

4. **Radiologic tests.** Renal ultrasound is sufficient to diagnose urinary obstruction in the majority of patients. Because of the risk of i.v. contrast dye, intravenous pyelogram (IVP) should be avoided.

   a. **Renal ultrasound** is the radiologic test of choice to evaluate for obstruction, characterized by dilatation of the urinary tract (hydronephrosis). The absence of hydronephrosis virtually excludes important urinary tract obstruction; hydronephrosis may be absent, however, in the following settings: (a) early obstruction (before the urinary tract has been able to dilate); and (b) obstruction due to the encasement of the urinary system by retroperitoneal fibrosis or tumor.

   Hydronephrosis that is not functionally significant may occur in pregnancy and in people with anatomic variants of the collecting system. If the functional importance of hydronephrosis is in doubt, a furosemide isotope renogram can evaluate the functional significance of the obstruction.

b. **Isotope renography** is performed by the intravenous injection of a radionucleotide and furosemide. Furosemide increases urinary flow and normally causes a rapid washout of the radionucleotide. Persistence of the isotope in the renal parenchyma suggests obstruction. Poor renal function limits the usefulness of this test because the diuretic response may be blunted, thus making interpretation of the test difficult.

c. **Noncontrast computed tomography (CT)** of the kidneys, ureters, and abdomen is often done following renal ultrasound to identify the cause and location of urinary obstruction.

d. **Cystoscopy and retrograde pyelography.** In instances of ARF with a high clinical suspicion of urinary tract obstruction (e.g., calculi, pyogenic debris, blood clots, bladder cancer), cystoscopy and retrograde or anterograde pyelography should be performed, even if ultrasonography is negative for obstruction.

C. **Intrinsic renal disease–large vessel disease**

1. **History.** Renal artery thrombosis or embolism, or bilateral renal vein thrombosis may present with flank pain. Predisposing disorders such as membranous nephropathy or antiphospholipid antibody syndrome may be present.

2. **Urine findings.**

a. **Urinalysis.** The urine dipstick is positive for heme.

b. **Urine sediment.** Red blood cells.

3. **Labs and radiology.** An elevated serum LDH may be present. Doppler ultrasound may be used to assess renal blood flow and to evaluate for renal vein thrombosis. CT is useful for detecting clots in the renal vein or inferior vena cava. Angiography may be required in emergent cases (e.g., acute anuria due to acute renal embolization).

D. **Intrinsic renal disease–small vessel disease.** Intrinsic renal disease due to small vessel disease is caused by either atheroembolic disease or thrombotic microangiopathy. The clinical and laboratory features of these disorders are as follows:

1. **Atheroembolic disease** is caused by the detachment of atheromatous plaques from the intimal surface of large vessels. These plaques travel distally and occlude small arteries or large arterioles of the kidney. Showers of cholesterol crystals or microemboli from the surface of ulcerated plaques may also occur, traveling distally to occlude small arterioles throughout the body (e.g., kidney, gut, or skin). The presentation and clinical findings of atheroembolic disease can be confused with those of polyarteritis nodosa, allergic vasculitis, subacute bacterial endocarditis, or left atrial myxoma.

The usual course is progressive renal insufficiency. However, milder forms of renal failure with some recovery of function have been described. No treatment is known. Prevention of the disease involves avoiding unnecessary invasive procedures (e.g., renal arteriogram in patients with clinical evidence of widespread atherosclerosis).

a. **History.** A history of ARF occurring after cardiovascular surgery, angiography, or administration of i.v. thrombolytics should raise a suspicion of atheroembolic disease as the cause of ARF, particularly in a patient with known atherosclerosis. Occasionally, the disease occurs spontaneously.

b. **Physical examination.** Skin manifestations of cholesterol emboli include discrete peripheral necrotic areas, blue-toe syndrome, and livido reticularis. Small cholesterol emboli to the gut and pancreas may cause abdominal pain.

c. **Laboratory investigation** may reveal an increased erythrocyte sedimentation rate, eosinophilia, and hypocomplementemia (C3 is reduced while C4 remains normal). Biopsy of the skin, muscle, or kidney reveals intravascular cholesterol crystals.

   d. Urinary evaluation

      (1) Urinalysis. Dipstick is frequently negative although heme and protein or both may be positive. Specific gravity is variable.

      (2) Urine sediment. Sediment is often bland, although red blood cells, granular casts, red blood cell casts, or all may be present.

      (3) Urine tests. Proteinuria is typically less than 1 g in 24 hours.

2. Thrombotic microangiopathies are characterized by a microangiopathic hemolytic anemia, thrombocytopenia, and variable renal and neurologic manifestations. These disorders begin with endothelial injury followed by secondary platelet thrombi formation in renal arterioles; renal cortical necrosis may result from the arterial lesions. The primary site of injury is the glomerulus or the vascular supply of the glomerulus; the proximal tubule and interstitium are relatively uninvolved.

   a. History and physical examination. HUS-TTP should be suspected in patients with anemia, ARF, thrombocytopenia, and neurologic signs such as confusion and seizures. Malignant hypertension causing a thrombotic microangiopathy is characterized by high blood pressure associated with papilledema and/or retinal hemorrhages; other organ involvement may manifest as chest pain, shortness of breath from pulmonary edema, and confusion from brain involvement. Scleroderma renal crisis should be considered in patients with scleroderma and an abrupt rise in serum creatinine associated with hypertension.

   b. Laboratory findings. Peripheral blood smear demonstrates increased red blood cell fragmentation (schistocytes) and thrombocytopenia. Indices of hemolysis (e.g., LDH) are elevated.

   c. Urine findings

      (1) On dipstick. Variable specific gravity; heme positive, protein positive, or both.

      (2) Urine sediment is characterized by granular casts, red blood cell casts, or both.

E. Intrinsic renal disease–glomerular disease from a nephrotic cause. Nephrotic glomerular disorders are characterized by a urine protein excretion of greater than 3 g in 24 hours. Nephrotic glomerular disorders are uncommonly associated with ARF, but it may occur in patients with minimal-change disease (especially in the elderly) and FSGS (especially from collapsing FSGS).

1. History and physical examination. Clinical symptoms and signs characteristic of a nephrotic disorder include pitting peripheral edema, hypertension, periorbital edema, and anasarca.

2. Laboratory findings. Typically hypoalbuminemia and hypercholesterolemia are present.

3. Urine findings. In cases of minimal-change-induced ARF, urine dipstick and sediment may also include features of ATN.

   a. Dipstick is strongly positive for protein. Heme is negative or trace.

   b. Urine sediment is typically bland; possibly with few RBCs. Oval fat bodies reflecting lipiduria may be present.

   c. Urine tests show proteinuria greater than 3 g in 24 hours.

F. Intrinsic renal disease–glomerular disease from a nephritic cause. Nephritic glomerular disorders (glomerulonephritis) frequently cause ARF. Nephritic glomerular disorders are characterized by hematuria and proteinuria (typically 1 to 2 g in 24 hours). RPGN should be suspected in a patient with glomerulonephritis who has a doubling of serum creatinine within a 3-month period.

1. History and physical examination. Clinical symptoms and signs that suggest that the glomerulonephritis is part of a systemic disease include palpable purpura, skin rash, arthralgias, arthritis, fever, cardiac murmurs, sinusitis, hemoptysis, abdominal pain, and acute neuropathy. Hemoptysis is an ominous symptom in an ARF patient and may indicate a life-threatening vasculitis, such as Goodpasture's syndrome or Wegener's granulomatosis.

2. **Urine findings.** Glomerulonephritis is characterized by hematuria and proteinuria. The identification of RBC casts confirms the presence of glomerular disease.

3. **Laboratory findings. Antineutrophil cytoplasmic antibodies** (ANCA) are helpful in determining the cause of glomerulonephritis. ANCA staining by immunofluorescence is either cytoplasmic (c-ANCA) or perinuclear (p-ANCA). Although c-ANCA and p-ANCA are sensitive screening tests, numerous conditions other than vasculitis and glomerulonephritis may result in c-ANCA or p-ANCA positivity. Therefore, all positive results must be confirmed with enzyme-linked immunosorbent assay (ELISA) tests for the more specific antigen targets proteinase 3 (PR3) and myeloperoxidase (MPO). The PR3-ANCA antibody is typically responsible for c-ANCA staining and the MPO-ANCA antibody is typically responsible for the p-ANCA staining.

   Of patients with active Wegener's disease, 90% are ANCA-positive (the majority are PR3-ANCA positive). Of patients with microscopic polyangiitis, 70% are ANCA positive (the majority are MPO-ANCA positive). Of patients with Churg-Strauss syndrome, 50% are ANCA positive (PR3- and MPO-ANCA detected with about equal frequency). More than 90% of patients with renal limited, idiopathic pauci-immune vasculitis are ANCA-positive (the majority are MPO-ANCA positive).

4. **Anti-GBM antibodies** are useful for the diagnosis of Goodpasture's disease, although the false negative rate may be as high as 40%.

5. Evaluation of **serum complement** (C3 and C4) may be helpful in the evaluation of patients with ARF and glomerulonephritis. Hypocomplementemia is common in postinfectious glomerulonephritis, lupus nephritis, membranoproliferative glomerulonephritis, and mixed cryoglobulinemia. Another cause of ARF associated with hypocomplementemia includes atherembolic renal disease. It is important to recognize that other, nonrenal conditions may lower serum complement levels (e.g., sepsis, acute pancreatitis, and advanced liver disease).

G. **Intrinsic renal disease–AIN.** Intrinsic renal disease due to interstitial nephritis may be secondary to medications, infections, or a systemic illness such as lupus. Drug-induced AIN may be divided into three categories: AIN from methicillin; AIN from a medication other than methicillin; and NSAID-induced AIN. The clinical presentation and findings of these three major forms of drug-induced AIN are described in Table 10-6. Renal failure typically persists for a mean of 1.5 months; however, complete recovery of renal function occurs in the majority of patients.

1. **History.** In NSAID-induced AIN, symptoms and findings do not occur until several months after initiation of drug therapy (average 6 months); fenoprofen is the culprit in half of cases. AIN from other medications typically occurs within a few weeks of drug therapy. Patients may complain of fever, rash, or flank pain.

2. **Physical examination.** Physical findings with acute drug-induced interstitial nephritis may be lacking, although fever and a maculopapular or

Table 10-6. Three types of drug-induced interstitial nephritis

Drug group	Age	Duration of therapy	Fever	Rash	Hematuria and pyuria	Eosinophilia	Nephrotic syndrome
Methicillin	Any age	2 weeks	80%	25%	90%	80%	No
Non-methicillin	Any age	3 weeks	<50%	<50%	50%	<50%	No
NSAIDs	>50 years	Months	10%	10%	<50%	20%	70%

petechial skin eruption may occur with any of the agents, particularly the penicillin derivatives and allopurinol.

3. **Laboratory findings.** Eosinophilia is common in methicillin-induced AIN, but is present in less than 50% of cases of AIN from NSAIDs and other drugs.

4. **Urine findings.** When AIN is caused by methicillin and other drugs, red and white blood cells are present in the majority of cases; also present are WBC casts, the urine is typically isotonic, and 20% of cases are oliguric. In NSAID-induced AIN, nephrotic-range proteinuria is present in 80% of cases (greater than 3 g in 24 hours); WBCs, RBCs, and eosinophils are present in less than 50% of cases.

The evaluation for urinary eosinophils should be performed with Hansel's secretion stain (methylene blue and eosin Y in methanol), which is superior to Wright's stain, because urinary eosinophils are readily identified by their brilliant red-pink granules. Hansel's stain is not influenced by urinary pH. In a recent review of four series of drug-induced AIN, the positive predictive value for eosinophils in the urine was only 50%; however, the negative predictive value was 90%.

H. **Intrinsic renal disease—ATN.** ATN typically occurs in hospitalized patients as a consequence of ischemia or nephrotoxins.

1. **History.** The evaluation of a patient with suspected ATN must focus on identifying a predisposing cause. The chart should be reviewed for a history of hypotensive episodes, fluid losses, aminoglycoside use, NSAID administration, or radiologic procedures associated with contrast administration.

2. **Physical examination.** Signs of sepsis or ongoing infection should be evaluated. Volume status should be determined (see **IV.2a**).

3. **Laboratory findings and urinalysis.** Distinguishing ATN from prerenal ARF is often very difficult; this is an important clinical problem because the vast majority of ARF in hospitalized patients is due to either ATN or prerenal ARF. In addition, prolonged prerenal ARF often predisposes to the development of ATN. Because the causative factors for prerenal ARF and ATN overlap, distinguishing between the two may become possible only by the outcome of therapy (e.g., if volume repletion reverses the ARF, then prerenal ARF was present).

In general, a urine sediment with muddy brown granular casts is characteristic of ATN. However, this finding may be lacking, and other clinical clues will be necessary to make the diagnosis. To distinguish between the two, numerous diagnostic indices and formulae have been developed based on their pathophysiologic differences.

Prerenal ARF is a hemodynamic condition in which tubular function is normal, whereas ATN is characterized by tubular dysfunction. This distinction is the basis for the following tests (Table 10-5):

  Urine specific gravity
  Urine osmolality
  Urine creatinine/plasma creatinine
  Urine sodium concentration
  Fractional excretion of sodium (FENa)
  Serum BUN to creatinine ratio

Prerenal ARF is characterized by the increased reabsorption of water and sodium by the nephron. The increased reabsorption of water increases urine specific gravity and osmolality. Tubular reabsorption of urea increases, thus increasing the serum BUN to creatinine ratio; creatinine, however, is not reabsorbed, and its concentration increases in the urine and increases the urine to plasma creatinine ratio. Sodium reabsorption increases, resulting in a low urine sodium concentration and fractional excretion of sodium (FENa). In ATN, these processes cannot occur. Therefore, urine specific gravity and osmolality are isotonic, the urine creatinine to plasma creatinine ratio does not increase above a

20:1 ratio, the serum BUN to creatinine ratio does not increase, and urine sodium and FENa are higher than in prerenal ARF. FENa is not always increased in ATN; the causes of ATN that are associated with a low urine sodium concentration and low FENa include radiocontrast nephropathy, rhabdomyolysis, and ATN superimposed on a prerenal state (e.g., sepsis, burns, hepatic failure, heart failure).

The use of loop diuretics in ARF is a confounding factor in the use of FENa to distinguish prerenal ARF and ATN. Distal acting diuretics (e.g., furosemide) increase urinary sodium excretion and increase FENa even if the patient is prerenal. A recent study evaluated the use of the fractional excretion of urea (FEUN) to distinguish prerenal ARF in the setting of diuretic use from ATN (both of which are typically associated with a FENa of greater than 2%). The basis of this test is that urea absorption increases in the proximal tubule in prerenal ARF and would not be affected by the use of diuretics, which act on the distal tubule. In the setting of loop diuretic use, FEUN was an excellent test to distinguish between these conditions. In prerenal ARF, the FEUN is less than 35% and in ATN it is greater than 50%. The use of FEUN in cases of ATN associated with a low FENa could not be assessed in this study because of the lack of patients with this condition. Keep in mind that FEUN cannot be used in the setting of osmotic diuretic use (e.g., mannitol), because as these agents affect proximal tubular absorption.

4. **Specific causes of ATN**
   a. **Aminoglycoside nephrotoxicity.** ARF occurs in up to 20% of patients on aminoglycosides, even with careful dosing and therapeutic plasma levels. The incidence of nephrotoxicity correlates better with total cumulative dose than with plasma levels. Predisposing factors are old age, preexisting renal disease, volume depletion, and combination with other agents (e.g., diuretics, cephalosporins, vancomycin). Nephrotoxicity is usually clinically apparent after 5 to 10 days of therapy; early findings are isosthenuria caused by nephrogenic diabetes insipidus, and magnesium and potassium wasting. Later findings include azotemia, which may not develop for the first time until after the drug has been discontinued; conversely, recovery of renal function after discontinuation of the nephrotoxic aminoglycoside is often delayed and may require weeks to months to be complete. ARF from aminoglycosides is typically nonoliguric.

   Table 10-7 shows a comparison of the clinical characteristics of aminoglycoside and radiocontrast nephropathy.
   b. **Radiographic contrast nephropathy.** Radiocontrast agents cause ARF through a direct nephrotoxic effect and by causing renal vasoconstriction. Risk factors include old age, high contrast dose, preexisting renal disease, (especially diabetes mellitus), volume depletion, and recent exposure to other agents, such as ACE inhibitors and NSAIDs. Renal failure develops 1 to 2 days after exposure and is typically nonoliguric and associated with a high urine specific gravity, bland urine sediment, and low FENa. Serum creatinine typically peaks at 3 to 4 days and returns to baseline after about a week.
      (1) **Prevention.** Nonionic contrast agents are less nephrotoxic and should be used in high risk patients, especially patients with preexisting renal dysfunction. Drugs that affect renal hemodynamics (NSAIDs, ACE inhibitors, etc.) and diuretics should be discontinued prior to the procedure if possible.

      Although numerous agents have been studied to prevent contrast nephropathy, the only therapy that has been proven to be clearly beneficial is hydration with **saline** before and after the contrast load.

      N-acetylcysteine (NAC) may be beneficial in the prevention of contrast nephropathy, and its administration prior to contrast is

Table 10-7. A comparison between aminoglycoside nephrotoxicity and contrast nephropathy

	Pathophysiology	Risk factors	Onset of renal failure	Urine output	Prevention
Aminoglycoside	Direct tubular toxin	Older age Volume depletion Diuretics Cephalosporins Vancomycin Older age Diabetes	5 to 10 days	Nonoliguric	Avoidance Correct drug dosing Nonionic, iso-osmotic contrast
Contrast	Vasoconstriction	Multiple myeloma ACE-inhibitors NSAIDs	1 to 2 days	Nonoliguric	NAC Isotonic saline

reasonable (600 mg b.i.d. the day prior and the day of the procedure). In a frequently cited prospective trial, NAC-treated patients had a significantly lower serum creatinine 48 hours after contrast administration. The benefit of NAC in the prevention of contrast nephropathy remains uncertain. However, while some studies have confirmed the benefit of NAC in the prevention of contrast nephropathy, others have not. In addition, new evidence suggests that NAC may interfere with the measurement of creatinine resulting in a lowering of serum creatinine without a true change in renal function. This new evidence may call into question the results of NAC studies which used serum creatinine as a primary endpoint.

The clinical significance of contrast nephropathy should not be underestimated. It has been demonstrated that the development of a 0.5 mg/dL increase in serum creatinine after contrast is associated with an adjusted odds ratio of death of 5.5 (see Table 9-3, mortality associated with ARF).

Agents tested and demonstrated to be ineffective in the prevention of contrast nephropathy include furosemide, mannitol, theophylline, dopamine, fenoldopam, and atrial naturatic peptide.

  c. **Rhabdomyolysis** is caused by muscle injury (traumatic or atraumatic) that leads to the systemic release of muscle contents including myoglobin. Myoglobin is a heme pigment that is directly nephrotoxic; the intratubular precipitation of myoglobin causes obstruction and also contributes to the development of renal failure. Rhabdomyolysis should be considered in patients with trauma, muscle pain, and dark brown urine. However, rhabdomyolysis is frequently atraumatic, and up to 50% of patients have no muscular complaints. Table 10-8 lists predisposing factors for rhabdomyolysis.

The characteristic **urine finding** is a heme positive urine with absence of red blood cells. Pigmented granular casts are typically present on urine sediment. Laboratory clues to the diagnosis include a rapid rise of serum creatinine, massively increased creatine phosphokinase, hyperphosphatemia, hyperuricemia, hypocalcemia, increased anion gap, and disproportionate hyperkalemia. Serum calcium is reduced due to the sequestration of calcium into injured muscle; this calcium is released from the tissue during the recovery phase and may cause hypercalcemia. Therefore, replacement of serum calcium should be avoided unless symptoms of hypocalcemia are present.

The only proven **therapy** in the treatment of rhabdomyolysis is early and vigorous infusion of intravenous isotonic saline. In crush injury, it is recommended that i.v. saline be administered even before extrication. Mannitol administration and urinary alkalinazation are often attempted in the treatment of rhabdomyolysis, although their efficacy has not been demonstrated to be superior to vigorous

Table 10-8. Causes of rhabdomyolysis

Direct muscle damage (e.g., crush injuries, polymyositis, prolonged immobilization associated with unconsciousness)

Muscle ischemia (e.g., arterial occlusion or embolism)

Excess energy consumption (e.g., seizures, hyperthermia, delirium tremens)

Decreased energy production (e.g., severe hypophosphatemia, hypokalemia, myxedema, genetic defect)

Drugs and toxins (e.g., alcohol, heroin, cocaine, amphetamines, poisonous insect and snake bites)

Severe infections (e.g., tetanus, Legionnaire's disease, influenza)

hydration with saline alone. Theoretically, forced diuresis with mannitol may aid in the washout of obstructing myoglobin pigment. Mannitol administration may be attempted only after the correction of volume deficits; saline and mannitol should be administered together with a goal urine output of 300 cc per hour. Urinary alkalinization may inhibit myoglobin precipitation; however, urinary alkalinizaion is difficult to achieve in practice and requires the administration of a large quantity of bicarbonate. Bicarbonate administration in rhabdomyolysis carries the risk of worsening hypocalcemia due to increased calcium and phosphorus precipitation into injured muscle.

   d. Acute uric acid nephropathy causes ARF due to the intratubular deposition of uric acid crystals. A very high serum uric acid concentration is present (e.g., greater than or equal to 15 mg per dL. The condition typically occurs during induction chemotherapy for malignancies with high cell turnover (e.g., leukemias and lymphoproliferative malignancies). Acute uric acid nephropathy and ARF occur in the tumor lysis syndrome, but may occur spontaneously in patients with high tumor burden. Clinical features of acute uric acid nephropathy are hyperuricemia, hyperkalemia, hyperphosphatemia, and a urine urate to creatinine ratio higher than 1. Preventive measures include allopurinol administration and vigorous hydration and forced diuresis with mannitol. Alkalinization of the urine has been traditionally recommended, but has not been proven more beneficial than saline administration alone; additionally bicarbonate therapy carries the risk of increased calcium precipitation.

V. ARF in special clinical circumstances

   A. Crystal-associated ARF. A number of important causes of ARF may be due to the formation of urinary crystals. Table 10-9 lists the causes of ARF associated with crystal formation.

   B. ARF in patients with acquired immunodeficiency syndrome (AIDS) (Table 10-10). The approach to the causes of ARF in AIDS patients is the same as that for other patients (i.e., classification into prerenal, intrinsic renal, and postrenal causes). ARF may develop in up to 20% of hospitalized patients with AIDS and is in most cases multifactorial. ATN is seen in AIDS because the patients are often acutely ill with multiple infections or malignancies. Their clinical course is often complicated by hypovolemia, multiorgan failure, compromised cardiovascular status, invasive diagnostic procedures complicated by bleeding, and the administration of multiple nephrotoxic drugs and radiocontrast agents. Although ATN is a major cause of morbidity and mortality in AIDS patients, it is also potentially reversible

Table 10-9. Urinary crystals associated with ARF

Type of ARF	Crystal	Shape/appearance
ATN from ethylene glycol	Calcium oxalate monohydrate or Calcium oxalate dihydrate	Needle-shaped Envelope-shaped
ATN from uric acid nephropathy	Uric acid	Diamond-shaped, yellow or brown
ARF from sulfadiazine (intratubular obstruction)	Sulfadiazine	Needle-shaped or shocks of wheat
ARF from acyclovir (intratubular obstruction)	Acyclovir	Needle-shaped, birefringent
ARF from indinavir (intratubular obstruction)	Indinavir sulfate	Needle-shaped, occasionally forming rosettes

Table 10-10. Acute renal failure in acquired immunodeficiency syndrome (AIDS) patients

Prerenal
Hypovolemia (diarrhea)
Hypotension (sepsis, bleeding)
Decreased effective arterial blood volume (hypoalbuminemia, cachexia,
  HIV nephropathy)
Vasoconstriction (radiocontrast agents)
Postrenal
Tubular obstruction due to crystalluria (intravenous acyclovir, sulfadiazine,
  indinavir, saquinavir, ritonavir)
Extrinsic ureteral compression (lymph nodes, tumors)
Intrinsic ureteral obstruction (fungus balls)
Bladder obstruction (tumors, fungus balls)
Renal
Hemolytic-uremic syndrome and thrombotic thrombocytopenic purpura
Postinfectious glomerulonephritis
Collapsing focal segmental glomerularsclerosis
Acute allergic interstitial nephritis (penicillins, sulfonamides)
Plasmacytic interstitial nephritis
Acute tubular necrosis (shock, sepsis, aminoglycosides, amphotericin)
Rhabdomyolysis (pentamidine, zidovudine)

and treatable. All supportive measures, including dialysis, should be used as warranted by the clinical situation. Importantly, ATN is avoidable in some cases when preventative measures are used (e.g., maintaining adequate hydration before use of radiocontrast agents and during use of antibiotics and antiretroviral therapy that precipitates crystalluria).

C. **ARF in bone marrow transplant patients.** ARF is a common complication of bone marrow transplant. [This procedure is now referred to as hematopoetic cell transplant (HCT), because other cells, such as stem cells, are transplanted as well as bone marrow.] Approximately 90% of patients have a doubling of serum creatinine after allogeneic HCT. This incidence is higher in patients who receive allogeneic as opposed to autologous transplantation. ARF also occurs in nonmyeloablative HCT, also known as "mini-allo" transplants. The incidence of ARF is high in HCT because of the life-threatening nature of the underlying diseases and the toxicity of the cancer drugs, immunosuppressive regimens, and antibiotics. Patients with ARF after HCT who require dialysis have a greater than 90% incidence of mortality.

Factors that predispose to ATN are vomiting and diarrhea due to radiochemotherapy or acute graft-versus-host disease; nephrotoxic drugs such as aminoglycosides and amphotericin B; and hemorrhagic and septic shock. Hepatic veno-occlusive disease, which is more common in allogeneic than autologous bone marrow transplants, is a syndrome that may resemble the hepatorenal syndrome. A sodium retention state occurs and leads to weight gain, edema, and a low FENa of less than 1%, despite the use of diuretics. Progressive hyperbilirubinemia and nonoliguric ARF occur.

By far, the most common time for development of ARF is 7 to 21 days after the transplant. The renal syndromes unique to bone marrow transplant patients are classified according to the time of presentation:
    Immediate (first few days)
        Tumor lysis syndrome
        Stored marrow toxicity

Early (7 to 21 days)
Hepatic veno-occlusive disease
Sepsis
ATN
Cyclosporin or FK506 toxicity
Late (6 weeks to 1 year)
Bone marrow transplant–associated hemolytic-uremic syndrome
Chronic cyclosporine nephrotoxicity

D. ARF in the setting of liver disease. In addition to hepatorenal syndrome, ARF in patients with liver disease may also occur in other clinical settings. Jaundice and ARF may be due to HUS, leptospirosis, mismatched blood transfusion, or falciparum malaria. Simultaneous ARF and acute liver failure suggests acetaminophen overdose, bacteremia, or carbon tetrachloride exposure. Glomerulonephritis and liver cirrhosis is associated with cryoglobulinemia, IgA nephropathy, membranous glomerulonephritis (associated with hepatitis B), and membranoproliferative glomerulonephritis (associated with hepatitis C).

E. Indications for renal biopsy. Renal biopsy is not performed in patients with prerenal ARF or the typical features of ATN. However, important indications for a renal biopsy in a patient with ARF exist.

    1. ARF of unknown etiology. In most cases, a stepwise approach reveals a cause of the ARF. However, in some patients with ARF, the diagnosis is not clear.

    2. Suspicion of **glomerulonephritis,** systemic disease (e.g., vasculitis), or **AIN** as the cause of ARF. A renal biopsy in such circumstances may provide the basis and justification for aggressive and life-saving therapy (e.g., high-dose steroids, cytotoxic agents, plasmapheresis, cessation of causative agent for AIN).

    3. ATN not recovering after 4 to 6 weeks of dialysis with no more recurrent insults. A renal biopsy may determine that a less favorable condition, such as diffuse cortical necrosis, has developed and that chronic hemodialysis may need to be instituted.

VI. Management

  A. Prerenal azotemia

    1. True volume depletion or hypovolemia. Therapy in this setting is directed toward correcting volume deficits. If volume depletion is due to hemorrhage, then the administration of packed red blood cells is indicated; otherwise, the administration of 0.9% normal saline (NS) is appropriate. When 1 L of 0.9 NS is given, approximately 250 mL remain in the plasma compartment, while 750 mL enter the interstitial compartment.

        The amount of intravenous fluid (IVF) and the rapidity of administration depend on the clinical situation. In a young, stable patient, IVF should be given in one-time boluses (e.g., 500 to 1,000 cc over 1 hour); **0.9NS should never be written as a continuous infusion.** Smaller boluses (e.g., 250 cc over 1 hour) may be prudent in elderly patients in whom cardiac status is unknown. After a bolus, the patient should be evaluated clinically for signs of hypovolemia or volume overload. Bedside evaluation includes monitoring of orthostatic changes in blood pressure and pulse and jugular venous pulsation (JVP). JVP is a gross indicator of pressure in the central venous area of the right heart. In a normovolemic patient, jugular venous pulsations are visible when the patient is supine but disappear when the patient assumes the sitting position. Jugular venous pulsations are not visible in the volume-depleted patient; thus, their reappearance following fluid administration suggests that the central venous pressure (CVP) has returned to normal. The presence of basilar crackles or a third heart sound implies too-vigorous fluid replacement, with resultant cardiopulmonary congestion. Intravenous boluses of fluid should continue until euvolemia is achieved. Electrolyte deficits (e.g., potassium) should be monitored and replaced if necessary.

In patients in whom vigorous resuscitation efforts are required, and cardiovascular tolerance to sudden fluid challenges is in doubt, some form of indwelling monitoring system is desirable. Hemodynamic monitoring may be achieved through the use of a **central venous catheter** or **Swan-Ganz catheter.**

   a. **Central venous catheter.** When rapid fluid administration is required, and severe heart or lung disease (or both) is absent, a catheter positioned in the central venous area of the right heart is a satisfactory guide to the speed of fluid administration. The CVP normally ranges between 2 and 12 cm of water. In volume-depleted states, values of zero or below can be expected. Before vigorous volume repletion is begun, a fluid challenge of 200 to 300 mL of normal saline should be attempted over a 10- to 20-minute period. In an otherwise uncomplicated volume-depleted patient, this amount of saline has little effect on the CVP reading. A CVP rise of more than 5 cm of water suggests cardiac failure, and the infusion should be immediately discontinued.

   b. **Swan-Ganz catheter.** When a volume deficit must be repaired in the presence of tricuspid stenosis, acute or chronic pulmonary disease, or an unstable cardiovascular system, the CVP does not give a reliable index of left ventricular performance. In this situation, a balloon-tipped Swan-Ganz catheter can be wedged in a pulmonary artery. This gives a measurement of pulmonary artery wedge pressure (PAWP), an indirect measurement of left ventricular end-diastolic pressure. The PAWP is a good guide to the adequacy and speed of fluid replacement. Because of the complications of infection, pulmonary infarction, and hemopneumothorax, this device should be inserted and placed only by trained professionals and should be removed as early as possible. In patients with liver encephalopathy and ARF, a clinical judgment of fluid balance may be difficult because of massive edema and ascites. The measurement of PAWP gives critical information about fluid balance: ARF in the presence of a low PAWP may respond to fluid administration.

2. **Arterial underfilling with an ECF excess.** Prerenal ARF in this setting is usually a secondary problem overshadowed by primary cardiac or liver disease. The management goal, therefore, is to treat the underlying cause; if the primary disease cannot be treated, then conservative management of symptoms is desirable.

   a. **Heart failure. Numerous medications may be employed to improve cardiac output in patients with cardiac disease.** In the outpatient setting of a patient with congestive heart failure (CHF), diuretic agents in combination with digitalis therapy may increase the cardiac output and improve renal perfusion, and thus lessen the azotemia. Cardiac unloading agents such as ACE inhibitors, ARBs, nitrates, and hydralazine may also improve cardiac function. However, with advanced heart failure that is refractory or only partially responsive to these agents, the physician may be forced to accept mild to moderate prerenal azotemia as a tradeoff. Such azotemia rarely leads to symptomatic uremia.

   In hospitalized patients with CHF who are diuretic resistant, fluid may be removed with continuous venovenous hemofiltration or intermittent ultrafiltration, without dialysis.

   b. **Liver disease.** Prerenal ARF associated with advanced hepatic cirrhosis and patients with type II HRS are often refractory to attempts to improve intravascular volume. Ordinarily, however, the management goal is to reduce symptoms and treat ascites and edema with a sodium-restricted diet (1 to 2 g of salt per day), an aldosterone antagonist (e.g., spironolactone 200 to 400 mg per day), and a loop diuretic (e.g., furosemide) while the usually mild prerenal state is ignored. Diuretic-resistant patients may be treated with intermittent large volume paracentesis, transjugular intrahepatic portosystemic stent shunt (TIPS), or liver transplantation. Treatment of hospitalized patients with type I HRS may include vasopressin analogs or somatostatin in an attempt to improve renal blood flow. These therapies have yet to be proven to impact mortality, which is greater than 90% in type I HRS. In reports from Europe, the ADH analogs ornipressin and terlipressin, with albumin infusion, have shown some promise in the treatment of HRS; however, these agents may have significant ischemic side effects. It remains to be determined if the benefits of these agents will outweigh the risk of use (neither medication is currently available in the United States). TIPS may be an option for some patients; improved mortality was demonstrated in one study; however, further studies must confirm this benefit. To date, liver transplant is the only definitive cure.

B. Postrenal failure. Foley catheter drainage is usually successful for acute obstruction secondary to prostatic hypertrophy. The decision regarding further therapy must be made in consultation with a urologist. Medical therapy with finesteride or an alpha blocker, or surgical removal of the prostate may be recommended.

With ureteral obstruction, cystoscopy and the placement of ureteral drainage catheters or stents may allow passage of obstructing stones, sludge, or pus, but if this fails, operative intervention is required.

C. Primary renal disease: vasculitis and glomerulonephritis. When renal failure develops in the course of a systemic or vascular disorder, it is usually a grave sign. A comprehensive discussion of the treatment of these systemic and vascular disorders is beyond the scope of this chapter. Obtaining a renal biopsy early after presentation is essential to make the diagnosis and to guide appropriate therapy. Theraputic options include immunosuppressive therapy with steroids and/or cyclophosphamide. A subset of patients may benefit from plasmapheresis (e.g., Goodpasture's syndrome).

D. Acute interstitial nephritis. When a therapeutic agent is identified as the cause of acute interstitial nephritis, removal of the agent is the obvious first step in therapy. Bacterial infectious etiologies should be treated with the appropriate antibiotics. When renal impairment is minor, nothing more need be done. If renal impairment has been present for weeks, or if renal involvement is severe, high-dose, short-term prednisone therapy (60 mg per day for 3 to 4 weeks) may speed recovery of renal function. Before initiating prednisone therapy, it is important to confirm the diagnosis with a renal biopsy.

E. Intrinsic renal disease, ATN. No specific therapy exists for the treatment of ARF due to ATN, although this is a widely investigated area of interest.

   1. What to avoid in ATN

      a. High-dose diuretics. No data support the use of high-dose diuretic therapy in established ATN. Furosemide and other loop diuretics are frequently used in oliguric ARF in an effort to convert it to nonoliguric ARF. Although the conversion of oliguric to nonoliguric renal failure may simplify fluid management, clinical trials have failed to demonstrate that the use of diuretics is associated with improved outcome in patients with ARF.

      b. Renal-dose dopamine. Dopamine is a selective renal vasodilatator. It elicits profound natriuresis and increases urine output. The renal selective dose is 1 to 3 mcg per kg per minute. No evidence suggests that renal-dose dopamine is beneficial in ARF. In fact, several studies have identified deleterious effects, such as, bowel ischemia and arrhythmias. Unless dopamine is required for circulatory support, it should not be used for ARF.

      c. Nephrotoxic drugs. Potentially nephrotoxic drugs and agents should be avoided in ARF, because they may perpetuate the renal injury. These agents and drugs include NSAIDs, ACE inhibitors, cyclosporine, tacrolimus, aminoglycosides, radiocontrast agents, and amphotericin B.

   d. Volume overload. The amount of IVF necessary for critically ill patients is unknown, and IVFs must be given judiciously in the setting of ATN, especially if the patient is oliguric. In general, IVFs should not contain potassium.

2. Supportive therapy in ATN

   a. Drug dosages. Drug dosages should be adjusted based on the measured or best estimate of creatinine clearance, not merely on the serum creatinine. Certain medication doses also must be adjusted if the ARF patient is receiving dialysis (intermittent hemodialysis or continuous renal replacement therapy).

   b. Nutritional support. ARF is a hypercatabolic state associated with increased protein breakdown. Nitrogen balance is extremely negative, especially in ARF associated with sepsis, post-surgery, and multiorgan dysfunction syndrome. Renal factors contributing to the negative nitrogen balance include uremia, acidosis, parathyroid hormone abnormalities, inadequate protein intake, and protein losses. In critically ill patients, supplemental nutritional support with enteral versus parenteral nutrition is associated with improved nutritional status, a reduction in infections and sepsis, and better survival. Thus, enteral feeding is the preferred method of nutritional support, although it is not always possible. The use of parenteral nutrition remains controversial, and randomized controlled clinical trials have yet to demonstrate a benefit in acutely ill patients with ARF. Opinion papers have suggested that protein intake not exceed 1.5 g of protein per kg of body weight, that early nutritional supplementation may not be beneficial, and that supplementation after 2 to 3 weeks of not eating is likely to be beneficial.

   c. Dialysis therapy. In general, the indications to start dialysis in ATN and ARF are not specific and should be individualized by nephrology consultation. Although not yet proven in clinical trials, a trend in clinical practice is to initiate dialysis early to avoid the potential consequences of uremia. Uremia that results in altered mental status or pericarditis is an absolute indication for dialysis.

   The common factors that are taken into consideration when making the decision to start dialysis are listed here. It should be kept in mind that these are guidelines, not absolute indications for the initiation of dialysis. The initiation of dialysis depends on the entire clinical picture, not just the presence or absence of one of these factors.

   Persistent oliguria (less than 400 mL per day)
   Serum creatinine higher than 6 mg per dL
   BUN greater than 100 mg per dL
   Pulmonary edema unresponsive to diuretics
   Hyperkalemia (serum potassium greater than 6.5 mEq per dL)
   Symptomatic uremia (e.g., encephalopathy, pericarditis)
   Severe metabolic acidosis

   The main modalities of dialysis are intermittent hemodialysis (IHD) and continuous renal replacement therapy (CRRT).

   (1) IHD is the same form of dialysis used in patients with end stage renal disease (ESRD). IHD is typically used in otherwise stable patients who can tolerate rapid fluid removal (e.g., 1 L per hour). IHD is mandatory in ambulatory patients.

   In this form of dialysis, the patient is connected to a dialysis machine for 4 hours at a time, daily or every second day. Fluid removal and urea clearance for the day is achieved during the period of a few hours. Rapid removal of solutes and fluids may cause hemodynamic instability. The technique requires a double-lumen catheter, tubing, a hemodialysis machine (blood pump, dialysate generation system, dialysate pump, and alarms and safety monitoring de vices), a dialysis membrane, and a dialysis nurse. Daily treatment for 4 hours, with a blood urea clearance of 200 mL per minute, can achieve a weekly urea clearance of 350 L.

The frequency of IHD and delivered dose of dialysis required in ARF is a matter of debate. In chronic end stage renal patients, IHD is typically performed on alternate days (three days per week) for approximately 4 hours at a time. The **dose** and **frequency** of dialysis for ARF may need to be much higher than in the chronic setting, because ARF patients are typically hypercatabolic and most temporary catheters have a high recirculation rate. A number of recent studies demonstrate that more urea clearance achieved by daily hemodialysis (HD) or continuous venovenous hemofiltration (CVVH), with increased ultrafiltration associated with a lower mortality rate. Thus, the available evidence seems to suggest that simple, alternate-day HD may be inadequate for a subset of patients with ARF, particularly those who are severely catabolic.

(2) CRRT. Currently, four main types of **CRRT** are used: slow continuous ultrafiltration (SCUF), CVVH, continuous venovenous hemodialysis (CVVHD), and continuous venovenous hemodiafiltration. Table 10-11 summarizes the different characteristic of each. The type of CRRT is individualized. A common approach is to start with CVVH and then add dialysate (CVVHDF), if clearance rates are too low. A recent, prospective randomized study demonstrated improved mortality in patients on CVVH who had an ultrafiltrate formation of 45 mL per kg per hour or 35 mL per kg per hour, compared with 20 mL per kg per hour. In a 70-kg man, this corresponds to 3,150 mL per hour 2,450 mL per hour, and 1,400 mL per hour respectively. Achieving ultrafiltrate formation rates greater than 2 liters per hour can be technically difficult.

In CRRT, the goal is for the patient to undergo continuous dialysis for 24 hours a day. In practice, interruptions in dialysis

Table 10-11. Comparison of intermittent hemodialysis (IHD) and various types of continuous renal replacement therapy (CRRT).

Type of renal replacement	Amount of ultrafiltrate formed/hour[a]	Use of replacement fluid[b]	Use of dialysate	Urea clearance (L/day)
Intermittent hemodialysis (IHD)	500 to 1,000 cc	No	Yes	40–60
Slow continuous ultrafiltration (SCUF)	50 to 100 cc	No	No	2–5
Continuous venovenous hemofiltration (CVVH)	1,000 to 2,000 cc	Yes	No	20–50
Continuous venovenous hemodialysis (CVVHD)	50 to 100 cc	No	Yes	20–55
Continuous venovenous hemodiafiltration (CVVHDF)	1,000 to 2,000 cc	Yes	Yes	25–75

[a]The ultrafiltrate formed has the same electrolyte composition as plasma; therefore, with high ultrafiltrate formation, increased losses of potassium, phosphorous, calcium, and magnesium may occur. These electrolytes may need to be replaced intravenously.
[b]Replacement fluid typically contains sodium, chloride, and calcium and replaces fluid lost in the ultrafiltrate and other sources (GI, etc.) to achieve the desired hourly net fluid loss. In IHD, net fluid loss is typically 500 to 1,000 cc per hour whereas in CRRT, net fluid loss is typically 50 to 100 cc per hour.

for patient procedures, radiologic testing, and dialysis membrane clotting are frequent and reduce the amount of time the patient is actually receiving dialysis. CRRT is the mandatory form of dialysis for hemodynamically unstable patients. Because the removal of solutes and fluid is slow and continuous, hemodynamic instability and hypotensive episodes are reduced. Minimization of hypotension theoretically avoids the perpetuation of renal injury. CRRT requires a double-lumen catheter (the same catheter that is used for IHD), tubing, a simple blood pump with safety devices, sterile replacement fluid, volumetric pumps to control replacement and ultrafiltration rate, continuous anticoagulation, and a high-flux dialysis membrane. ICU nurses typically monitor therapy.

   (3) **Intermittent versus continuous dialysis.** Many nonrandomized studies have compared IHD and CRRT. Prospective randomized studies are difficult to carry out, because hemodynamically unstable patients who cannot tolerate IHD are almost always started on CRRT. Alternatively, confining a mobile patient to bed to receive CRRT may be unethical. Thus, randomization may be biased. CRRT is believed to be the modality of choice in very ill patients, and IHD is used in less ill patients. At present, IHD and CRRT are regarded as equivalent methods for the treatment of ARF. The choice of IHD or CRRT should be made in consultation with a nephrologist and tailored for the individual patient. The decision may also depend on facility-specific issues, such as experience, nursing resources, and technical proficiency. The cost of CRRT is greater than IHD. At present, indications for CRRT in ARF include hemodynamic instability, cerebral edema, hypercatabolism, and severe fluid overload. Table 10-12 lists a comparison of IHD and CRRT. CRRT is similar in solute clearance to a GFR of 15 to 20 mL per minute. A day of CRRT is roughly equivalent to one HD treatment. Thus, drug-dosing adjustments must be made in CRRT.

   (4) **Type of dialysis membrane.** Some studies have demonstrated that the dialysis of ARF patients with biocompatible membranes is associated with improved mortality; therefore, biocompatible membranes are used for dialysis in ARF. Biocompatible membranes are made of synthetic polymers and include polyamides, polycarbonate, and polysulfone. The adverse effects of bioincompatible

Table 10-12. Analysis of continuous renal replacement therapy versus intermittent hemodialysis

Advantages
   Hemodynamic stability (may relate in part to decreased body temperature)
   Unlimited alimentation
   Avoidance of rapid fluid and electrolyte shifts
   Aggressive correction of acid-base status
   Massive fluid removal
   Potential elimination of mediators (e.g., cytokines) by membrane absorbance
Disadvantages
   Immobilization
   Lactate load[a]
   Continuous anticoagulation[b]

[a]Lactate should be avoided in patients with severe liver disease who cannot metabolize lactate. The lactate load may be avoided by making a custom dialysate that contains bicarbonate instead.
[b]CRRT may be performed without anticoagulation; however, frequent clotting of the membrane may occur.

cellulosic membranes (e.g., cellulose, cuprophane, hemophane, cellulose acetate) include activation of complement, increased production of cytokines, and hypotension.

(5) Temporary vascular access. The primary vascular sites used for insertion of temporary dialysis catheters are the internal jugular and femoral. The internal jugular access is required in patients who are mobile. Femoral access is indicated when the cardiopulmonary condition of the patient limits attempts at thoracic catheterization; it is useful in bedridden patients. The subclavian vein may be used if other access sites are unavailable; however, use of subclavian catheters entails a major risk of stenosis or thrombosis of the subclavian vein or its branches.

(6) Peritoneal dialysis is uncommonly used as a mode of dialysis therapy in ARF in developed countries despite the fact that it is not technically difficult and can be used with minimally trained staff. It may be an option in locations where IHD or CRRT is not available. It is indicated in patients with minimally increased catabolism without an immediate or life-threatening indication for dialysis. It is ideal for hemodynamically unstable patients. For short-term dialysis, a rigid dialysis catheter is inserted into the peritoneum, through the anterior abdominal wall, 5 to 10 cm below the umbilicus. Exchanges of 1.5 to 2.0 L of standard peritoneal dialysis solutions are infused into the peritoneum. The major risks are bowel perforation during insertion of the catheter and peritonitis. Acute peritoneal dialysis offers the same potential advantages to the pediatric patient that CRRT offers to the adult with ARF.

Suggested readings

Alkhunaizi AM, Schrier RW. Management of acute renal failure: new perspectives. *Am J Kidney Dis* 1996;28:315–328.

Carvounis CP, Nisar S, Guro-Razman S. Significance of the fractional excretion of urea in the differential diagnosis of acute renal failure. *Kidney Int* 2002;62:2223–2229.

Beutler JJ, Koomans HA. Malignant hypertension: still a challenge. *Nephrol Dial Transplant* 1997;12:2019–2023.

DuBose TD Jr., Warnock DG, Mehta RL, et al. Acute renal failure in the twenty-first century: recommendations for management and outcomes assessment. *Am J Kidney Dis* 1997;29:793–799.

Edelstein CL, Ling H, Schrier RW. The nature of renal cell injury. *Kidney Int* 1997;51:1341–1351.

Edelstein CL, Ling H, Wangsiripaisan A, Schrier RW. Emerging therapies for acute renal failure. *Am J Kidney Dis* 1997;30:S89–S95.

Esson ML, Schrier RW. Diagnosis and treatment of acute tubular necrosis. *Ann Int Med* 2002;137:744–752.

Jennette JC, Falk RJ. Diagnosis and management of glomerulonephritis and vasculitis presenting as acute renal failure. *Med Clin North Am* 1990;74:893–908.

Parikh CR, McSweeney PA, et al. Renal dysfunction in allogeneic hematopoietic cell transplantation. *Kidney Int* 2002 Aug;62(2):566–573.

Proceedings of the First International Congress on Continuous Renal Replacement Therapy. *Am J Kidney Dis* 1996;28:S1–S121.

Proceedings of the First International Course on Critical Care Nephrology. *Kidney Int* 1998;53:S1–S190.

Rao TK. Renal complications of HIV disease. *Med Clin North Am* 1996;80:1437–1451.

Rossert J. Drug-induced acute interstitial nephritis. *Kidney Int* 2001;60:804–817.

Schlondorff D. Renal complications of nonsteroidal anti-inflammatory drugs. *Kidney Int* 1993;44:643–653.

Star RA. Treatment of acute renal failure. *Kidney Int* 1998;54:1817–1831.

The Patient with Chronic Kidney Disease

Michael Conchol and David M. Spiegel

Patients with end-stage renal disease (ESRD) have decreased quality of life, high morbidity, and an annual mortality of about 22%. The number of persons with kidney failure who are treated with dialysis and transplantation is projected to increase from 340,000 in 1999 to 651,000 in 2010 (1). The high morbidity and mortality seen in dialysis patients may decrease significantly if patients were healthier at the time of initiating renal replacement therapy.

This chapter presents an overview of the current recommendations designed to retard the progression of chronic kidney disease (CKD); to optimize the medical management of comorbid medical conditions, such as cardiovascular disease (CVD), diabetes, and lipid disorders; and to decrease the complications secondary to progression of kidney disease, including hypertension, anemia, secondary hyperparathyroidism, and malnutrition. These recommendations are derived from the recent clinical practice guidelines published by the Kidney Disease Outcomes Quality Initiative (K/DOQI) of the National Kidney Foundation (NKF) (2).

I. **Definition and staging of chronic kidney disease.** The definition of chronic kidney disease (CKD) is:
   A. **Kidney damage** for 3 months or longer, as defined by structural or functional abnormalities of the kidney, with or without decreased glomerular filtration rate (GFR), manifest by either:
      1. Pathological abnormalities; or
      2. Markers of kidney damage, including abnormalities in the composition of the blood or urine, or abnormalities in imaging tests
   B. **GFR** of less than 60 mL per minute per 1.73 m^2 for 3 months or longer, with or without kidney damage.

   In a recent NKF report, CKD was divided into stages of severity (Table 11-1.) Importantly, the staging system is based on calculated GFR and not on the measurement of serum creatinine. Stage 1 CKD is recognized by the presence of kidney damage at a time when GFR is conserved; this includes patients with albuminuria or abnormal imaging studies. For example, a patient with type II diabetes and normal GFR, but with microalbuminuria, is classified as Stage 1 CKD. The definition for microalbuminuria is 30 to 300 mg per day (24-hour excretion) and for clinical proteinuria: more than 300 mg per day (24-hour excretion). Stage 2 CKD takes into account patients with evidence of kidney damage with decreased GFR (60 to 89 mL per minute per 1.73 m^2). Last, all patients with a GFR of less than 60 mL per minute per 1.73 m^2 are classified as having CKD irrespective of whether kidney damage is present.

   The staging of chronic kidney disease is useful because it endorses a model in which primary physicians and specialists share responsibility for the care of patients with CKD. This classification also offers a common language for patients and the practitioners involved in the treatment of CKD. For each stage of CKD, K/DOQI provides recommendations for a clinical action plan (Table 11-1).

   An essential requirement for the classification and monitoring of CKD is the measurement or estimation of GFR. Serum creatinine is not an ideal marker of GFR, because it is both filtered at the glomerulus and secreted by the proximal tubule. Creatinine clearance (CrCl) is known to overestimate GFR by as much as 40% in normal individuals and by even more in

Table 11-1. National Kidney Foundation kidney disease outcomes quality initiative classification, prevalence, and action plan for stages of chronic kidney disease[2]

Stage	Description	GFR, mL per min per 1.73 m³	Prevalence, n (%)	Action
—	At increased risk	≥60 (with chronic kidney disease risk factors)	—	Screening: chronic kidney disease risk reduction
1	Kidney damage with normal or increased GFR	≥90	5,900,000 (3.3)	Diagnosis and treatment; treatment of comorbid conditions; slowing progression; CVD risk reduction
2	Kidney damage with slightly decreased GFR	60–89	5,300,000 (3.0)	Estimating progression
3	Moderately decreased GFR	30–59	7,600,000 (4.3)	Evaluating and treating complications
4	Severely decreased GFR	15–29	400,000 (0.2)	Preparation for kidney replacement therapy
5	Kidney failure	<15 (or dialysis)	300,000 (0.1)	Kidney replacement (if uremia present)

National Kidney Foundation: K/DOQI Clinical Practice Guidelines for Chronic Kidney Disease: evaluation, classification, and stratification: *Am J Kidney Dis* 2002; 39 (Suppl 1): S1–S266.

patients with CKD (3). Estimates of GFR based on 24-hour CrCL require timed urine collections, which are difficult to obtain and often involve errors in collection. Classic methods for measurements of GFR, including the gold-standard inulin clearance, are cumbersome, require an intravenous infusion and timed urine collections, and are not clinically feasible. In adults, the normal GFR based on inulin clearance and adjusted to a standard body surface area of 1.73 m^2 is 127 mL per minute per 1.73 m^2 for men and 118 mL per minute per 1.73 m^2 for women, with a standard deviation of approximately 20 mL per minute per 1.73 m^2. After age 30, the average decrease in GFR is 1 mL per minute per 1.73 m^2 per year (2).

Equations based on serum creatinine but factored for gender, age, and ethnicity are the best alternative for estimation of GFR. The most commonly used formula is the Cockcroft-Gault equation. This equation was developed to predict CrCl, but has been used to estimate GFR (4):

$$CrCl = \frac{(140 - age)(weight\ in\ kg)}{(Serum\ creatinine)(72)} \times 0.85\ if\ female$$

The Modification of Diet in Renal Disease (MDRD) Study equation was derived on the basis of data from more than 500 patients with a wide variety of kidney diseases and GFRs up to 90 mL per minute per 1.73 m^2. Thus, the abbreviated MDRD equation is recommended for routine use and requires only serum creatinine, age, gender, and race (2):

$$GFR\ (mL/min\ per\ 1.73\ m^2) = 186 \times (SCR)^{-1.154} \times (age)^{-0.203}$$

$$\times (0.742\ if\ female) \times (1.210\ if\ African\text{-}American)$$

The calculations can be made using available web-based and downloadable medical calculators (www.kdoqi.com).

The MDRD study equation has many advantages. It is more accurate and precise than the Cockcroft-Gault equation for persons with a GFR of less than approximately 90 mL per minute per 1.73 m^2. This equation predicts GFR as measured by using an accepted method (urinary clearance of ^{125}I-iothalamate). It does not require height or weight and has been validated in kidney transplant recipients and African-Americans with nephrosclerosis. It has not been validated in diabetic kidney disease, in patients with serious comorbid conditions, in normal persons, or in individuals older than 70 years of age (2).

II. **Prevalence of CKD.** The Third National Health and Nutrition Examination Survey (NHANES III) included 15,625 participants age 20 years or older and was conducted, between 1988 to 1994, by the National Center for Health Statistics (NCHS) of the Centers for Disease Control and Prevention. The goal of this survey was to provide nationally representative data on the health and nutritional status of the civilian, noninstitutionalized United States (U.S.) population. The results, when extrapolated to the U.S. population of adults age older than 20 years (n = 177 million), revealed the following findings relevant to CKD (5):

A. 6.2 million individuals had a serum creatinine equal to or greater than 1.5 mg per dL, which is a 30-fold higher prevalence of reduced kidney function compared with the prevalence of treated ESRD during the same time interval.

B. 2.5 million individuals had a serum creatinine equal to or greater than 1.7 mg per dL.

C. 800,000 individuals had a serum creatinine equal to or greater than 2.0 mg per dL.

D. Of individuals with elevated serum creatinine, 70% have hypertension.

E. Only 75% of patients with hypertension and elevated serum creatinine received treatment, with only 27% having a blood pressure (BP) reading lower than 140/90 mm Hg and 11% having their BP reduced to lower than 130/85 mm Hg.

In a further analysis of NHANES III data, estimated GFR was calculated from the serum creatinine using the MDRD study equation (2). The prevalence of the different stages of CKD clearly shows that the CKD population is several times larger than the ESRD population. The challenge for the medical community is to identify earlier stages of CKD and institute correct treatment strategies to decrease complications and slow the progression to ESRD.

III. **Mechanism of kidney disease progression.** Diabetes and hypertension are responsible for the largest proportion of ESRD. Glomerulonephritis represents the third most common cause of ESRD. Despite the many diseases that can initiate kidney injury, a limited number of common pathways are available for kidney disease progression (6). A general theme of many of these pathways is that adaptive changes in the nephron lead to maladaptive consequences. One of the best developed of these themes is the hyperfiltration that occurs in remaining nephrons after loss of renal mass. Elevated glomerular pressures drive this hyperfiltration. Glomerular hyperfiltration has initial adaptive effects by maintaining GFR, but later may lead to glomerular injury. Abnormal glomerular permeability is common in glomerular disorders, with proteinuria being the clinical consequence. Evidence has accumulated that this proteinuria might be a factor inciting tubulointerstitial disease (6). The extent of tubulointerstitial damage is a prime risk factor for subsequent renal disease progression in all forms of glomerular diseases studied (7). In experimental models and in humans trials, an association has been consistently demonstrated between the reduction of proteinuria and renoprotection.

IV. **Risk factors for progression to ESRD.** The quantity of protein excreted in the urine is one of the strongest predictors of renal disease progression and response to antihypertensive therapy in almost all studies of CKD (8). Thus, the greater the proteinuria, the higher the risk for progression.

As described in the previous section, an important risk factor for most glomerular diseases is the extent of tubulointerstitial disease on renal biopsy (7).

A. **Ethnicity** is a risk factor for many renal diseases. For example, African-American patients with diabetes have a twofold to threefold higher risk for developing ESRD compared with white patients (9). Some of this increased risk is attributable to such modifiable factors as suboptimal health behaviors, suboptimal glucose and BP control, and lower socioeconomic status (9). Human immunodeficiency virus (HIV)-associated nephropathy is also more common in African-American patients compared with white patients.

B. **Gender** is an additional risk factor for the development and progression of certain types of renal disease. Overall, the incidence of ESRD is greater in males than females.

C. **Smoking** has been associated with proteinuria and renal disease progression in both type 1 and 2 diabetes, as well as in IgA nephropathy, lupus nephritis, and polycystic kidney disease. Smoking cessation has been associated with a slower rate of progression of renal failure in type 1 diabetic patients (10).

D. **Finally,** heavy consumption of **non-narcotic analgesics**, particularly phenacetin, has been associated with an increased risk of CKD.

V. **Retarding progression to ESRD**

A. **Anti-hypertensive therapy.** Hypertension is a risk factor for the progression of kidney disease, and it is the second most common cause of ESRD. The opinion of the seventh report of the Joint National Committee (JNC VII) recommended that blood pressure be lowered to levels below 130/80 mm Hg in patients with diabetes or chronic kidney disease (11).

An increasing amount of evidence has demonstrated that the inhibition of the renin-angiotensin system by either inhibiting angiotensin II generation with angiotensin converting enzyme (ACE) inhibitors, or blocking the angiotensin type 1 A receptor with angiotensin receptor blockers (ARBs) has renoprotective effects above and beyond the effects of these therapies on reducing blood pressure.

1. **Studies in patients with diabetic kidney disease with established nephropathy**
   a. **Type 1 diabetic patients with established nephropathy**
      A pronounced benefit of ACE inhibitors in type I diabetics who already had overt nephropathy has been demonstrated in the largest study to date. Four hundred and nine patients with overt proteinuria and a plasma creatinine concentration equal to or greater than 2.5 mg per dL were randomized to therapy with either captopril or placebo. Further antihypertensive drugs were then added as necessary, although calcium channel blockers and other ACE-inhibitors were excluded. At approximately 4 years of nearly equivalent BP control, patients treated with captopril had a slower rate of increase in the plasma creatinine concentration and a lesser likelihood of progressing to ESRD or death (12).
   b. **Type 2 diabetic patients with established nephropathy**
      (1) **The Reduction of Endpoints in type 2 diabetes with the Angiotensin II Antagonist Losartan (RENAAL)** study examined the effects of losartan versus non-ACE inhibitors or ARB antihypertensive therapy in 1,513 patients with type 2 diabetes and nephropathy, followed for a mean of 3.4 years (13). The results of this study demonstrated a beneficial effect of losartan, beyond its effects on lowering BP, on the time to doubling of serum creatinine concentration and onset of ESRD.
      (2) **In the Irbesartan Diabetic Nephropathy Trial (IDNT)**, 1,715 patients with nephropathy secondary to type 2 diabetes were randomly assigned to receive irbesartan, amlodipine, or placebo. The mean duration of follow up was 2.6 years. This study revealed that patients assigned to irbesartan had a 33% reduction of risk for the doubling of serum creatinine compared with placebo and a 37% decrease compared with patients on amlodipine (14).
   c. **Studies in patients with diabetic kidney disease with microalbuminuria**
      (1) **Meta-analysis of published trials.** Diabetic nephropathy trialists have examined 12 selected studies involving 698 patients to compare the effects of ACE inhibitors versus placebo in type 1 diabetic patients with microalbuminuria and normal BP (15). Results showed that ACE inhibitors were more likely associated with regression of microalbuminuria. This effect persisted despite adjustment for any changes in blood pressure.
      (2) **The United Kingdom Prospective Diabetes Study (UKPDS)** examined the efficacy of atenolol and captopril in reducing the risk of both macrovascular and microvascular complications in type 2 diabetic patients with hypertension. This study found that both captopril and atenolol were equivalent in reducing the renal endpoints of progression of albuminuria, overt nephropathy, a twofold increase in serum creatinine, and the development of ESRD (16).
      (3) The Appropriate Blood Pressure Control in Diabetics (**ABCD**) trial was a prospective randomized trial of 950 type 2 diabetic patients examining whether intensive versus moderate BP control affected the incidence of progression of type 2 diabetic complications (17). The hypertensive patients (n = 470) were randomized to intensive BP control (DBP goal of 75 mm Hg) versus moderate blood pressure control (DBP goal of 80 to 89 mm Hg) and

to either nisoldipine or enalapril as the initial antihypertensive medication. Blood pressure control of 138/86 or 132/78 mm Hg with either nisoldipine or enalapril as the initial antihypertensive medication appeared to stabilize renal function in hypertensive type 2 diabetic patients without overt albuminuria over a 5-year period. The enalapril-treated patients had significantly fewer heart attacks than the nisoldipine-treated patients. The more intensive BP control decreased all cause mortality. The effects of intensive versus moderate diastolic BP control were also studied in 480 normotensive type 2 diabetic patients (18). Over a 5-year follow-up period, intensive (approximately 128/75 mm Hg) BP control in normotensive type 2 diabetic patients: (a) slowed the progression to incipient and overt diabetic nephropathy; (b) decreased the progression of diabetic retinopathy; and (c) diminished the incidence of stroke. Cardiovascular events occurred more commonly in the nisoldipine group (19).

(4) The **Heart Outcomes Prevention Evaluation (HOPE)** study included 3,577 people with diabetes (20). Of the patients recruited in the study, 1,120 had microalbuminuria. Patients were randomized to the ACE inhibitor ramipril or placebo. Patients treated with ramipril had a 25% reduction in myocardial infarction, stroke, or cardiovascular death. In the ramipril group, the risk of developing overt nephropathy decreased by 24%.

(5) **Irbesartan Microalbuminuria Study.** The effects of the ARB irbesartan were examined in 590 hypertensive patients with type 2 diabetes and microalbuminuria (21). The primary endpoint was time from baseline visit to the first detection of overt nephropathy. This study revealed that irbesartan had a renoprotective effect independent of its BP lowering effect.

d. **Studies in patients with nondiabetic kidney disease**

(1) The **African-American Study of Kidney Disease and Hypertension (AASK)** was designed to study the effect on progression of hypertensive kidney disease of: (a) two different mean arterial pressure goals usual (MAP: 102 to 107 mm Hg) and lower (MAP: equal to below 92 mm Hg) and (b) treatment with three different antihypertensive drug classes: an ACE inhibitor (ramipril), a dihydropyridine calcium channel blocker (amlodipine), and a betablocker (metoprolol) (22). This study concluded that lowering BP below the achieved 141/85 mm Hg was not associated with added beneficial effects and that ACE inhibitors are more effective antihypertensives in slowing the progression of hypertensive nephrosclerosis.

(2) In the **Ramipril Efficacy in Nephropathy (REIN)** study, patients were stratified before randomization by the level of 24 hour urinary protein, with stratum 1 having 1 or more and less than 3 g per 24 hour proteinuria, and stratum 2 having 3 or more g per 24 hour proteinuria (23). The patients were then randomized to receive ramipril or placebo, with other medications added to achieve a target diastolic blood pressure (DBP) of lower than 90 mm Hg. An analysis of the results of this study demonstrated a beneficial effect of ramipril on slowing GFR decline that was more than expected from the reduction in BP.

The care of diabetic and nondiabetic renal disease has been significantly advanced by this series of controlled trials. The results of these studies clearly demonstrate the renoprotective effects of ACE inhibitors and ARBs in both reducing proteinuria and slowing the progression of renal disease. The effects of these medications may be related to decreases in glomerular capillary pressure or other effects of angiotensin II on fibrosis and growth. These agents should be considered the drugs of first choice in patients with CKD, and the BP goal should be lower than 130/80 mm Hg.

   e. **Combined therapy with ACE inhibitors and ARBs in nondiabetic renal disease**

   (1) **COOPERATE study.** This study was a randomized, double-blind study designed to test the efficacy and safety of combination therapy with an ACE inhibitor (trandolapril) and an angiotensin receptor blocker (losartan), compared with monotherapy with each drug in 263 patients with nondiabetic kidney disease (24). Combination therapy was associated with a marked antiproteinuric effect, and fewer patients reached the combined primary endpoint of time to doubling of serum creatinine or ESRD compared with either of the monotherapy groups.

   f. **Combined therapy with ACE inhibitors and ARBs in diabetic renal disease**

   (1) In the **Candesartan and Lisinopril Microalbuminuria (CALM)** study, the effects of candesartan or lisinopril or both on BP or urinary albumin excretion was examined in patients with microalbuminuria, hypertension, and type 2 diabetes (25).

   Combination therapy reduced BP and albumin excretion more than either agent alone.

   In summary, these studies provide some evidence that combining an ACE inhibitor with an ARB may be more effective than either agent alone in reducing proteinuria and improving renal survival. An increase in adverse events does not appear to exist with combination therapy. However, at present, it is not clear in some studies whether maximizing the dose of either agent is better than the combination or whether the effect of combination therapy is independent of BP reduction.

VI. **Managing complications of chronic kidney disease**

   A. **Anemia.** The anemia of chronic renal failure develops during the course of CKD. The degree of anemia is better evaluated using hemoglobin values rather than hematocrit. A direct correlation exists between the level of hemoglobin and GFR. In the NHANES III data, this association exists at GFR levels of less than 90 mL per minute per 1.73 m^2, but was most marked when the GFR was less than 60 mL per minute (2).The etiology of the anemia of CKD is multifactorial, with the major factor being a decline in erythropoietin synthesis by the kidneys. Anemia is associated with worse outcomes in CKD patients. Low hemoglobin levels have been associated with an increase in cardiovascular morbidity and mortality. The increase in cardiovascular endpoints is likely related to the association between low hemoglobin and increased left ventricular mass index. Hemoglobin has been shown to be one of the most important predictors of left ventricular hypertrophy. In the RENAAL study, after control of BP in type 2 diabetic patients, anemia was recognized as one of the independent risk factors that predicted renal outcomes (26). K/DOQI guidelines recommend patients with CKD be evaluated for anemia when the GFR is less than 60 mL per minute per 1.73 m^2. Erythropoietin levels are not helpful in assessing the anemia of renal disease. The iron status of patients should be assessed, including measurements of serum ferritin, iron, and transferrin saturation (2). Transferrin saturations and ferritin levels should exceed 20% and 100 ng per mL, respectively, to optimize erythropoiesis.Early treatment with erythropoietin (EPO) can prevent severe anemia and may improve the long-term survival of patients with ESRD. The ideal hemoglobin for CKD patients has not been definitively determined. NKF-DOQI guidelines recommend a target hemoglobin of 11 to 12 g per dL.

   B. **Phosphate control.** Phosphate control in CKD is important to preserve the bone mineral content and avoid hyperparathyroidism. Calcium-containing phosphate binders should be instituted when the GFR falls below 30 to 50 mL per minute. The use of vitamin D analogs, primarily 1,25,dihydroxy-vitamin D_3, is more controversial. These analogues can clearly help suppress parathyroid gland overactivity, but often at the expense of higher serum phosphate levels and the risk of hypercalcemia, both of which can worsen extraskeletal calcifications. Recommendations for patients with CKD include (2):

1. Maintain serum phosphorus between 3.0 and 4.6 mg per dL
2. Restrict dietary phosphorus to 800 to 1,000 mg per day when serum phosphorus is greater than 4.6 mg per dL
3. Restrict dietary phosphorus to 800 to 1,000 mg per day when serum levels of intact PTH are greater than 65 mg per mL
4. Monitor serum phosphorus every 3 months if patients are on a phosphorus restricted diet
5. The target range for corrected serum calcium (for every 1 g decrease in serum albumin, the serum calcium should be corrected by 0.8 mg) is 8.8 to 9.5 mg per dL
6. If serum calcium is greater than 10.2 mg per dL, reduce or discontinue vitamin D, and/or switch to a noncalcium-based phosphate binder
7. Serum calcium-phosphorus product should be less than 55 mg^2 per dL^2

C. **Acid-base control.** Acidosis is common in almost all forms of CKD. The main mechanism responsible for the acidosis is a decrease in total ammonia excretion, leading to a decrease net hydrogen secretion and a fall in serum bicarbonate. This net positive acid balance results in dissolution of bone, ultimately worsening uremic osteodystrophy. Other adverse consequences of metabolic acidosis include protein malnutrition and the suppression of albumin synthesis. Early treatment of acidosis with oral bicarbonate therapy may help prevent some of the bone disease of chronic uremia. K/DOQI recommends maintaining a serum bicarbonate level of greater than 22 mEq per L (2). Care must be taken, however, not to precipitate or worsen hypertension with the added sodium intake.

VII. **Managing cardiovascular comorbidity.** Cardiovascular disease remains the most common cause of death in patients with ESRD, and CKD patients are more likely to die from cardiovascular disease than are expected to progress to ESRD. The CKD population has a higher incidence of traditional cardiovascular risk factors, including diabetes, hypertension, and dyslipidemias. In addition, overwhelming scientific evidence has shown that decreased GFR and proteinuria are independent risk factors for cardiovascular disease. Consensus exists in the nephrology community that the CKD population should undergo aggressive risk factor management. This includes strict control of BP and lipids, as well as smoking cessation. K/DOQI clinical practice guidelines on the management of dyslipidemias in CKD have recommended drug therapy for patients with a low-density lipoprotein (LDL) level equal to or greater than 100 mg per dL after 3 months of therapeutic lifestyle changes. Statins are recommended as initial drug therapy for high LDL, and fibrates (e.g., gemfibrozil) are recommended for an elevated fasting triglyceride.

VIII. **When to refer to a nephrologist.** Several studies have shown that delayed referral to a nephrologist is common and is associated with adverse consequences, including greater morbidity and mortality, more severe uremia, increased use of percutaneous vascular access with associated morbidity, reduced use of the preferred arteriovenous fistula for vascular access, restricted patient choice of treatment modality, prolonged and more costly hospitalization at initiation of dialysis, and higher rates of emotional and socioeconomic problems. An early referral allows the patient to develop an effective relationship with a multidisplinary team consisting of a nephrologist, vascular surgeon, nurse, dietitian, social worker, and mental health professional. This relationship allows for a more informed consideration by patients of renal replacement options including transplantation, initiation of renal replacement therapy to maintain optimal patient health, timely placement of a dialysis access, supervision of dietary modification, and support services regarding unmet psychological, social, and financial needs. A nephrologist should participate in the care of patients with a GFR of less than 30 mL per minnute per 1.73 m^2.

References

1. United States Renal Data System. Excerpts from the 2000 U.S. Renal Data System Annual Data Report: Atlas of End Stage Renal Disease in the United States. *Am J Kidney Dis* 2000;36:S1–S279.
2. National Kidney Foundation: K/DOQI Clinical Practice Guidelines for Chronic Kidney Disease: evaluation, classification, and stratification. *Am J Kidney Dis* 2002;39 (Suppl 1):S1–S266.
3. Shemesh O, Golbetz H, Kriss JP, Myers BD. Limitations of creatinine as a filtration marker in glomerulopathic patients. *Kidney Int* 1985;28:830–838.
4. Cockcroft DW, Gault MH. Prediction of creatinine clearance from serum creatinine. *Nephron* 1976;16:31–41.
5. Jones C GM, Kusek JW, et al. Serum creatinine levels in the US population: Third National Health and Nutrition Examination Survey. *Am J Kidney Disease* 1998;32:992–999.
6. Remuzzi G, Bertani T. Pathophysiology of progressive nephropathies. *N Engl J Med* 1998;339:1448–1456.
7. Nath K. The tubulointerstitium in progressive renal disease. *Kidney Int* 1998;54:992–994.
8. Keane W. Proteinuria: its clinical importance and role in progressive renal disease. *Am J Kidney Dis* 2000;35:S97–S105.
9. Krop J, Coresh J, Chambless L, et al. A community-based study of explanatory factors for the excess risk for early renal function decline in blacks vs. whites with diabetes. *Arch Intern Med* 1999;159:1777–1783.
10. Orth SR, Ritz E, Schrier RW. The renal risks of smoking. *Kidney Int* 2003;51:1669–1677.
11. The JNC 7 Report. *JAMA* 2003;289:2560–2572.
12. Lewis EJ, et al. Effect of ACE inhibition on nephropathy in type 1 diabetes. *N Engl J Med* 1993;329:1456–1462.
13. Brenner BM, Cooper ME, De Zeeuw D, et al. Effects of losartan on renal and cardiovascular outcomes in patients with type 2 diabetes and nephropathy. *N Engl J Med* 2001;345:861–869.
14. Lewis EJ, Hunsiker LG, Clarke WR, et al. Renoprotective effect of the angiotensin receptor antagonist irbesartan in patients with nephropathy due to type 2 diabetes. *N Engl J Med* 2001;345:851–860.
15. Kshirsagar AV, Joy MS, Hogan SL, et al. Effect of ACE inhibitors in diabetic and nondiabetic chronic renal disease: a systematic overview of randomized placebo-controlled trials. *Am J Kidney Dis* 2000;35:695–707.
16. UK Prospective Diabetes Study Group. Efficacy of atenolol and captopril in reducng risk of macrovascular and microvascular complications in type 2 diabetes: UKPDS 39. *Br Med J* 1998;317:713–720.
17. Estacio R, Jeffers B, Gifford N, Schrier RW. Effect of blood pressure control on diabetic microvascular complications in patients with hypertension and type 2 diabetes. *Diabetes Care* 2000;23 suppl 2:B54–64.
18. Schrier RW, Estacio R, Esler A, Mehler P. Effect of aggressive blood pressure control in normotensive type 2 diabetic patients on albuminuria, retinopathy and strokes. *Kidney Int* 2002;61:1086–1097.
19. Estacio R, Jeffers B, Gifford N, et al. Effect of blood pressure control on diabetic microvascular complications in patients with hypertension and type 2 diabetes. *N Engl J Med* 1998;338:645–652.
20. Mann JF, Gestein H, Pogue J, et al. Renal insufficiency as a predictor of cardiovascular outcomes and the impact of ramipril: the HOPE randomized trial. *Ann Int Med* 2001;134:629–636.

21. Parving HH, Lehnert H, Brochner-Mortensen J, et al. The effect of irbesartan on the development of diabetic nephropathy in patients with type 2 diabetes. *N Engl J Med* 2001;345:870–878.
22. Wright JT, Bakris G, Greene T, et al. Effect of blood pressure lowering and antihypertensive drug class on progression of hypertensive kidney disease. Results from the AASK Trial. *JAMA* 2002;288:2421–2431.
23. The GISEN Group: randomized placebo-controlled trial of effect of ramipril on decline in glomerular filtration rate and risk of terminal renal failure in proteinuric, non-diabetic nephropathy. *Lancet* 1997;349:1857–1863.
24. Nakao N, Yoshimura A, Morita H, et al. Combination treatment of angiotensin II receptor blocker and angiotensin-converting enzyme inhibitor in non-diabetic renal disease (COOPERATE): a randomized controlled trial. *Lancet* 2003;361:117–124.
25. Mogensen CE, Neldam S, Tikkanen I, et al. Randomized controlled trial of dual blockade of renin-angiotensin system in patients with hypertension, microalbuminuria, and non-insulin dependent diabetes: the candesatan and lisinopril microalbuminuria (CALM) study. *Br Med J* 2000;321:1440–1444.
26. Keane WF, Brenner BM, de Zeeuw D, et al. The risk of developing end stage renal disease in patients with type 2 diabetes and nephropathy: the RENAAL study. *Kidney Int* 2003;63:1499–1507.

The Patient Receiving Chronic Renal Replacement with Dialysis

David M. Spiegel

The number of individuals kept alive by dialysis therapy in the United States continues to increase each year. This life-prolonging therapy continues to make end stage kidney failure the only major organ system failure that does not result in certain death without organ transplantation. However, the morbidity and mortality associated with end stage kidney disease (ESRD) remains high. Increased understanding of the disease process, new insights into pathogenic mechanisms, and new therapeutic options are emerging that may improve survival rates and quality of life for patients with ESRD.

I. **The need for renal replacement therapy (RRT).** RRT is required when kidney function deteriorates to the point where the accumulation of waste products begins to interfere with life functions. As kidney function deteriorates, a number of physiologic alterations occur, many of which are ultimately detrimental. Renal replacement therapy is indicated when these changes can no longer be controlled by medications and diet, or when the accumulation of waste products starts to interfere with life functions. The progressive deterioration of kidney function through end stage kidney failure has been defined as chronic kidney disease (CKD). Appropriate care designed to slow the progression of CKD, control factors known to contribute to the morbidity and mortality of kidney failure, and appropriate preparation for RRT during the stages of CKD ensures that patients are in the best overall condition at the time they start dialysis. (See Chapter 11.)

II. **Preparing for RRT**

   A. **Access creation.** Preparation for dialysis therapy is critical for the smooth transition from CKD care to RRT. Poor planning for RRT is a major cause of increased morbidity and mortality at the initiation of dialysis therapy. The use of temporary or tunneled dialysis catheters contributes to dialysis mortality by increasing the incidence of sepsis, acting as a stimulus for chronic inflammation, and damaging the central veins, thereby preventing or shortening the survival of more permanent vascular access once created.

   1. **Hemodialysis (HD).** Permanent access for HD requires either a native arterial-venous fistula (AVF) or an artificial AV graft. Both types of accesses are placed surgically. Native AVFs are always preferable to artificial grafts, because they have a significantly lower incidence of infection and a longer event-free survival. Vein mapping by ultrasound or venography may increase the likelihood of successful AVF placement by identifying suitable veins for access creation. In ideal candidates, an AVF may mature in as little as 4 weeks. However, in patients with less than ideal veins, AVFs can take 6 months or longer to mature. Therefore, access planning should start 6 to 12 months before dialysis is anticipated. As a general rule, the longer an AVF matures prior to first use, the better the chances for long-term success. For artificial grafts, surgery should be performed 4 to 6 weeks before the anticipated start of dialysis. Usually the access is placed in the nondominant arm, in the most distal position available.

   2. **Peritoneal dialysis (PD).** PD catheters are surgically inserted into the peritoneal cavity. Several types of catheters are now available and the time from placement to first use may vary greatly. Most nephrologists allow 7 to 10 days before using a catheter that is externalized at the

time of implantation. Many PD catheters are left in a subcutaneous tunnel for several months before being externalized. This option may allow better in-growth of the catheter in a sterile environment and allows for externalization at the time of training.

III. **Modality selection.** Current evidence suggests that both PD and HD provide equal RRT for most patients. Modality selection should be based on patient preference, which is largely related to lifestyle decisions. Proper education, starting early in the course of CKD, is the best means of ensuring that patients are able to make rational and educated decisions.

A. **Hemodialysis**

1. **In-center HD.** The largest percentages of dialysis patients in the United States are dialyzed via this modality. As a general rule, patients dialyze on a 3 times per week basis for approximate 4 hours each session. At the beginning and throughout the treatment, vital signs are measured. Two needles are placed in the AVF or graft so that blood can be circulated through the artificial kidney at a rate of 300 to 500 mL per minute. Excess fluid is removed by a transmembrane pressure gradient, while toxins are removed by diffusion down their concentration gradient. At the end of the treatment, the needles are removed and bleeding stopped by the application of local pressure. Although most patients participate very little in their actual dialysis care, some facilities promote "self-care," where in patients actively participate by taking their blood pressure (BP), responding to machine alarms, and even performing needle placement.

2. **Home HD.** The number of patients on home HD in the United States remains small. Traditionally, this therapy has required a partner to help with the treatment, especially in emergencies. However, newer machines designed for home use are making it possible for some patients without partners to receive the benefits of home HD. The average training time before patients are able to perform HD at home is about 6 weeks. Once trained, patients generally do quite well, having the lowest mortality rate of any group of U.S. dialysis patients. Part of this low mortality may be related to patient selection, since traditionally only the healthiest patients were selected for home HD.

3. **New HD therapies.** Emerging HD therapies offer some advantages over current treatment and may ultimately improve the quality of life of dialysis patients, along with increasing survival. These therapies include daily home HD, nocturnal HD, and daily in-center HD. In both daily home and daily in-center HD, patients dialyze 2 to 3 hours, 6 days per week. Nocturnal dialysis is typically 6 to 8 hours, 6 days per week, although fewer treatments per week are being studied. In all these therapies, the advantages are that patients dialyze more frequently and achieve higher clearances than with traditional HD. The increased dialysis frequency allows for better fluid and BP control. Noncontrolled trials also suggest that patients feel better, experience a higher quality of life, and are more socially adjusted. Some studies have found a reduced requirement for erythropoeitin, although this has not been universal. Patients on nocturnal HD generally have greatly reduced need for phosphate binders (see **IV.A.6.c.(3)**). Although these therapies are more expensive than traditional HD, emerging evidence suggests that the total cost of patient care may be decreased, because patients on these more frequent therapies have a decreased need for supplemental medications and experience fewer hospitalizations.

B. **Peritoneal dialysis**

1. **Continuous ambulatory PD (CAPD),** along with automated PD (APD) accounts for 15% to 18% of all dialysis in the United States. With this dialysis modality the semi-permeable lining of the peritoneal cavity is used as a dialysis membrane such that toxins diffuse out of the blood into a sterile dialysate fluid that has been instilled into the abdominal

cavity. The process of draining out the old PD dialysate and instilling fresh dialysate into the peritoneal cavity is referred to as an exchange. As patients perform the PD exchanges at home, PD allows patients a more flexible schedule than HD, because the exchanges can be done around most schedules. Another advantage of PD is that patients in remote areas do not have to travel to a dialysis center.

   2. APD uses a machine to perform the dialysis exchanges, usually overnight, thus allowing patients greater daytime flexibility. This is especially useful for people in school or young children.

IV. Renal replacement therapy. The appropriate time to initiate dialysis for a patient cannot be clearly defined. Most nephrologists base their decision upon clinical laboratory data and a subjective patient assessment. By the time the glomerular filtration rate (GFR) falls below 10 mL per minute, most patients require dialytic intervention. However, many patients appear to function quite well until the GFR approaches 5 mL per minute. As a general rule, patients with diabetes require earlier intervention (GFR less than 15 mL per minute) than do those with other etiologies for their renal failure. Clearly, dialysis must be initiated before the uremic symptoms of peripheral neuropathy, encephalopathy, malnutrition, or serositis (including pericarditis) become evident. Although many of these complications resolve with adequate dialysis, peripheral neuropathy and malnutrition may be exceedingly difficult to reverse. Some nephrologists believe that early initiation with dialysis may improve long-term outcome, although this has not been shown to be true.

A. Hemodialysis

   1. Technical aspects. Although the basic principles of HD (diffusion-based mass transfer of solute and pressure gradient–driven water removal) have not changed a great deal in the last 20 years, the technology has dramatically improved. Most patients dialyze three times per week. For each treatment, two large-bore needles are inserted into the vascular access for removal and return of blood. The patient must remain confined to their dialysis machine for the duration of the treatment. Today, most dialysis units use volumetric machines designed to remove a precise amount of fluid. These volumetric machines permit the use of larger, highly porous dialyzers with high water and solute permeability. This new design not only allows for significantly more removal of larger molecules than older dialyzers, but also increases the efficiency of urea removal.

   2. Adequacy. What constitutes optimal HD remains controversial. Urea kinetic modeling is a useful tool to quantify dialysis and thereby prevent underdialysis. Care must be taken to ensure that the modeling is based on delivered dialysis. Additionally, as dialysis times are shortened, plasma urea rebound due to delayed intercompartmental shifts must be considered. Currently, a delivered dialysis dose, as measured by a urea removal, of less than 65% or a Kt/V (where K equals the dialyzer clearance of urea, t is the treatment time, and V is the urea volume of distribution) of less than 1.2 is considered inadequate (1). To ensure adequate dialysis, the recommended targets have been set at a URR of greater than or equal to 70% [$URR = 100 \times (1 - C_t/C_0)$, where C_t is the postdialysis BUN and C_0 is the pre-dialysis BUN] or a K_t/V of greater than or equal to 1.3 (determined by formal urea kinetic modeling or the Kt/V natural logarithm formula (1).

   3. Blood pressure control. Cardiovascular mortality remains the leading cause of death in ESRD patients. Whereas the condition of patients at the time they start dialysis clearly plays a role in their long-term outcome, optimal BP control while on dialysis remains critical. The timing of BP determination in HD patients is controversial. Most patients experience a fall in BP during their dialysis treatment, often correlated with the amount of fluid removed. Therefore, post-dialysis BP is usually lower than pre-dialysis BP. In most studies that have closely evaluated BP in dialysis patients, it is clear that within 8 to 12 hours post-dialysis, BP has returned to pre-dialysis levels. It is therefore generally recommended that of the two, the pre-dialysis BP better reflects overall hypertensive risk. However, due to the fall in BP with dialysis, it is generally accepted that a slightly higher than normal BP be accepted for patients pre-dialysis. Although there are no definitive studies, and the topic remains controversial, many nephrologists aim for a pre-dialysis target of less 140 to 160/95 mm Hg.

In the United States, 50% to 80% of dialysis patients are receiving antihypertensive therapy. Some evidence suggests that many of these patients could have their BP adequately controlled without or with significantly less antihypertensive medications if adequate dialysis was provided along with vigilant control of fluid volume. Although all antihypertensive medications except diuretics are available to treat dialysis patients, the use of both angiotensin converting enzyme (ACE) inhibitors and beta-blockers are increasing due to their cardioprotective advantage. Carvedilol has recently been shown to decrease mortality in a prospective study of dialysis patients with dilated cardiomyopathy (2).

4. **Anemia.** Anemia occurs in most dialysis patients and almost certainly contributes to cardiac hypertrophy. Studies have shown that the anemia of ESRD is largely due to a deficiency of erythropoietin (EPO) and can be corrected by administration of exogenous EPO. Initial doses usually range from 120 to 180 units per kg per week intravenously, or 80 to 120 units per kg per week subcutaneously (1). Dose adjustments are then made on a monthly or every-other-week basis. Adequate iron stores are also required. The correction of anemia in dialysis patients has been shown to improve patients' quality of life and exercise physiology. Short-term studies have shown a decrease in cardiac hypertrophy when the anemia of CRF was partially corrected. As with hypertension, some data suggest that adequate dialysis is associated with improved hemoglobin values and a decreased EPO requirement. The optimal level of hemoglobin for dialysis patients remains to be determined. Clear survival benefits have been achieved by increasing the hemoglobin to greater than 11 gm per dL. Some retrospective studies suggest that improved survival can be achieved by hemoglobin levels in the normal range. However, one prospective randomized trial was stopped early due to failure to show improved benefit in a large group of dialysis patients with underlying heart disease whose hemoglobin values were normalized (3). A smaller European randomized trial showed no difference in survival between patients with hemoglobin values maintained between 11 to 12 and 13 to 14 mg per dL in patients without heart disease (4).

5. **Rehabilitation and psychosocial adjustment.** When compared to the normal U.S. population, patients on HD have a much lower employment rate and a much higher percentage of disability recipients. Efforts to improve these figures through vocational rehabilitation have been only marginally successful. However, on quality of life questionnaires, most HD patients rate their quality of life only slightly below the general population. Despite their overall high self-rating on quality of life questionnaires, many dialysis patients suffer from depression and anxiety disorders. A social worker is a critical member of all dialysis facility teams and can play a vital role in helping patients adjust to dialysis and deal with feelings of depression and anxiety.

6. **Complications.** Despite its life-saving nature, HD remains a poor substitute for normal renal function and is fraught with a number of complications, both technical and secondary to kidney failure itself.

   a. **Technical complications**

      (1) **Vascular access.** Despite recent advances, vascular access remains the Achilles heel of HD. Although some arteriovenous fistulas last 5 to 20 years, many patients have poor native vessels and

therefore have shortened AVF survival rates. These patients often must rely on artificial grafts, which are predisposed to thrombosis, pseudoaneurysm formation, and infection. The average survival of new grafts is about 2 years. Early intervention for failing grafts, along with new radiologic techniques, has improved the average survival rate (5). Intervention can take several forms, including the measurement of static or dynamic venous pressures or indirect measures of access blood flow rate.

(2) **Hypotension.** Despite improvements in dialysis equipment, hypotension remains a common problem during HD. Use of bicarbonate dialysate, higher dialysate sodium concentrations, and volumetric machines have helped to decrease its frequency. However, hypotension continues to occur for a number of reasons including autonomic insufficiency, rapid ultrafiltration (fluid removal) that exceeds the rate of vascular refilling, or myocardial dysfunction.

(3) **Allergic reactions.** These can occur to the dialyzer material or the sterilant. They can range from mild itching to anaphylaxis.

(4) **Other.** Air embolism, ruptured dialyzer, improper dialysate mixture, or failures of the water purification system are a cause of rare but often life-threatening complications. Care and proper maintenance of dialysis machines and water treatment facilities, with special attention to the dialysis technique and to the safety and alarm mechanisms, help prevent these complications.

b. **Complications associated with inadequate dialysis**

(1) **Uremic pericarditis.** Although often thought of as a pre-dialysis problem, occasionally HD patients develop pericarditis. This often occurs in the setting of an acute illness, catabolic states, or at a time of vascular access difficulty, resulting in inadequate dialysis.

(2) **Uremic neuropathy.** This complication is often overlooked by many nephrologists, because it is generally a peripheral neuropathy starting in the feet or hands. It must be differentiated from diabetic neuropathy, which is common in the dialysis population. Because the two conditions can co-exist, chronic inadequate dialysis must considered as a possible cause for any peripheral neuropathy.

c. **Long-term complications**

(1) **Cardiovascular.** Cardiovascular death remains the major cause of mortality in patients with ESRD. Many factors contribute, including hypertension, anemia, smoking, hypercholesterolemia, and the presence of an arteriovenous shunt. Most of these factors are present long before the development of ESRD. Although the aggressive treatment of these risk factors seems prudent, good clinical studies in ESRD patients are lacking. New evidence shows that kidney failure, and possibly the abnormal mineral metabolism that results, increases the deposition of calcium in the media of blood vessels in patients. This calcium deposition appears to be an active process, much like the calcium deposition in bone. This medial vascular calcification has been associated with increased mortality presumably due to alterations in normal vascular physiology. Typical findings in patients with excessive vascular calcification are a widened pulse pressure and linear calcium deposition on plain films. In patients on dialysis, evidence of cardiac dysfunction and vascular calcification predict poor outcome (6,7).

(2) **Infectious.** Infections remain a common cause of morbidity and mortality in HD patients. Infection of temporary catheters and artificial AV grafts are common. When they become infected, temporary catheters generally must be removed. Evidence suggests that changing the catheter over a guidewire, along with antibiotic therapy, may allow for resolution of the infection. Staphylococcal organisms remain the most common, followed by other gram-positive

bacteria. Work on a staphylococcal vaccine for dialysis patients is ongoing. Endocarditis is a very serious complication that may result from a catheter or graft infection. Native vein fistulas have a lower infection rate than all forms of temporary or artificial graft material and are the access of first choice. In addition to the vascular access as a route of infection, improper reprocessing of dialyzers can lead to sepsis, often from waterborne organisms.

(3) **Bone disease.** Bone disease is common in long-term dialysis patients. The morphology of the bone pathology has changed over the past 10 years. Hyperparathyroid bone disease (i.e., osteitis fibrosa), remains the most common. It results from overactivity of the parathyroid glands as a result of hyperphosphatemia and low 1,25-vitamin D_3 levels. Rapid bone turnover, increased osteoclastic activity, and ultimately fibrosis of the marrow space characterize this bone disease. It can be mild to severe, pure or mixed with aluminum (Al) bone disease. Aluminum is directly toxic to bone. Dialysis patients can acquire Al either through oral Al-containing phosphate binders or via a contaminated water supply. It accumulates due to lack of renal excretion and deposits at the mineralization front of growing or remodeling bone. This impairs bone mineralization and leads to a condition of weakened bone with increased unmineralized matrix or osteoid (osteomalacia). A histologic pattern increasingly found in bone biopsies from dialysis patients has been termed adynamic bone. This bone is characterized by very low bone turnover with few osteoblasts or osteoclasts. Whereas severe hyperparathyroidism can cause hypercalcemia, both adynamic and Al bone disease also predispose patients to hypercalcemia. Treatment for the abnormalities of mineral metabolism in ESRD has traditionally been limited to oral phosphate binders and intravenous or oral vitamin D preparations. The recent cloning of the calcium sensing receptor has allowed for a new class of therapeutic agents called calcimimetics. These small organic compounds bind to the calcium sensing receptor and modify its affinity for calcium. Through a second intracellular messenger, the net effect is a reduction in parathyroid hormone release (8). Work is ongoing in an attempt to determine whether the abnormalities in bone mineral metabolism or the current treatment of bone disease are linked in any way to the abnormal vascular calcification seen in dialysis patients. A final form of bone and osteoarticular disease seen in long-term dialysis patients is beta-2-microglobulin (β_2M) amyloidosis. β_2M is a small protein that accumulates in the blood of dialysis patients and precipitates at osteoarticular surfaces to form amyloid. Symptoms include pain, swelling, bone cysts, and fractures. Recent data suggest that highly permeable dialysis membranes may delay the onset of disease symptoms.

(4) **Malnutrition inflammation syndrome.** Large-scale studies have demonstrated that the nutritional state of a dialysis patient, as measured by the serum albumin, has a major impact on their long-term survival. Traditionally, it was believed that a low albumin reflected inadequate protein and calorie intake to maintain lean body mass. Whereas some patients do suffer from true malnutrition, it is now recognized that albumin is an important inverse acute phase reactant, and the utility of a low serum albumin as a marker of mortality probably reflects in large part the presence of an active inflammatory process rather than specific nutritional deficiencies. Although the cause of the chronic inflammation is evident in some patients, in many patients a clearly identifiable cause cannot be found. The finding of a low serum albumin

and elevated levels of inflammatory markers has been termed the malnutrition-inflammation syndrome. Identifying and correcting reversible causes of both inflammation and malnutrition is essential to maintaining optimal health in patients with ESRD.

(5) **Skin disorders.** Pruritus remains one of the most troubling complaints of dialysis patients. Causes include an elevated calcium-phosphorus product, dry skin, and hyperparathyroidism. Some relief may be achieved with antihistamines and phosphate control. In severe cases, treatment with ultraviolet (UV) light has been effective. Other skin conditions in dialysis patients include bullous dermatitis and porphyria cutanea tarda.

(6) **Acquired renal cystic disease.** Many patients undergoing maintenance dialysis develop cysts in their native kidneys that tend to increase in size and number over time. Although these cysts are generally an incidental finding, complications have been reported including polycythemia, spontaneous rupture, and retroperitoneal bleeding. Dialysis patients with acquired renal cystic disease appear to have a 100-fold increase in the incidence of renal cell carcinoma. However, deaths from renal cancer remains uncommon in the ESRD population, and routine screening has not been advocated due to the high rate of false positive studies that might lead to unnecessary surgery in this high-risk population. Patients with hematuria, flank pain, or abnormal weight loss should be evaluated.

B. Peritoneal dialysis

1. **Technical aspects.** Technically, PD is much less complex than HD. A sterile electrolyte and dextrose solution (dialysate) is allowed to flow into the peritoneal cavity through a previously implanted catheter using gravity or via a low-pressure pump. Following a specified period (dwell time), the fluid is drained out of the peritoneal cavity and fresh fluid is again infused. The peritoneal lining acts as the semi-permeable membrane across which diffusion occurs. The process of fluid infusion and drainage (exchanges) can be performed manually (CAPD) or by a machine (APD). A new, nondextrose dialysate solution is now available in the United States. Its advantages include a long duration of osmotic activity due to its poor peritoneal transport and the lack of a glucose load to the patient that occurs when the dextrose in traditional PD fluid is absorbed across the peritoneal membrane (9).

2. **Adequacy.** Because the quantity of PD that can be delivered is limited by the fixed peritoneal membrane kinetics and the amount of dialysate that can be comfortably infused and carried, it seems prudent to deliver as much dialysis as is reasonably possible. For many patients on PD, residual kidney function plays a vital role in their ability to achieve adequate creatinine clearances. Many experts have advocated minimum targets for creatinine clearance of 50 L per week per 1.73 m^2 for patients with low peritoneal membrane transport rates, and 60 L per week per 1.73 m^2 for patients with more rapid transport rates. Urea clearance is less affected by residual renal function, the K_t/V urea of 2.0 has been advocated for all CAPD patients (1).

3. **Blood pressure control.** As in HD, BP control is important for the long-term well being of PD patients. Many patients on PD are able to discontinue their antihypertensives and maintain a normal BP. This may be attributable to the steady-state volume control achieved by this continuous dialysis modality.

4. **Anemia.** Correction of anemia using EPO is important in improving the quality of life for PD patients. EPO is generally administered subcutaneously in PD patients. Adequate correction of anemia can generally be achieved with once or twice weekly injections. The lower overall dose of

EPO needed to correct the anemia in PD patients, compared with HD patients, reflects the difference in routes of administration (subcutaneous is more effective than intravenous) and the small ongoing blood losses in HD patients.

5. **Nutritional aspects.** Nutrition is critically important in PD patients. Protein requirements for PD patients are considered to be slightly higher than for HD patients due to the ongoing loss of protein in the spent dialysate. Many patients on PD gain weight over the first 1 year to 18 months. This phenomenon probably results from an increase in fat mass due to excess calorie intake, part of which comes from the high glucose content of the peritoneal dialysate solution. However, long-term PD patients, like HD patients, tend to lose lean body mass. It is unclear how this relates to the adequacy of PD or to underlying inflammatory processes.

6. **Rehabilitation and psychosocial adjustment.** Although PD allows individual patients more control over their health care and a more flexible dialysis schedule, the percent of PD patients in the work force and the percent on disability are no different from those on HD. On quality of life questionnaires, PD patients as a group rate their quality of life about the same as HD patients. Unfortunately, no prospective studies are available, and the variability in patient selection is certainly a major factor in these outcomes.

7. **Complications.** As in HD, PD has a number of associated complications. They can be divided into infectious and long-term complications. However, unlike HD, inadequate PD tends to result in malnutrition and technique failure, with pericarditis and peripheral neuropathy being less common, although they do occur.

   a. **Infectious.** Peritonitis remains the most frequent complication of PD. Technical improvements, including disconnect "flush before fill" systems, have reduced the peritonitis rates in most centers. Most episodes of peritonitis are treatable in the outpatient setting; however, severe infections require hospitalization and occasionally catheter removal. This is particularly true when peritonitis is caused by a fungal infection or *Pseudomonas aeruginosa*. Exit site infections are also common in PD and usually result from gram-positive organisms. These infections can generally be treated with antibiotics and increased local care. However, some infections, particularly those secondary to *Staphylococcus aureus* may require catheter removal. Although no consensus on proper exit site care has emerged, most experts agree that the catheter should exit the skin in a downward direction. Tunnel infections usually result from exit site infections and are frequently caused by *S. aureus*. Early diagnosis is often difficult. An episode of peritonitis, with the same organism causing an exit site infection, may be the presenting symptoms. In some centers, ultrasound has been useful in detecting the fluid around the subcutaneous tunnel that indicates a tunnel infection. Tunnel infections usually necessitate catheter removal.

   b. **Long-term complications.** Although acute hemodynamic complications are less frequent with PD due to the continuous nature of the technique, cardiovascular disease remains the most common cause of death. Aggressive treatment of lipid abnormalities seems warranted, although outcome studies are not available. Renal osteodystrophy also occurs in PD patients. The morphology is similar to that seen in HD patients, with a slightly higher incidence of adynamic bone disease. $\beta_2 M$ amyloid also occurs in PD patients, although theoretically its onset may be delayed due to the higher clearance of $\beta_2 M$ by the peritoneal membrane when compared to conventional HD. Acquired renal cystic disease and renal cell cancer appear to have the same increased incidence in PD as in HD. A number of long-term complications are unique to PD. These include a leak of PD fluid from the peritoneal space to either the pleural space or into the subcutaneous tissues, resulting in either pleural effusions or hernias, respectively. Sclerosing peritonitis resulting in ultrafiltration failure is an uncommon complication of PD; when it occurs, it is usually in the setting of repeated episodes of peritonitis. A much more common cause of failure of patients on PD is a gradual loss of residual renal function that results in a fall in total clearance, often leading to inadequate dialysis.

V. **Mortality.** Despite major advances in renal transplantation and the technology of HD and PD, the diagnosis of ESRD carries an increased mortality compared to age-matched controls. Whereas much of the increased mortality can be related to the underlying medical conditions that resulted in renal failure, some can be directly attributable to the current practice of dialysis and transplantation. Dialysis in any form provides only a very small percent of the clearance achieved by the normal kidneys. Although the hormones produced by the normal kidney, such as erythropoietin and 1,25-dihydroxy vitamin D_3 and its analogues, have been available for some time, their optimal use remains to be determined. The appropriate target hemoglobin remains unknown, as does the optimal use of vitamin D analogues and the new calcimimetic agent.

A. **Hemodialysis versus peritoneal dialysis.** In the United States, the gross annual mortality among dialysis patients is about 20% to 22%. This figure is 25% to 50% higher than that reported in much of Europe and Japan, and has raised questions about the delivery of dialysis in this country. However, differences in case mix remain a large confounding variable. The risk of death is higher for patients with diabetes as well as those with increasing age. For all age and race groups, the life expectancy on dialysis is significantly shorter than that of the general population. As an example, a white man in the United States, at age 45, has a life expectancy of 32 years compared to white male dialysis patients, whose life expectancy is about 7.4 years. For a black woman, the numbers are similar: normal population 33 years versus dialysis patient 8.4 years (10). However, most studies comparing survival on HD versus PD have found little difference in overall mortality.

B. **Dialysis versus transplantation.** There is no doubt that a successful renal transplant improves an individual's quality of life and rehabilitation potential. For diabetic patients and the young, renal transplantation also significantly increases the average life expectancy of those with ESRD.

References

1. *NKF-K/DOQI Clinical Practice Guidelines.* 2000 Update. New York: National Kidney Foundation, Inc., 2001.
2. Cice G, Ferrara L, D'Andrea A, D'Isa S, et al. Carvedilol increases two-year survival in dialysis patients with dilated cardiomyopathy: a prospective, placebo-controlled trial. *J Am Coll Cardiol* 2003;May 7;41(9):1438–1444.
3. Besarab A, Bolton WK, Browne JK, Egrie JC, et al. The effects of normal as compared with low hematocrit values in patients with cardiac disease who are receiving hemodialysis and epoetin. *N Engl J Med* 1998;339:584–590.
4. Furuland H, Linde T, Ahlmen J, Christensson A, Strombom U, Danielson BG. A randomized controlled trial of haemoglobin normalization with epoetin alfa in pre-dialysis and dialysis patients. *Nephrol Dial Transplant* 2003; Feb;18(2):353–361.
5. Schwab SJ, Raymond JR, Saeed M, Newman GE, Dennis PA, Bollinger RR: Prevention of hemodialysis fistula thrombosis. Early detection of venous stenoses. *Kidney Int* 1989;36:707–711.
6. Foley RN, Parfrey PS, Harnett JD. Left ventricular hypertrophy in dialysis patients. *Sem Dialysis* 1992;5:34–41.
7. Blacher J, Guerin AP, Pannier B, Marchais SJ, London GM. Arterial calcifications, arterial stiffness, and cardiovascular risk in end stage renal disease. *Hypertension* 2001;38:938–942.

8. Lindberg JL, Moe SM, Goodman WG, Coburn JW, et al. The calcimimetic AMG 073 reduces parathyroid hormone and calcium X phosphorus in secondary hyperparathyroidism. *Kidney Int* 2003;63:248–254.

9. Davies SJ, Woodrow G, Donovan K, Plum J, et al. Icodextrin improves the fluid status of peritoneal dialysis patients: results of a double-blind randomized controlled trial. *J Am Soc Nephrol* 2003; Sep;14(9):2338–2344.

10. U.S. Renal Data System. USRDS 2003 Annual Data Report: Atlas of End-Stage Renal Disease in the United States, Bethesda, MD.: National Institutes of Health, National Institute of Diabetes and Digestive and Kidney Diseases, 2003.

The Patient with Renal Transplantation

Eric Gibney, Chirag Parikh, and Alkesh Jani

I. **Introduction and epidemiology.** The prevalence of end stage renal disease (ESRD) in the United States and developed nations continues to increase at an alarming rate. In the year 2000, there were more than 375,000 U.S. patients with ESRD. Currently, hemodialysis (HD), peritoneal dialysis (PD), and renal transplantation are the only available therapies for ESRD, with in-center HD being the most common. Comparisons of renal transplant recipients to dialysis patients awaiting kidney transplant have shown that renal transplantation, in most cases, is the ideal treatment of ESRD. Advantages include longer patient survival, less morbidity, cost savings, and improved quality of life compared with dialysis. Furthermore, substantial improvement has occurred in both short- and long-term graft survival, which can be expected to widen the advantage of transplantation over HD. The life expectancy for the average living donor kidney has now exceeded 20 years. This good news is tempered by the reality that demand for transplant kidneys far exceeds the supply of available organs. The waiting list for kidney transplants is over 56,000 as of December 2003. Currently, less than 15,000 kidney transplants are performed each year, and this number is growing less rapidly than the waiting list. Due to the high morbidity and mortality associated with ESRD, the unfortunate outcome is that many patients die before receiving a transplant.

II. **Patient selection.** Few contraindications to receiving a kidney transplant exist. However, patients should not receive a transplant if they have an active infection, ongoing active immunologic disease that led to renal failure, metastatic malignancy, inability to follow a medical regimen due to medical or psychologic reasons, or are at high operative risk due to other conditions. Although there is no definite age limit to receive a kidney transplant, the benefits of transplantation may be attenuated by comorbid conditions. Therefore, elderly patients should be screened thoroughly and counseled regarding the risks of transplantation. Human immunodeficiency virus (HIV) infection has historically been a contraindication to transplantation, but successful kidney transplantation has occurred in patients free of opportunistic infections with undetectable viral replication and sustained CD4 counts of greater than 200.

A. **Recipient evaluation.** The goals of evaluating a potential recipient should be to identify potential barriers to transplantation, identify treatable conditions that would attenuate the risk of the operation or immunosuppression, and to explain benefits and risks. Attention is given to the cause of ESRD and its tendency to recur in renal transplants. Comorbid conditions and the effects of immunosuppression on these conditions are considered. Patient older than 50, diabetes, abnormal electrocardiogram, angina, or congestive heart failure (CHF) have been demonstrated as predictors of cardiac death and nonfatal cardiac events. Noninvasive strategies such as thallium perfusion imaging and dobuatmine stress echo have demonstrated the ability to predict cardiac events and may prevent high-risk patients from requiring angiography. Screening for malignancy should follow age-appropriate guidelines. In patients with malignancies, a 2 to 5 year remission may be required before transplantation, depending on tumor type and invasiveness. Although obesity is a risk for wound-related complications, long-term outcomes are similar to nonobese patients unless cardiovascular disease exists. Psychosocial screening is usually performed. Testing generally includes evaluation for HIV and Hepatitis B and C. Imaging or functional evaluation of the kidneys and lower urinary tract may be necessary in certain patients. After a patient has been accepted as a candidate, ABO and human leucocyte antigen (HLA) typing is performed, along with a determination of serologic status for cytomegalovirus (CMV) and varicella. The candidate's blood is also screened with a panel reactive antibody test (PRA) for cytotoxic antibodies against common HLA antigens. A patient on the waiting list for longer than 1 year should be seen periodically to update their condition.

  B. Donor evaluation. Although the risks of donation are small, these risks need to be carefully explained to a potential **living donor.** Mortality is uncommon, but has occurred in 0.02% of donors (2 per 10,000). Infection, bleeding, and other postoperative complications occur in approximately 0.5% to 3% of patients. Progression to ESRD has occurred, but does not appear to be more common than in the general population. Mild blood pressure elevation and proteinuria may occur after donation, but the long-term consequences are currently unclear. After ABO compatibility and a negative cross match are assured, the donor evaluation process can begin. If there are multiple candidates, the donor with fewer HLA mismatches is usually selected. Donors are carefully screened for kidney disease to prevent the possibility of loss of function in the remaining kidney. Depending on severity, hypertension, proteinuria, obesity, kidney stones, and structural or functional renal disease may be contraindications to donation. Testing for latent diabetes mellitus with a glucose tolerance test may be performed if there is a family history or perceived risk for future diabetes. When recipients are affected by hereditary disorders such as polycystic kidney disease or hereditary nephritis, the condition must be ruled out before a living, related donation. If a donor is thought to be acceptable, imaging of the kidneys is performed using magnetic resonance angiography (MRA) or other modalities, allowing the team to assess for structural or vascular anomalies and suitability for laparoscopic donation. A **cadaveric or deceased donor** also must be evaluated. The presence of metastasis, unknown cause of death, HIV, or widespread infection precludes donation. Donors with Hepatitis C are sometimes accepted for Hepatitis C–positive recipients. A combination of factors such as hypertension, advanced age, elevated creatinine, oliguria, or dependence on pressor support may exclude a donor. Pre-implantation biopsies can be performed on an individual basis when there is concern about the function of a donor kidney.

  C. Predictors of outcome. Recipient factors, donor factors, and donor–recipient compatibility all influence long-term graft survival. Although it is difficult to eliminate confounding variables, the United States Renal Data Systems 2002 report found that recipients who are younger, have low levels of PRA, have spent less time on dialysis, and who are employed or college educated have superior graft survival. Recipients who have been transplanted preemptively also have superior long term graft survival. Race and ethnicity may affect graft survival for both donors and recipients, with non-black donor kidneys and non-black, non-Hispanic recipients of grafts having the longest graft survival. Kidneys from living related or unrelated donors survive longer on average than cadaveric kidneys. Other donor qualities that positively affect outcomes include younger age and shorter cold ischemia time. The presence of hypertension, stroke as a cause of death, older age, or terminal creatinine greater than 1.5 may qualify a kidney as an *expanded criteria donor* kidney due to influence on poorer graft survival. Finally, factors of donor and recipient compatibility also affect outcomes: Better HLA matching, CMV serologic status matching, and equivalent donor–recipient body mass index all have positive effects on long-term graft survival.

III. Immunology and pharmacotherapy
  A. Immunology. A basic review of the mechanisms of immune recognition and response to an allograft is helpful to better understand the kidney

transplant patient as well as the pharmacologic agents used to prevent allograft rejection.

1. **Major histocompatibility complex (MHC).** Cells in the tissues of mammals, birds, and bony fish express MHC surface molecules, which are crucial for the immune system to be able to recognize and respond to a foreign antigen. In humans, these MHC molecules are located on the short arm of chromosome 6 and encode for HLA proteins. MHC molecules serve two basic functions: they identify self from non-self, and coordinate the T-cell receptor recognition of the antigen-MHC complex. The MHC molecules are divided into two groups: class I and class II. MHC class I molecules appear on the surface of all cells and are known as HLA-A, -B, and -C. MHC class II molecules appear on antigen presenting cells (APC) and are termed HLA-DR, -DP, and -DQ. One MHC *haplotype* is inherited from each parent as a locus containing each of the six genetically linked HLA molecules. In kidney transplantation, only the HLA-A, -B, and -DR are determined due to their immunogenicity. A "zero-antigen mismatched kidney" has no mismatches in either locus for HLA A, -B, and -DR, although mismatches may be present at HLA-C, -DP, -DQ, or at other minor antigens. Although advances in immunosuppression have narrowed advantages for well-matched transplants, a two haplotype-identical transplant from a family member or a zero antigen-mismatched cadaveric transplant confers a graft survival benefit compared to transplants with lesser degrees of matching.

2. **Antigen-presenting cells (APCs).** APCs are distributed in a ubiquitous manner in body tissues and allow T cells to recognize foreign antigens. Monocytes, macrophages, dendritic cells, and activated B cells can all serve as APCs. Either by phagocytosis or through surface immunoglobulin (B cells), APCs capture foreign antigens, degrade and process them into peptides, and express these foreign peptides on MHC class II surface molecules. Through T-cell receptor interactions and various downstream events, the T cell is then able to coordinate an immune response to this foreign antigen.

3. **T cells** are processed in the thymus and are central to cellular immunity and allograft recognition and rejection. These properties make them a common target of drugs designed to prevent rejection. Central to the immune response is the ability of the T cell to recognize foreign antigens through a surface T-cell receptor (TCR). These receptors recognize antigens through either indirect or direct pathways. The indirect pathway involves TCR recognition of a foreign antigen that is presented by a self-MHC molecule located on an APC surface. The direct pathway refers to the ability of some T-cell populations to recognize foreign MHC that is not presented with self MHC on an APC. There are two major classes of T cells: T helper cells, which express CD4 surface molecules (CD4+), and cytotoxic T cells, which express CD8. (CD8+). CD4+ cells recognize MHC class II molecules on the surface of APCs, whereas CD8+ cells are restricted to the recognition of MHC class I. CD4+ cells are activated after the recognition of a foreign antigen (e.g., foreign MHC from a kidney transplant). They then initiate an immune response to foreign peptides by secreting cytokines important in B cell proliferation and activation and cytotoxic T-cell activation. CD8+ T cells kill cells bearing foreign antigen through the use of cytotoxic molecules such as perforins, granzymes, and Fas, which triggers apoptosis in the targeted cell.

4. **T-cell and APC interactions.** T cells and APCs have a number of important interactions central to allograft recognition and rejection. **Signal 1** is the term for initial binding of the T cell to the APC through interactions between the TCR/CD3 complex and foreign peptide expressed in MHC. Signal 1 is a calcium-dependent process and results in calcineurin activation. Although signal 1 alone will cause anergy, the addition of **signal 2,** also known as costimulation, will lead to an immune response.

The best understood costimulation signal is between CD28 on the T-cell surface and B7 on the APC surface. CD28/B7 activation leads to intracellular signaling, interleukin-2 (IL-2) production, and T-cell activation. Whereas B7 is expressed on resting T cells, the T-cell surface molecule cytotoxic T lymphocyte antigen-4-immunoglobulin (CTLA4) is expressed only on activated T cells. CTLA4 binds preferentially to B7 and eventually inactivates the immune response, thereby providing potent negative feedback. Another costimulatory molecule, CD40, is found on APCs and activated B cells. It binds to CD40 Ligand (CD40L) on T cells. The CD40/CD40L pathway is important in immunoglobulin production and class switching by B cells.

   5. **B cells** develop at multiple sites of the body, including the liver, spleen, and lymph nodes. In response to T-cell signals for activation and proliferation, they produce immunoglobulins. A naive B cell produces immunoglobulin M (IgM) and, after class switching, is able to produce IgG, IgA, or IgA. Depending on their class, antibodies mediate opsonization for phagocytosis or antibody-dependent cellular cytotoxicity, and can fix complement. B cells and antibodies are important in the processes of hyperacute rejection (immediate allograft destruction due to preformed antibodies), and donor-specific antibodies have been implicated in both acute humoral rejection and chronic allograft dysfunction.

B. Pharmacotherapy. In the past two decades, the number of immunosuppressive agents available has increased greatly. Commonly used agents, their mechanism of action, and common toxicities appear in Table 13-1. Agents can be used for *induction* therapy at the time of transplant, as *maintenance* therapy to prevent rejection of the allograft, or for the treatment of *acute rejection*.

   1. **The calcineurin inhibitors,** cyclosporine A (CsA) and tacrolimus (FK506), are a mainstay of maintenance immunosuppression. Cyclosporine and tacrolimus have similar side effects, but hyperlipidemia, hypertension, hirsutism, and gingival hyperplasia are more common with cyclosporine, and post-transplant diabetes mellitus and neurotoxicity are more common with tacrolimus. Both agents cause significant nephrotoxicity. Tacrolimus has also been advocated as the maintenance agent of choice for steroid-resistant acute rejection.

   2. **One target of rapamycin (TOR) inhibitor,** sirolimus, is currently used in renal transplantation for maintenance therapy and for calcineurin inhibitor withdrawal. Important toxicities include hypertriglyceridemia, hypercholesterolemia, cytopenias, and diarrhea. Sirolimus may also increase the toxicity of cyclosporine.

   3. **The antiproliferatives,** either mycophenolate mofetil (MMF) or azathioprine, can be used in combination with calcineurin inhibitors and corticosteroids for maintenance immunosuppression. MMF often causes diarrhea and gastrointestinal discomfort, can be associated with cytopenias, and may be associated with an increased risk of tissue-invasive CMV. Azathioprine, a purine analog, provides less selective lymphocyte inhibition and can be associated with cytopenias and neoplasias.

   4. **Corticosteroids** are used during induction, as maintenance therapy, and for the treatment of acute rejection. Their effectiveness is complicated by a variety of well-known side effects, including hypertension, glucose intolerance, weight gain, cataracts, poor wound healing, osteoporosis, and osteonecrosis. Although corticosteroid withdrawal and avoidance have been explored (**V.C.2**), they remain a mainstay of current immunosuppression.

   5. **Antibody therapies** are available for many indications in kidney transplantation, including acute humoral rejection, steroid-resistant acute rejection, and induction in patients with elevated PRA, repeat transplant, positive B-cell cross match, ABO incompatibility, or other situations involving high immunologic risk. *Muromonab/CD3 (OKT3)* is a

Table 13-1. Commonly used drugs in renal transplantation

Class and Drugs	Mechanism	Toxicity	Indication
Calcineurin Inhibitors			
Cyclosporine	Binds cyclophilin and blocks calcineurin's action	Hypertension, hyperlipidemia nephrotoxicity, neurotoxicity hirsuitism, gingival hyperplasia	M
Tacrolimus	Binds to FKBP, inhibiting calcineurin's action	PTDM, neurotoxicity side effects similar to cyclosporine	M
TOR inhibitors			
Sirolimus	Binds to FKBP and inhibits mTOR effects, cytokine signaling, cell cycling, and CD28 mediated costimulation	Elevated cholesterol and triglycerides, cytopenias, acne, arthralgia, CsA toxicity, pneumonitis	M, CIW
Antiproliferatives			
Azathioprine	6-MP release in vivo, interferes with DNA synthesis, cell cycling	Cytopenias, diarrhea, hepatotoxic, neoplasias	M
Mycophenolate mofetil	Inosine monophosphate dehydrogenase inhibitor, blocks de novo purine synthesis	Diarrhea, GI discomfort, cytopenias, invasive CMV	M
Corticosteroids	Multiple sites of action; cytokine production, T-cell proliferation, leucocyte traffic, others	HTN, PTDM, hyperlipidemia, obesity, infection, osteoporosis, AVN	I, M, AR
Antibody therapies			
Muromonab/CD3	Mouse monoclonal Ab against CD3 on TCR	Cytokine release syndrome Pulmonary edema, leucopenia	I, AR
Antithymocyte Globulin ATGAM	Rabbit polyclonal Ab against thymocytes Horse polyclonal Ab against thymocytes	Allergic reaction, leucopenia Thrombocytopenia	I, AR
Daclizumab	Humanized (90%) monoclonal Ab against CD-25, the alpha subunit of IL-2 receptor	Low incidence of side effects: fever, chills, allergy	I
Basiliximab	Partially humanized (75%) monoclonal Ab, same target as daclizumab		I

M: Maintanence, I: Induction, AR: Acute Rejection, CIW: Calcineurin Inhibitor Withdrawal, 6-MP: 6 Mercaptopurine, HTN: Hypertension, AVN: Avascular Necrosis, PTDM: Post-Transplant Diabetes Mellitus, TCR: T-cell Receptor, Ab: antibody.

murine monoclonal Ab against the CD3 complex of the TCR. Given intravenously for 7 to 14 days, it is available for induction therapy and for the treatment of acute rejection. Toxicities include a cytokine release syndrome that can sometimes be complicated by capillary leak and pulmonary edema. Aseptic meningitis, serum sickness, profound immunosuppression, and lymphoproliferative disorders are less common side effects. *Polyclonal antibody preparations (anti-lymphocyte globulin, anti-thymocyte globulin)* are also available for induction and acute rejection. These compounds are developed by injecting human lymphoid or thymic extracts into animals (horse, rabbit, etc.) and purifying the antibodies produced. These preparations neutralize lymphocytes by multiple antibody-mediated mechanisms, with a sustained effect on proliferation. Toxicities are related to immunosuppression, heterogeneity of preparations, allergic or anaphylactoid responses to nonhuman preparations, and cytopenias. Finally, *daclizumab* and *basiliximab* are 90% and 75% humanized monoclonal antibodies to the CD25 portion of the IL-2 receptor. These agents are used for induction therapy and prevention of acute rejection. Administration has decreased the incidence of acute rejection with minimal side effects.

6. **Drug interactions.** Although it is not possible to list all possible drug interactions, it is important for the clinician to be aware of general types of interactions when initiating new therapies or witnessing unexpected toxicities. In general, interactions can result from changes in absorption, metabolism, or excretion, or through additive or synergistic toxicity with agents that have similar side effects. Agents that can decrease the absorption of immunosuppressive agents include antacids, cholestyramine, and food, and promotility agents can increase absorption. The metabolism of tacrolimus and cyclosporine occurs through cytochrome p450-3A4, so agents that affect this system can alter calcineurin-inhibitor levels or alter the metabolism of the interacting agent, thus leading to toxicity or inadequate levels. Examples of these agents include azole antifungals, calcium channel blockers, anticonvulsants, some antimicrobials, and grapefruit juice. Statin clearance may be decreased due to cytochrome p450 interactions, resulting in myopathy and rhabdomyolysis. Antimicrobials and other agents should be dosed according to renal function as in any patient, with added attention to agents that affect cyclosporine or tacrolimus metabolism. Drugs that cause synergistic or additive toxicities include allopurinol, trimethoprim-sulfamethoxazole, angiotensin converting enzyme (ACE) inhibitors or ganciclovir with azathioprine; all potentially cause myelosuppression. Also, nonsteroidal anti-inflammatory drugs (NSAIDs) and ACE inhibitors may have additive effects on glomerular hemodynamics when used with calcineurin inhibitors. Anticoagulation or antiplatelet therapies require more cautious monitoring due to frequent thrombocytopenia and multidrug therapy in many transplant patients. Although this summary is not exhaustive, cautious attention to these possibilities can prevent morbidity from drug interactions.

IV. **Transplantation**

A. **Induction.** With few exceptions, renal transplant recipients receive a brief course of high-dose steroids at the time of transplantation, followed by a taper to the initial maintenance dose. For patients at high risk for acute rejection, antibody therapy may be given during induction. These patients include those with high panel-reactive antibodies (PRA), previous transplants, African Americans, and multiple HLA-mismatches. Available antibodies therapies include anti-thymocyte globulin, muromonab/CD3 (OKT3), and IL-2 receptor antagonists (see section **IV.B.5**).

B. **Donor nephrectomy.** Living donor kidneys can be harvested in either an open or laparoscopic approach, each with its own advantages and disadvantages. The left kidney is most often selected due to its longer renal vein and better accessibility. Laparoscopic donation rates have increased due to technical advancement and donor preferences. In general, laparoscopic donation has the advantages of a shorter hospital stay, quicker return to work, and less pain, but can come with higher costs, longer operative time, and a learning curve to decrease rates of morbidity and warm ischemia time to equal that of open nephrectomy. Cadaveric kidneys are removed together with a patch of aorta and inferior vena cava as part of a multiorgan harvesting procedure. The organs are then separated and stored in hypothermic preservation solution until implantation.

C. Transplant surgery. The transplanted kidney is placed in either the right or left iliac fossa. The renal vein and artery are both connected through and end-to-side anastamosis, the donor vein usually being connected to the external iliac vein and the donor artery to either the external iliac, common iliac, or internal iliac artery. The ureter is implanted into the bladder, and the bladder mucosa is usually pulled over the ureter to create a tunnel that prevents reflux and urine leak. A ureteral stent is often placed at the time of surgery to ensure patency and prevent urine leak. Lymphatics are ligated to prevent postoperative lymphocele formation. Routine closure does not involve the use of drains except in anticoagulated patients; their presence may indicate concern for the vascular or ureterovesicular anastamosis. A Foley catheter is placed at the time of surgery and maintained for up to 5 days postoperatively. Kidney transplantation in the absence of donor ischemia or technical complications is usually accompanied by prompt urine formation.

V. Postoperative management

A. Immediate postoperative care of the transplant recipient involves the close monitoring of urine output, fluid administration, and vital signs. Many centers use algorithms that replace the urine output with $1/2$ normal saline plus a small amount of hypotonic fluid to account for insensible losses. Hourly central venous pressure (CVP) measurements are often done as part of routine monitoring, with target CVP of 5 to 10 mm Hg. The brisk diuresis that can ensue in a transplant patient can cause disturbances in potassium, magnesium, calcium, and phosphorus. The effect of elevated parathyroid hormone, along with a suddenly functioning kidney, also contributes to these abnormalities. Insulin requirements may increase in diabetic patients or those without prior diabetes due to the presence of steroids, calcineurin inhibitors, and improved clearance of insulin by the transplanted kidney. An uncomplicated patient with a functioning kidney can usually ambulate by postoperative day 1 or 2, and the diet can be advanced as tolerated. By postoperative day 5, the Foley catheter can be removed, and the patient can be discharged if they are free of other complications.

B. Complications can occur as a result of technical problems related to surgery, infections, disorders of renal function, or other routine postoperative complications. Surgical complications include problems with each of the aspects of the transplant: the vascular anastamoses, urologic complications, lymphocele, and wound complications.

   1. Urologic complications include urine leak, obstruction, and reflux. Routine stenting at many centers may be responsible for a decrease in the incidence of urologic complications. *Urine leak* can occur in approximately 2% of transplants. It is usually due to ureteral necrosis caused by an interruption of blood supply, but it can be at the site of bladder implantation or the calyces. The clinical presentation is one of decreased urine output, pain, fever, abdominal tenderness, swelling, and a perinephric fluid collection by ultrasonography. Fluid aspiration reveals a high creatinine that far exceeds the plasma creatinine. The diagnosis can be confirmed through a nuclear scan demonstrating extravasation into local tissues. Temporary Foley catheterization and ureteral stenting, followed by surgical repair, is the usual management. *Ureteric obstruction* is usually secondary to ureteral ischemia but can be due to multiple other factors. Imaging by ultrasound, cystogram, or other studies usually leads to a diagnosis; the obstruction can be relieved by ureteral repair, stenting, or nephrostomy. *Vesicoureteral reflux* into the transplanted ureter is less common since the introduction of submucosal tunneling of the ureter through the bladder.

2. **Arterial or venous thrombosis** are uncommon but may occur as a result of preexisting hypercoagulability or technical difficulty; these should be suspected when sudden deterioration develops in a previously functioning transplant. Although venous thrombosis can occasionally be reversed surgically or by anticoagulation, vascular thromboses most often lead to graft loss.

3. **Lymphocele** presents often as an asymptomatic cystic fluid collection. Lymphoceles may, however, cause graft obstruction and reduced renal function, pain, or lower extremity edema due to the compression of the femoral vein. Lymphoceles are distinguished from urine leaks when fluid aspiration yields a fluid creatinine equal to serum creatinine. The aspirated fluid should also be sent for cell count and Gram stain to rule out hematoma or abscess. Lymphoceles can be aspirated, but may require operative repair (marsupialization) if they are recurrent.

4. **Wound complications** may stem from the problems already described, or due to infection. Clinical suspicion is necessary, as immunosuppression both masks the symptoms and increases the risk of wound infections. Prompt drainage and antibiotic administration are central to treatment.

5. **Infections** in the first postoperative month are similar to those in other postoperative patients but occur frequently in immunosuppressed patients. Pneumonia, urine and wound infections, and infections related to dialysis catheters are common culprits. Infections of fluid collections (lymphocele, urinoma, hematoma) may also occur. Opportunistic and other infections are discussed in section **VI**.

C. **Maintenance immunosuppression**

1. **Conventional therapy.** Since 1995, the available options for maintenance immunosuppression have been expanded with the introduction of MMF, tacrolimus, cyclosporine microemulsion, and sirolimus. In the United States, standard therapy consists of a calcineurin inhibitor, an antiproliferative or TOR inhibitor, and corticosteroids. The calcineurin inhibitors tacrolimus and cyclosporine have similar efficacy in patient and graft survival, but with slightly different toxicity profiles. Tacrolimus also has lowered both the incidence and severity of acute rejection in head-to-head comparisons. Our center maintains target trough levels of cyclosporine that are highest (300 ng per mL) in the first month, with gradual tapering to 200 to 250 ng per mL by 6 months and 150 to 200 ng per mL after 12 months. Similarly, target tacrolimus levels are 12 to 16 ng per mL in the first month, 8 to 12 ng per mL for months 1 through 5, and 5 to 7 ng per mL after 6 months. Target levels may need to be lower in patients receiving sirolimus; these levels are often individualized based on match, rejection history, and the presence of infection. MMF and sirolimus have largely supplanted azathioprine in clinical use, as both result in less acute rejection. Corticosteroids are the third agent used in combination regimens; they are usually tapered rapidly over the first 2 to 3 weeks post-transplant to minimize side effects. They are then gradually tapered to 5 to 10 mg daily by month 6. The availability of multiple agents has allowed clinicians to choose a regimen that best fits a patient's profile of immunologic risk and perceived susceptibility to side effects. For example, patients with second transplants or poor matching, who are at greater risk for rejection, may be placed on tacrolimus. An obese patient with a family history of diabetes but with low immunologic risk, however, may be placed on cyclosporine or chosen for a steroid withdrawal protocol in an attempt to reduce the risk of post-transplant diabetes mellitus.

2. **Alternative regimens.** The toxicities of corticosteroids and calcineurin inhibitors have led to interest corticosteroid withdrawal or avoidance and calcineurin inhibitor withdrawal. A meta-analysis of late steroid withdrawal, however, has been associated with acute rejection and graft loss, particularly in African Americans. In contrast, trials of early withdrawal or avoidance of steroids in low-risk patients have shown promise but lack long-term results. Until larger trials with long-term follow-up are available, steroid withdrawal remains controversial outside the realm of clinical studies. Calcineurin inhibitor withdrawal is another goal due to nephrotoxicity and other side effects. A meta-analysis of studies revealed that calcineurin-inhibitor withdrawal was again associated with an increased risk of acute rejection, especially in African-Americans. However, more recent trials with sirolimus-based regimens have allowed for calcineurin inhibitor withdrawal in low to moderate risk patients and led to Food and Drug Administration (FDA) approval for this indication. Similarly, calcineurin avoidance in sirolimus-containing regimens has been studied with relatively promising results.

VI. **Renal complications.** In addition to delayed graft function, acute rejection, recurrent disease, and chronic allograft nephropathy, renal transplant patients are susceptible to renal failure from all the causes that affect the general population. In the initial 48 hours after transplantation, technical causes related to surgery or delayed graft function are most common. After 48 hours, the approach to a patient with renal dysfunction should rule out hypovolemia, medication toxicity, and obstruction, and should attempt to uncover causes of acute tubular necrosis such as hypotension, sepsis, or radiocontrast. Evaluation for acute rejection should take place if clear causes are not found.

A. **Delayed graft function (DGF).** DGF is defined as the requirement for dialysis in the first 7 days after transplantation. It occurs in approximately 20% of cadaveric transplants but is uncommon in living donor transplants. Although technical factors or other events that affect kidney function can cause DGF, it is most commonly a result of post-ischemic ATN, caused by donor hypovolemia or hypotension, or prolonged cold or warm ischemia during harvesting and preservation. DGF adds to the cost and length of hospitalization and is associated with poorer short- and long-term graft survival. To determine the cause of graft dysfunction in the early postoperative period, a renal ultrasound should be performed to rule out technical causes, and the timing of renal biopsy, to rule out acute rejection, should be guided by the patient's immunologic risk.

B. **Acute rejection.** Rejection refers to an immunological response by the recipient to the transplanted organ. Several types of acute rejection occur. **Hyperacute rejection** is rare and is caused by preformed antibodies against donor antigen, leading to immediate graft destruction after perfusion. **Accelerated acute rejection** usually occurs 2 to 3 days after transplant, and often is an antibody-mediated process that takes place in presensitized patients with prior transplants, transfusions, or pregnancies. **Acute cellular rejection** is a T-cell mediated response that may occur at any time, but is most common from 5 to 7 days post-transplant until 4 weeks after transplant, with a gradual lessening of risk in the first 6 months. Clinically, the spectrum of low-grade fever, a swollen, tender allograft, and oliguria are not seen commonly with modern immunosuppression. Thus, frequent lab monitoring and a high incidence of suspicion are necessary to diagnose acute rejection. Acute rejection typically presents as a decrease in renal function, as measured by the serum creatinine. However, rejection can occur without discernable changes in renal function, a process referred to as subclinical rejection. Some centers perform routine "protocol biopsies" to evaluate for subclinical rejection and other graft abnormalities. Current regimens incorporating newer agents have lowered the incidence of acute rejection in the first year to less than 20%, have improved 1 year cadaveric allograft survival to nearly 90%, and may be responsible for some of the improvement in long-term outcomes. The diagnosis of acute rejection requires an ultrasound-guided renal biopsy, with application of the Banff criteria to grade the severity of rejection or disclose other pathology. Pathologic features are interstitial infiltration with lymphocytes, tubulitis, and endarteritis. Treatment of acute rejection is usually a 3 to 5 day course of high-dose intravenous steroids, with OKT3 or antithymocyte globulin reserved for steroid-refractory or more severe rejection. Whereas most acute rejection can be reversed, its occurrence remains a powerful predictor of long-term graft survival. Patients who do not experience acute rejection may experience graft survival that is two to three times longer than those who experience rejection episodes. The term **acute humoral rejection** is reserved for antibody-mediated rejection. It is distinguished by peritubular capillary staining with the complement-split product C4d, neutrophilic glomerulitis, donor-specific antibodies, and occasional fibrinoid necrosis of vessels. This process is often resistant to steroids and antibody therapies, and portends a worse prognosis than cellular rejection. It has been managed with plasmapheresis, intravenous immunoglobulin (IVIG), immunoadsorption, and tacrolimus or MMF rescue, but optimal therapy is not established.

C. **Recurrent disease.** The diagnosis of recurrent disease is guided by the clinical scenario and knowledge of which diseases tend to recur in renal transplants. In patients with glomerulonephritis, for example, recurrent disease is the third most common cause of graft loss, after chronic allograft nephropathy and death with a functioning allograft. Recurrent nephritis may present as proteinuria, nephrotic syndrome, microscopic hematuria, and loss of function. It can be differentiated from other causes (chronic allograft dysfunction, *de novo* glomerular disease) through renal biopsy. In the transplanted patient, the important variables are the frequency of recurrence and frequency of graft loss due to recurrence. For example, focal and segmental glomerulosclerosis (FSGS) and type 1 membranoproliferative glomerulonephritis (MPGN) recur in 30% to 60% and 20% to 30% of patients, and commonly may lead to graft loss. Alternatively, IgA nephropathy, type II MPGN, type 1 diabetes recur in 50%, 50% to 100%, and up to 100% of recipients respectively, but are uncommon causes of graft loss. Systemic lupus erythematosus (SLE) may also recur microscopically in renal allografts but rarely is clinically important. Oxalosis is a systemic disease that commonly causes graft loss unless concomitant liver transplant is performed, whearas cystinosis does not usually recur in allografts. Autosomal dominant polycystic kidney disease (ADPKD) does not recur in an allograft from a donor lacking the PKD mutation. Although recurrent disease caused only 3% of first graft losses in a recent European report, 48% of patients who lost one graft due to recurrence lost a second graft to recurrent disease.

D. **Chronic allograft nephropathy (CAN)** is a syndrome that appears clinically as progressive renal failure, proteinuria, and hypertension. Pathologically, its features are tubular atrophy, interstitial fibrosis, and glomerular, vascular, and mesangial matrix changes. The etiology for this disorder is unknown, but a combination of immunologic and nonimmunologic factors have been implicated, thus explaining replacement of the term "chronic rejection." Despite advances in the treatment of acute rejection and other areas of transplantation, up to 40% of grafts experience CAN, and it is the most common cause of graft loss after 1 year. The importance of immune mechanisms in the development of CAN is underscored by the reality that acute rejection episodes, anti-donor HLA antibodies, poor matching, and C4d staining all correlate with the incidence of chronic allograft nephropathy. However, important nonimmune risks also correlate with the development of CAN. These include donor age, prolonged ischemia times, size mismatching, hypertension, hyperlipidemia, proteinuria, and smoking. Some of these risks implicate low nephron dose and hyperfiltration injury as a contributing factor. The allograft response to injury may cause the release of proinflammatory and profibrotic growth factors and cytokines, such as transforming growth factor beta (TGF-β), platelet derived growth factor (PDGF), and others, worsening the cascade of CAN. Premature senescence (aging) has also been implicated. Although calcineurin-inhibitor–induced nephrotoxicity has similar effects on renal function, there are conflicting results on their use and the risk of CAN. Treatment of CAN is not currently well-defined; control of blood pressure and lipids are advocated, and ACE-inhibition appears safe and helpful in retrospective analysis. Immunosuppressive strategies are not generally effective, but trials of novel regimens aimed at preventing CAN are ongoing.

VII. Medical care of the transplanted patient. The success of renal transplantation and the growing population of transplant recipients are unfortunately accompanied by the complications from comorbid diseases and side effects of long-term immunosuppression. Patients often die with functioning grafts due to cardiovascular disease, infections, and malignancy, and these and other conditions contribute to a spectrum of common disorders in transplantation.

A. Infectious diseases. In the transplanted patient, typical signs and symptoms of infection may be absent, and coinfections are common, thus necessitating increased scrutiny. Infections after renal transplantation occur in patterns that are important to recognize. Immediately after transplant, patients are at risk for common postoperative infections: wound infections, pneumonia, line, and urinary infections. The first 6 months after transplant is marked by a risk of opportunistic infections due to more intense immunosuppression, especially after antibody induction. For this reason, patients usually receive prophylaxis against *Pneumocystis carinii* pneumonia (PCP) for at least 6 months, and for cytomegalovirus (CMV) for 3 to 6 months if they are at risk (see section **VII.A.2**). Some centers provide prophylaxis for fungal infections. After 6 months, the risk of opportunistic infections is lower but remains present, and patients remain at risk for more frequent and severe infections by community-acquired pathogens.

1. Immunosuppression during infection. No clear guidelines exist for decreasing immunosuppression during infection. Furthermore, many infections carry an increased risk of acute rejection due to upregulation of immune surveillance and activity. In general, mild infections treated with appropriate antimicrobials, can be managed without a change in immunosuppression. However, more severe infections may require decreasing or stopping antiproliferative medications (sirolimus, MMF, azathioprine) and reducing calcineurin-inhibitor dosing. Severe or life-threatening infections should include attention to the requirement for stress-doses of corticosteroids, which are often adequate to decrease the risk of rejection during an illness. Reduction of immunosuppression is best done with careful monitoring of graft function along with the consultation of transplant physicians.

2. Cytomegalovirus (CMV) is a human herpes virus that is common in the general population but usually does not lead to serious morbidity without immunosuppression. A potential organ recipient who has not been exposed to CMV is at risk for a primary infection if transplanted with a CMV$^+$ organ, and a recipient who has been exposed before transplant is at risk for reactivation or superinfection, especially if receiving antibody induction. Thus, the risk of CMV infection is tied to the serologic status of the donor and recipient, with rates as high as 50% to 70% in Donor$^+$/Recipient$^-$ patients not receiving prophylaxis, and 20% to 30% in patients who were exposed prior to transplant. CMV infection is uncommon in Donor$^-$/Recipient$^-$ transplants. Therefore, Donor$^+$/Recipient$^-$ patients and Recipient$^+$ patients who receive antibody therapies should receive prophylaxis for CMV for 3 to 6 months. Options for oral agents include ganciclovir, valganciclovir, and valacyclovir. CMV infection leads to morbidity related directly to infection, but also increases the risk of acute rejection, graft loss, and death. Clinically, the disease often presents as low-grade fever, leucopenia and/or thrombocytopenia, and malaise. Tissue invasion can occur in 5% to 15% of infections, with syndromes of pneumonitis, hepatitis, esophagitis, and diarrhea being most common. PCR-based testing is the most sensitive diagnostic technique, but other options exist, including biopsy of affected tissues. Standard therapy is intravenous ganciclovir, a nucleoside analog, although ganciclovir-resistance can develop.

3. **BK virus nephropathy (BKV nephropathy, polyomavirus).** Human BK virus is a polyoma virus that is present as a latent infection in most of the population and has tropism for the genitourinary tract. During immunosuppression, the virus can reactivate. In renal transplant patients, BK virus most commonly causes a syndrome of decreased renal function and interstitial nephritis that appears clinically and pathologically similar to acute rejection. Ureteral stenosis and ulceration may also occur, and infection is a risk for allograft loss. When BKV nephropathy is present, "decoy cells" are usually shed in the urine, and polymerase chain reaction (PCR)-based testing usually demonstrates viuria and viremia. Immunohistochemical techniques and the presence of viral inclusions can be used to confirm the diagnosis through renal biopsy. It is important to suspect BKV nephropathy when presumed acute rejection does not respond to steroids or occurs after 6 months, because increasing the intensity of immunosuppression may lead to graft loss. Lessening the intensity of immunosuppression may stabilize graft function, but increases the risk of acute rejection. IVIG therapy may have advantages because it can theoretically improve both acute rejection and viral infection. Cidofovir may have activity against the virus, but it can cause severe nephrotoxicity, thus underscoring the importance of finding new antiviral agents.

4. **Hepatitis B and C.** Although the incidence of Hepatitis B in patients with ESRD has been declining due to immunization, isolation techniques, and the screening of transfused blood, Hepatitis C infections are relatively common, affecting up to 7% of recent U.S. cadaveric transplant recipients. No consensus has been formed on the management or outcome of either disease in respect to renal transplant. For Hepatitis B, patients with antigenemia usually receive evaluation and liver biopsy prior to transplant, because antiviral therapies may be more effective before transplantation. For Hepatitis C, the effect on outcomes and management are somewhat controversial. Data suggest that Hepatitis C infection increases the risk of graft loss, death, and post-transplant diabetes mellitus, and that donor seropositivity may also affect graft loss and death. Although many patients have mild, indolent disease, there are reports of rapid progression to cirrhosis and liver failure after renal transplantation. A complicating factor is that interferon therapy may increase the risk of acute rejection. Thus, decisions about the timing and treatment of Hepatitis C should be considered prior to transplantation, and post-transplant interferon therapy should only be undertaken with careful monitoring and collaboration among caregivers.

5. **Other infections.** Urinary infections are common after renal transplantation, and pyelonephritis of the transplanted kidney can lead to decreased renal function. Pulmonary infections from both common and uncommon pathogens are the most common cause of tissue-invasive infection. Although the list of pathogens affecting patients is too long to mention, differential diagnosis should include fungal diseases such as *Cryptococcus, Candida*, and endemic fungi, mycobacterial disease, *Nocardia, P. carinii*, viral pathogens, and others.

6. **Immunization.** Potential transplant recipients should receive immunization against influenza, pneumococcus, Hepatitis B, and varicella if they are seronegative. After transplant, many centers wait 6 months before any immunizations because of theoretical risks of stimulating the immune system and increasing the risk of rejection. Also, the vaccines may

be less effective during this period. The oral polio, typhoid, varicella, yellow fever, and bacillus Calmette-Guerin (BCG) vaccines are live vaccines that are contraindicated after renal transplant due to their ability to cause disease in immunocompromised hosts. However, the live measles-mumps-rubella (MMR) vaccine can be given after 6 months if indicated. Vaccination for influenza, pneumococcus, Hepatitis A and B, and tetanus/diphtheria should be given as indicated.

B. **Cardiovascular disease** is the most common cause of death in patients with a functioning allograft. Ischemic coronary artery disease, congestive heart failure (CHF), and left ventricular hypertrophy are all more common in patients with kidney disease than in the general population, and cerebrovascular disease is another important cause of morbidity and mortality. Thus, efforts at improving outcomes after renal transplantation have been appropriately shifted to focus on cardiovascular risks. Efforts at preventing cardiovascular events begin with pre-transplant evaluation, risk-stratification, and intervention when necessary. After renal transplant, attention is given to the modification of existing risk factors and a careful evaluation and treatment of new symptoms or disease.

1. **Hypertension.** Since the introduction of calcineurin inhibitors, hypertension has been present in 70% to 90% of patients after renal transplant. Hypertension not only represents a modifiable cardiovascular risk factor, but also is correlated with graft loss, especially in African-Americans. Clinicians should aim for a target blood pressure below 130/80 mm Hg, as indicated by current recommendations for patients with chronic kidney disease. The choice of agents after renal transplantation is controversial and complicated by the interpretation of fluctuations in renal function that occur with diuretics, angiotensin converting enzyme (ACE) inhibitors, and angiotensin receptor blockers (ARBs). In general, beta-blockers and dihydropyridine calcium channel blockers are used in the early post-transplant period due to their lack of drug interactions and effects on renal function. Many patients require diuretics because of salt retention due to corticosteroids, calcineurin inhibitors, and other blood pressure medication. ACE inhibitors and ARBs are often avoided early after transplantation due to effects on renal hemodynamics and serum creatinine. These agents appear to be safe and effective in patients with chronic allograft nephropathy, however, and may be an important addition to attenuate hypertension and cardiovascular risk.

2. **Hyperlipidemia.** Lipid abnormalities occur in at least 50% of transplant patients and represent an important modifiable cardiovascular risk factor. Hypertriglyceridemia, high low-density lipoprotein (LDL), and low high-density lipoprotein (HDL) often occur as part of a metabolic syndrome that is common after transplantation. Corticosteroids, calcineurin inhibitors, and sirolimus may all play important roles in worsening lipid profiles. Despite concerns about rhabdomyolysis due to drug interactions, we now have prospective data from randomized, controlled trials indicating that statins (specifically, fluvastatin) prevent cardiac death and nonfatal myocardial infarction after renal transplantation without effects on graft survival. Other therapies such as niacin, fibrates, and binding resins have been used as well. As always, attention to drug interactions must be given, especially regarding the risk of rhabdomyolysis (statins, fibrates, calcineurin inhibitors) and decreased or enhanced absorption (binding resins, ezetimibe).

3. **Diabetes mellitus**
   a. **Background.** Diabetes is a major independent risk factor for cardiovascular disease, is present in 30% to 40% of patients prior to transplant, and develops after transplant in 2.5% to 20% of nondiabetic patients. Complications from diabetes have important effects on patient outcomes, leading to cardiovascular and infectious morbidity, renal allograft loss and decreased function, as well as decreased patient

survival. In patients with diabetes preceding transplant, control may be worsened by corticosteroids, calcineurin inhibitors, and the decreased half-life of endogenous and exogenous insulin due to improved kidney function. The rigorous control of diabetes is likely to decrease diabetic complications, based on accumulated evidence in other populations. A target glycosylated hemoglobin target of 6.5 to 7.0 is likely to be associated with improved outcomes.

    b. Post transplant diabetes mellitus (PTDM) also called new onset diabetes after transplantation, complicates a substantial percentage of renal transplants and is associated with poorer patient outcomes. Risks for PTDM include increasing age, obesity, family history of diabetes, African-American or Hispanic race or ethnicity, Hepatitis C infection, and abnormal glucose tolerance. Corticosteroids have well-known adverse effects on insulin resistance, and calcineurin inhibitors are diabetogenic, likely due to a combination of beta cell toxicity and the promotion of insulin resistance. The definition of PTDM has varied in the past, but consensus has established that it should be defined similarly to the general population: a fasting glucose of greater than 126 mg per dL, symptoms of diabetes with any glucose above 200 mg per dL, or a 2-hour oral glucose tolerance test value above 200 mg per dL. Fasting plasma glucose should be routinely monitored after transplant, because the incidence of PTDM is high. Prevention of diabetes through weight loss and exercise in patients at risk should be attempted, and treatment of new onset diabetes should follow established guidelines.

  4. Other cardiovascular risk factors. Smoking is obviously an important modifiable cardiovascular risk factor, and evidence is accumulating that smoking also influences deterioration of renal function and is a risk for graft loss. At any stage in the transplant process, counseling, formal smoking cessation programs, and pharmacologic agents should be offered to encourage smoking cessation.

    Anemia is present in many patients both before and after transplant, and may be underrecognized and undertreated. Anemia is correlated with left ventricular hypertrophy and cardiovascular disease; therefore, diagnosis and treatment based on cause is probably appropriate.

    Homocysteine is increased in renal transplant patients and is also correlated with cardiovascular events. It is not yet clear if lowering homocysteine levels with high-dose B-vitamins and folic acid will lead to decreased events.

C. Malignancy is an important complication of immunosuppression, probably due to effects on immune surveillance of abnormal tumor cell populations and viral-mediated cancers. The intensity of immunosuppression, including exposure to antilymphocyte antibodies, is an important factor in determining the risk for malignancy. Nonmelanoma skin cancers, especially squamous cell carcinomas, have a particularly high incidence and aggressiveness in transplant patients compared with the general population. Human papilloma virus (HPV) has been partially implicated in these cancers. Thus, patients with transplants are counseled to avoid the sun, use protective sunscreens and clothing, and see a dermatologist at least once yearly. After skin cancers, post-transplant lymphoproliferative disorders (PTLD) are the next most common malignancy. These lymphomas are associated with Epstein Barr virus (EBV) infection and usually contain EBV DNA. Risks are increased after T-cell–depleting antibody therapies. These malignancies are often managed with a reduction in immunosuppression and antiviral treatment, but aggressive tumors, particularly when monoclonal, may require systemic chemotherapy. Similarly, women are at increased risk of cervical squamous cell carcinomas related to HPV infection; they require yearly Pap smears, with increased frequency of surveillance and attention if there are any abnormalities. Vulvar, perineal, and anogenital cancers are also more frequent after transplantation. Hepatitis B and C may lead to hepatocellular carcinoma, and Kaposi's sarcoma, caused by human herpes virus 8, is another viral-mediated cancer that affects transplant patients. Solid tumors, such as breast, lung, and colon cancer are approximately twice as common in transplant patients than the general population. Given the risks of malignancy in transplantation, age-appropriate screening should occur prior to placement on the waiting list, and should continue for the patient's lifetime.

D. Bone disease

1. **Preexisting bone disease.** The clinical picture after renal transplantation is often complicated by the presence of preexisting bone disease. Most commonly, secondary hyperparathyroidism leads to osteitis fibrosa, imparting a risk of bone loss and fracture. Other causes of preexisting bone disease include adynamic (low-turnover) bone disease, aluminum related osteomalacia, and β_2-microglobulin (β_2M)-associated arthropathy. Furthermore, diabetic patients have decreased in bone mineral density compared to other populations. While aluminum and β_2M-related bone disease are no longer common, many patients will undergo transplant with established bone loss and increased fracture risk.

2. **Post-transplant bone disease.** It is well established that up to 9% of bone density is lost in the first 6 to 12 months after transplantation. Furthermore, osteopenia and osteoporosis are present in a substantial number of transplanted patients after long-term follow-up. Renal transplant patients carry an increased risk of fracture of 3% to 4% per year for the first 3 years after transplant, declining somewhat after that time. Fracture risk is increased in men and women and is particularly increased in older women. Many factors contribute to the milieu that supports bone loss. Steroids are known to induce osteopenia and osteoporosis through effects on calcium absorption and excretion, aggravation of secondary hyperparathyroidism, hypogonadism, and effects on bone turnover. Cyclosporine, secondary hyperparathyroidism, renal phosphate wasting, uremia, and gonadal hormones are other contributing factors to bone loss. Another syndrome affecting transplant patients is avascular osteonecrosis, especially of the femoral head, which is associated with steroid use. Patients present with bone pain but may be asymptomatic. Often patients require operative intervention, including replacement of the affected joint.

3. **Management.** The timing and frequency of measuring bone mineral density is not well-defined, but should be performed at some established interval due to the risk of fractures. The control of secondary hyperparathyroidism before transplant is important. After transplant, calcium and vitamin D supplements are recommended unless hypercalcemia is present. Parathyroidectomy is usually reserved for patients with symptomatic or persistent hypercalcemia or with persistent (longer than 1 to 2 years) hyperparathyroidism. Trials of bisphosphonates have been shown to reduce bone loss, especially when given immediately after transplant, but indications are not defined and concerns remain regarding the promotion of adynamic bone disease. Weight-bearing exercise is a low-cost intervention that should be recommended for all patients.

E. Hematologic disease. Hematologic disorders are common after transplantation and have multifactorial origins. Anemia and post-transplant erythrocytosis are common. Leucopenia and thrombocytopenia often are seen as complications of antiproliferative medication, CMV or other viral infections, or any of a number of primary diseases.

1. **Anemia** is all too common after renal transplantation, occurring in 30% to 40% of patients in some series. Furthermore, it has been correlated with an increased risk of cardiovascular events and death and thus may be an important prognostic factor. It is more common in the early post-transplant period, but it is also present in high frequency in patients with

decreased renal function. An obvious factor involved in the presence of anemia is the decreased renal production of erythropoietin (EPO), especially when graft function is impaired. Iron deficiency, ACE inhibitors, ARBs, MMF, and azathioprine have also been associated with anemia after transplantation. Recurrent or *de novo* hemolytic uremic syndrome (HUS) can be a dramatic cause of anemia and graft loss and may be associated with calcineurin inhibitors and other medications. Although prospective data is needed, it seems prudent to correct anemia depending on the underlying etiology, including administration of EPO to those with impaired renal function.

2. **Post-transplant erythrocytosis (PTE),** defined as a hematocrit above 51%, occurs in 10% to 15% of renal transplant patients. The etiology of the disorder is not clear, but EPO– and non-EPO– dependent mechanisms have been implicated. It is more common in smokers, those without acute rejection episodes, and patients with diabetes. This condition can usually be managed by treatment with ACE inhibitors or ARBs. Occasionally, phlebotomy may be necessary if the hematocrit cannot be lowered below 56% to 60%.

F. **Pregnancy.** Years of experience in renal transplantation have allowed some understanding of pregnancy after transplantation. Most women are counseled to avoid pregnancy for some period after the transplant, usually 6 months to 2 years. Fertility is improved after transplantation, and attention to contraception should be given. Intrauterine devices (IUDs) should be avoided, but other contraception options can be used unless there are specific contraindications. In mothers at high risk for primary CMV infection, pregnancy should probably be delayed until an antibody response has occurred and viremia has cleared. Renal function, if normal at the time of conception, is probably not adversely affected during pregnancy. However, the risk of a pregnancy-related deterioration in renal function is increased when renal insufficiency is present. Glucose intolerance may also complicate pregnancy, leading to gestational diabetes or increased insulin requirements in those with diabetes. Immunosuppression should be maintained at levels similar to nonpregnant women, but levels should be checked frequently, because changes in pharmacokinetics are unpredictable. Prednisone is unlikely to be teratogenic, and calcineurin inhibitors and azathioprine have minimal to small risks. Animal data indicate that MMF may be teratogenic, and MMF has limited experience in pregnancy. Sirolimus has similar limited experience in pregnancy. Fetal outcomes after renal transplantation include a significant risk of pre-term delivery (50%) and growth restriction (40%), but these outcomes may be more closely related to renal impairment than the transplant *per se*. After delivery, breast feeding may not be recommended in patients taking calcineurin inhibitors, but discussion of the risks and benefits should occur on an individual basis.

Suggested readings

Chan L, Gaston R, Hariharan S. Evolution of immunosuppression and continued importance of acute rejection in renal transplantation. *Am J Kidney Dis* 2001; 38(6 Suppl 6):S2–9.

Hariharan S, Johnson CP, Bresnahan BA, et al. Improved graft survival after renal transplantation in the United States, 1988 to 1996. *N Engl J Med* 2000;2;342(9):605–612.

Kasiske BL, Chakkera HA, Louis TA, Ma JZ. A meta-analysis of immunosuppression withdrawal trials in renal transplantation. *J Am Soc Nephrol* 2000;11(10):1910–1917.

Oberbauer R, Kreis H, Johnson, et al. Long-term improvement in renal function with sirolimus after early cyclosporine withdrawal in renal transplant recipients: 2-year results of the Rapamune Maintenance Regimen Study. *Transplantation* 2003;76(2):364–370.

Primer on Transplantation, 2nd ed. Norman DJ, Turka LA, eds. Mt. Laural, NJ: American Society of Transplantation, 2001.

Wolfe RA, Ashby VB, Milford EL, et al. Comparison of mortality in all patients on dialysis, patients on dialysis awaiting transplantation, and recipients of a first cadaveric transplant. *N Engl J Med* 1999;2;341(23):1725–1730.

USRDS 2002 Annual Data Report. *Am J Kidney Dis* 2003;41(4),Suppl 2.

Chan L, Wang W, and Kam I. Outcomes and complications of renal transplantation. In: Schrier RW ed. *Diseases of the kidney and urinary tract,* 7th ed. Philadelphia: Lippincott Williams & Wilkins, 2001.

The Patient with Kidney Disease and Hypertension in Pregnancy

14

Phyllis August and
Marshall D. Lindheimer

In most instances, pregnancy in women with renal disorders is successful, provided kidney function is well preserved and hypertension absent.

I. **The kidney and blood pressure in normal pregnancy.** The anatomy and function of the kidneys and lower urinary tract are altered during gestation. Physiologic alterations in volume homeostasis and blood pressure (BP) control also occur, and recognizing this is a prerequisite for the appropriate interpretation of data from pregnant patients with renal disease or hypertension (Table 14-1).

A. **Anatomic and functional changes in urinary tract.** Kidney length increases approximately 1 cm during normal gestation. The major anatomic alterations of the urinary tract during pregnancy, however, are seen in the collecting system, where calyces, renal pelves, and ureters dilatate, often giving the erroneous impression of obstructive uropathy. The dilation is accompanied by hypertrophy of ureteral smooth muscle and hyperplasia of its connective tissue, but whether bladder reflux is more common in gravidas is unclear. The cause of the ureteral dilation is disputed. Some researchers favor hormonal mechanisms, whereas other researchers believe that it is obstructive in origin. Clearly, as pregnancy progresses, assumption of a supine or upright posture may cause ureteral obstruction when the enlarged uterus entraps the ureters at the pelvic brim (Fig. 14-1). These morphologic changes have considerable clinical relevance. Stasis in the dilated urinary tract may contribute to the propensity of pregnant women with asymptomatic bacteriuria to develop frank pyelonephritis. The widened ureters contain substantial volumes of urine, which may lead to collection errors in tests that require timed urine volumes. These errors may be avoided by the following simple protocol. Gravidas to be tested should receive a water load and remain in bed positioned in lateral recumbency for 1 hour before the start of the collection. This procedure minimizes inaccuracies by standardizing the procedures and by producing a modest water diuresis, so that residual urine is diluted and of recent origin. Acceptable norms of kidney size should be increased by 1 cm if estimated during pregnancy or the immediate puerperium, and reductions of renal length noted several months postpartum need not be attributed to renal disease. Rarely, ureteral dilation is of sufficient magnitude to cause a "distention" syndrome (characterized by abdominal pain, and on occasion small increments in serum creatinine levels presenting in late gestation; these resolve with the placement of ureteral stents). Also, because dilation of the ureters may persist until the twelfth postpartum week, elective ultrasonographic or radiologic examination of the urinary tract should be deferred, if possible, until after this time.

B. **Renal hemodynamics.** The changes in renal hemodynamics in gestation are the most striking and clinically significant of all the urinary tract alterations of pregnancy.

1. **Glomerular filtration rate (GFR) and renal plasma flow (RPF)** increase to levels 30% and 50% above nongravid values during pregnancy. Increments in GFR that are already present during the early days after conception reach a maximum during the first trimester. The basis for the increase in GFR and RPF is unknown. Animal studies suggest that renal vasodilation (mediated by nitric oxide) leading to increased glomerular

Table 14-1. Renal changes in normal pregnancy

Alteration	Manifestation	Clinical relevance
Increased renal size	Renal length approximately 1 cm greater on radiographs	Postpartum decreases in size should not be mistaken for parenchymal loss
Dilation of pelves, calyces, and ureters	Resembles hydronephrosis on renal ultrasound or intravenous pyelography (more marked on right)	Not to be mistaken for obstructive uropathy; elective evaluation should be deferred to the twelfth postpartum week; upper urinary tract infections are more virulent; retained urine leads to collection errors
Increased renal hemodynamics	Glomerular filtration rate and renal plasma flow increase 35% to 50%	Serum creatinine and urea nitrogen values decrease during normal gestations; >0.8 mg/dL creatinine already suspect; protein, amino acid, and glucose urinary excretion all increase
Changes in acid-base metabolism	Renal bicarbonate threshold decreases	Serum bicarbonate is 4 to 5 μmol/L lower in normal gestation
Renal water handling	Osmoregulation altered	Serum osmolality decreases 10 mOsm/L (serum sodium decreases 5 mEq/L) during normal gestation
	Osmotic thresholds for thirst and AVP decrease; the metabolic clearance of AVP increases markedly; high levels of vasopressinase circulating	Increased metabolism of AVP may cause transient diabetes insipidus in pregnancy

AVP, arginine vasopressin.

plasma flow is a contributing, but not the sole, factor. RPF is greatest at midgestation, declining somewhat in the third trimester. Although increments in GFR measured by the infusion of inulin appear to be sustained until term, 24-hour creatinine clearance declines during the last 4 weeks of pregnancy, accompanied by increases in serum creatinine levels of 15% to 20%.

The increase in GFR has important clinical implications. Because creatinine production is unchanged during pregnancy, increments in its clearance result in decreased serum levels. Using the Hare method, one group of investigators observed that true serum creatinine, which averaged 0.67 mg per dL in nongravid women, decreased to 0.46 mg per dL during gestation [to convert to SI units (μmol per L), multiply serum creatinine (mg per dL) by 88.4]. In studies that also measured creatinine chromogen (which yielded results resembling those reported in most clinical laboratories), values were 0.83 mg per dL in nonpregnant women and decreased to 0.74, 0.58, and 0.53 mg per dL in the first, second, and third trimester of pregnancy, respectively. Thus, values considered normal in nongravid women may reflect decreased renal function during pregnancy.

A   **B**

Figure 14-1. Intravenous pyelogram. **A:** Ureteral dilation of pregnancy. The right ureter is sharply cut off at the pelvic brim where it crosses the iliac artery (the iliac sign). **B:** Relationship between the ureters and iliac arteries can be demonstrated in postmortem studies. Note the iliac sign at the pelvic brim on the right. (From Dure-Smith P. Pregnancy dilation of the urinary tract. *Radiology* 1970;96:545. Reprinted with permission.)

For example, in gravid women, concentrations of serum creatinine exceeding 0.8 mg per dL or of serum urea nitrogen that are greater than 13 mg per dL suggest the need for additional evaluation of renal function.

2. **Other consequences of the increased renal hemodynamics.** Increased GFR and RPF also alter urinary solute content. For example, excretion of glucose, most amino acids, and several water-soluble vitamins increases, and these increments in the nutrient content of urine may be a factor in the enhanced susceptibility of gravidas to urinary tract infections (UTIs). Urinary protein excretion also increases during gestation, but the fate of albumin excretion is more complex and disputed.

C. **Acid-base regulation in pregnancy.** Renal acid-base regulation is altered during gestation. The bicarbonate threshold decreases, and early-morning urines are often more alkaline than those in the nongravid state. In addition, plasma bicarbonate concentrations decrease approximately 4 μmol per L, averaging 22 μmol per L. This change most likely represents a compensatory renal response to hypocapnia, because pregnant women hyperventilate, and their P_{CO_2} averages only 30 mm Hg. The mild alkalosis (arterial pH averages 7.44) found in pregnancy is in accord with this view. Because steady-state P_{CO_2} and HCO_3 levels are already diminished, pregnant women are, in theory, at a disadvantage when threatened by sudden metabolic acidosis (e.g., lactic acidosis in preeclampsia, diabetic ketoacidosis, or acute renal failure); however, they respond with appropriate increments in urinary titratable acid and ammonia after an acid load, and proton regeneration is already evident at blood pH levels higher than those in similarly tested nonpregnant women. Finally, when managing gravidas with pulmonary disorders, it should be noted that a P_{CO_2} of 40 mm Hg, normal in nonpregnant women, signifies considerable carbon dioxide retention in pregnancy.

D. Water excretion. After conception, a rapid decrease in plasma osmolality levels of 5 to 10 mOsm per kg below that of nongravid subjects occurs. If this decrease occurred in a nonpregnant woman, she would cease secreting antidiuretic hormone and enter a state of water diuresis; however, gravidas maintain this new osmolality, diluting and concentrating urine appropriately when the woman is subjected to water loading or dehydration. This suggests a resetting of the osmoreceptor system, and, indeed, clinical studies demonstrate that the osmotic thresholds for both thirst and arginine vasopressin (AVP) release are decreased in pregnant women. Furthermore, the plasma of pregnant women contains large quantities of a placental enzyme (vasopressinase) capable of destroying substantial quantities of AVP *in vitro*; moreover, the *in vivo* production and metabolic clearance of antidiuretic hormone are increased fourfold after midgestation.

The changes in osmoregulation and AVP metabolism may be responsible for two unusual syndromes of transient diabetes insipidus that complicate pregnancy. One, in which polyuria is responsive to both AVP and deamino-8-D-arginine vasopressin (dDAVP), probably occurs in women with unapparent partial central diabetes insipidus whose disease is brought to the fore by the increment in hormonal disposal rates during late gestation. The other disorder, in which the marked polyuria continues despite large doses of AVP, is responsive to dDAVP, an analogue resistant to inactivation by vasopressinase. These gravidas may have excessively high circulating levels of the aminopeptidase enzyme due to increased activation.

E. Volume regulation. Most healthy women gain approximately 12.5 kg during the first pregnancy and 1 kg less during subsequent pregnancies. Generations of physicians have considered these averages as upper limits of permissible weight gains, forgetting that a mean has plus and minus deviations. As a result, many gravidas were scolded for excessive weight gain, and their salt, calories, or both were restricted. Most of the increment is fluid, with total body water increasing 6 to 8 L, 4 to 6 L of which is extracellular. Plasma volume increases 50% during gestation, the largest rate of increment occurring during midpregnancy, whereas increments in the interstitial space are greatest in the third trimester. A gradual cumulative retention of approximately 900 mEq of sodium occurs in pregnancy; this is distributed between the products of conception and the maternal extracellular space. These alterations in maternal intravascular and interstitial compartments produce apparent hypervolemia, yet the gravida's volume receptors sense these changes as normal. Thus, when salt restriction or diuretic therapy limits this physiologic expansion, maternal responses resemble those in salt-depleted nonpregnant women. This is one compelling reason for the reluctance to recommend sodium restriction or diuretics during pregnancy. Pregnant women are now advised to salt their food to taste, and some researchers believe that a liberal sodium intake is beneficial during gestation. Another physiologic adaptation that appears to influence sodium balance during pregnancy is the marked stimulation of the renin-angiotensin-aldosterone system. Aldosterone levels are markedly increased during pregnancy, despite normal blood pressure and normal potassium balance. It is likely that the increased aldosterone secretion is a compensatory mechanism to counteract the increase in sodium excretion that would be expected as a result of the large increase in GFR and renal plasma flow. Arterial vasodilation that causes relative arterial underfilling, as occurs in pregnancy, is known to stimulate the renin-angiotensin-aldosterone system. Moreover, increases in aldosterone balance the natriuretic effects of the large increases in progesterone during pregnancy.

F. Blood pressure regulation. Mean BP starts to decrease early in gestation, with diastolic levels in midpregnancy averaging 10 mm Hg less than measurements postpartum. In later pregnancy, BP increases, gradually approaching nonpregnancy values near term. Because cardiac output rises quickly in the first trimester and remains relatively constant thereafter, the decrease in pressure is due to a marked decrement in peripheral vascular resistance. The slow rise toward nonpregnant levels after a midtrimester nadir is interesting, because it demonstrates that increasing vasoconstrictor tone is a feature of late gestation in normal women as well as in women in whom preeclampsia is developing. The cause of the decrease in peripheral resistance during pregnancy is obscure. Studies of arterial compliance in pregnancy demonstrate early rises, perhaps due to alterations in vessel ground substance. Elevations of plasma estrogen and progesterone to concentrations that may relax smooth muscle occur, and increments in vasodilating prostaglandins may also be present during gestation. Hormonally mediated increases in endothelial nitric oxide production may also contribute to the vasodilation in pregnancy. Despite lower BP, the levels of all components of the renin-angiotensin system are increased during pregnancy. Exaggerated hypotensive responses to converting enzyme inhibition in normal gravidas suggest that the increased renin-angiotensin system in pregnancy is a normal physiologic response to decreased BP and increased sodium excretion.

Lack of awareness of the fluctuation in BP during normal gestation may lead to diagnostic errors. For example, women with mild essential hypertension often experience a decrease in BP during early pregnancy, and BP may even approach normal levels. They may be then erroneously labeled preeclamptic in the last trimester, when frankly elevated pressures occur.

G. **Mineral metabolism.** Serum calcium levels decrease in pregnancy, in conjunction with a decrement in circulating albumin concentrations. Ionized calcium levels, however, remain in the normal nonpregnant range. Striking changes relating to calcium regulatory hormones also occur during normal pregnancy. Production of 1,25, dihydroxy-vitamin D_3 increases as early as the first trimester, reaching circulating levels that are approximately two times nonpregnant values. Gastrointestinal absorption of calcium increases, resulting in an "absorptive hypercalciuria," with 24-hour urine excretion often exceeding 300 mg per day (in appropriately nourished individuals). Intact parathyroid hormone levels are lower during normal pregnancy.

II. **Clinical evaluation of renal function in pregnancy**
 A. **Examination of the urine.** The association of proteinuria with eclampsia was first noted in the 1840s, and the science of prenatal care advanced dramatically when physicians began to systematically examine the urine of gravidas, primarily for albuminuria. In certain instances, latent renal disease is first uncovered by the detection of excessive protein excretion or microscopic hematuria during a routine prenatal evaluation.

Healthy nonpregnant women excrete considerably less than 100 mg of protein in the urine daily, but due to the relative imprecision and variability of testing methods used in hospital laboratories, proteinuria is not considered abnormal until it exceeds 150 mg per day. During pregnancy, protein excretion increases, and excretion up to 300 mg per day may still be normal. On occasion, a healthy gravida can excrete more than that amount. The problem is compounded by the fact that approximately 5% of healthy adolescents and young adults have postural proteinuria, which may become apparent only during pregnancy. In addition, postural proteinuria may increase near term, when gravidas tend to assume a more lordotic posture, which augments protein excretion. Another cause of increased proteinuria in pregnancy may be the compression of the renal veins by the enlarged uterus, especially when gravidas lie supine. Thus, when the gravida is tested for postural proteinuria (see Chapter 8), she should be positioned in lateral recumbency.

Few attempts have been made to quantitate the urine sediment in pregnancy. The excretion of both red and white blood cells may increase during normal gestation, and one to two red blood cells per high-powered field is acceptable in a urinalysis.

B. Renal function tests. The clearance of endogenous creatinine, the most satisfactory approximation of GFR in nongravid subjects, is equally useful for assessing renal function in gravidas. Gravidas, as well as nonpregnant women, show little variation (approximately 10% per day) in urinary creatinine excretion and, presumably, in creatinine production, which in a given woman is similar both during and after gestation. The lower limit of normal creatinine clearance during gestation should be 30% greater than the average of 110 to 115 mL per minute for nongravid women.

Acid excretion and urinary concentration and dilution are similar in gravid and nonpregnant women. Thus, tests such as ammonium loading (rarely indicated in gestation) give values similar to those in nongravid women. When examining urinary diluting ability, the clinician should be aware that supine posture can interfere with this test. Therefore, studies to detect minimal urinary osmolal concentrations should be performed with the patient lying on her side. However, although lateral recumbency is the required position for prenatal measurement of most renal function parameters, this posture interferes with tests of concentration. For example, a urine osmolality that was 800 mOsm per kg after overnight dehydration may decrease to 400 mOsm per kg within 1 hour through fluid mobilization from the extremities during bed rest, thus resulting in volume-induced inhibition of AVP secretion, a mild osmotic diuresis, or both. These observations demonstrate the importance of upright posture, such as quiet sitting, when maximum urinary concentration is measured in pregnancy.

C. Role of renal biopsy in pregnancy. Percutaneous renal biopsy is seldom performed during gestation. In fact, pregnancy was once considered a relative contraindication to the procedure because of early reports of excessive bleeding and other complications in gravid women. This view, however, stemmed from the period when many biopsies were performed in hypertensive patients at a time predating the understanding of the coagulation abnormalities that may occur in preeclamptic women. It is now evident that if the renal biopsy is performed in women with well-controlled BP and normal coagulation indices, morbidity is similar to that of nonpregnant patients. Our opinion is that renal biopsy should be considered only when renal function suddenly deteriorates remote from term and no obvious cause is present. This is because certain forms of rapidly progressive glomerulonephritis, when diagnosed early, may respond to aggressive treatment such as steroid pulses and, perhaps, plasma exchange. Another situation in which biopsy is recommended is symptomatic nephrotic syndrome. Although some might consider a therapeutic trial of steroids in such cases, we prefer to determine beforehand whether the lesion is likely to respond to steroids, because pregnancy is itself a hypercoagulable state prone to worsening by such treatment. On the other hand, proteinuria alone in a normotensive woman with well-preserved renal function who has neither marked hypoalbuminemia nor intolerable edema would lead us to examine the patient at more frequent intervals and defer the renal biopsy to the postpartum period. This is because the consensus among most investigators is that prognosis is determined primarily by the level of renal function and the presence or absence of hypertension rather than by the type of renal lesion (see section **III.D**). We take a similar position in the management of pregnancies with asymptomatic microscopic hematuria alone, when neither stone nor tumor is suggested by ultrasonography. Finally, renal biopsies should not be performed after gestational week 30, because at this stage the fetus will probably be delivered in any case, and the decision usually has to be made quickly and independent of biopsy results.

III. Renal disease in pregnancy
A. Asymptomatic bacteriuria. UTI is the most common renal problem occurring in pregnancy. The urine of gravidas supports bacterial growth better than that of nonpregnant women because of its increased nutrient content. This, as well as ureteral dilation, stasis, and occasional obstruction,

would be expected to increase the susceptibility of pregnant women to UTI. Surprisingly, this is not the case, and, with the exception of certain high-risk groups (diabetic patients and gravidas with sickle cell trait), the prevalence of asymptomatic bacteriuria during gestation varies between 4% and 7%, a value similar to that in sexually active nonpregnant women. The natural history of asymptomatic UTIs is, however, quite different in pregnancy.

Although in the nonpregnant state asymptomatic bacteriuria is quite benign, progression to overt cystitis or pyelonephritis occurs in up to 40% of affected gravidas. Therefore, screening all pregnant women for the presence of asymptomatic bacteriuria and treating those with positive urine cultures is important.

1. **Method of urine collection.** Pregnant women contaminate midstream urine specimens more frequently. The incidence can be reduced by the use of multiple vulval washings combined with carefully supervised collection procedures. In some women, suprapubic aspiration is required to differentiate contamination from true infection. Pregnancy is not a contraindication to this procedure.

   If the urine is sterile at the beginning of pregnancy, it usually remains so until term. Still, a small number (1% to 2%) of gravidas whose original urine cultures are negative subsequently have bacteriuria. Abnormal urinalysis and the presence of dysuria do not differentiate between contamination and true infection. For example, dysuria occurs in 30% of gravidas whose urines are sterile, and the urine may be infected and still contain fewer than two leukocytes per high-power field.

2. **Method of treatment.** The optimum way to manage asymptomatic UTI in pregnancy has not been precisely defined. In the earlier literature, some authors recommended continuous antibiotic treatment from the time the bacteriuria was detected until delivery. This was based on the belief that the relapse rate was high, and that most bacteriuric women have renal parenchymal involvement as opposed to bladder infection. However, it is now apparent that one-half of these infections involve only the bladder, and the majority of these patients are cured by standard short-course (or even single-dose) therapy. More than 90% of the uropathogens involved are aerobic gram-negative rods, usually *Escherichia coli*, and we recommend a 4–7-day course of the antibiotic to which the cultured organism is sensitive, preferably a short-acting sulfa drug, nitrofurantoin, amoxicillin, or a cephalosporin. This approach, when combined with surveillance for recurrent bacteriuria, has been shown to be quite effective.

3. **Importance of postpartum evaluation.** Asymptomatic UTI has been linked to premature labor, hypertension, and anemia during gestation, but these assertions have not been proved. On the other hand, an increased incidence of occult urinary tract pathology is present in these gravidas. Therefore, women with bacteriuria during pregnancy may benefit from evaluation of their urinary tract postpartum, especially those in whom the infection is resistant to therapy.

B. **Symptomatic bacteriuria.** The clinical approach to symptomatic UTI during gestation differs from that for asymptomatic bacteriuria.

   1. **Acute pyelonephritis.** Pyelonephritis was a cause of maternal death in the preantibiotic era, and 3% of pregnant patients in a more recently reported series developed septic shock. At one time, symptomatic UTIs complicated almost 2% of all gestations, but prenatal screening combined with rapid treatment of asymptomatic bacteriuria has reduced this incidence to approximately 0.5%. The bacteriology of these infections resembles that in asymptomatic patients (predominantly *E. coli*), and most cases present after midpregnancy. The clinical presentation of pyelonephritis in pregnancy can be dramatic. As noted before, the disease caused maternal deaths in the preantibiotic era, and upper UTIs in gravidas are associated with exaggerated effects of endotoxemia,

including shock, respiratory distress syndrome, marked renal dysfunction, and hematologic and liver abnormalities. Symptomatic UTIs have also been implicated in the etiology of intrauterine growth retardation, prematurity, congenital anomalies, and fetal demise. Thus, although treatment of cystitis may take place in an outpatient setting, treatment of pyelonephritis should be aggressive and is best performed in the hospital.

Most patients with pyelonephritis respond quickly, with defervescence within 48 to 72 hours. However, in contrast to patients with cystitis or asymptomatic bacteriuria, these women are likely to experience relapse. Thus, gravidas with acute pyelonephritis should receive the therapeutic dose of antibiotics for 2 to 3 weeks. Subsequently, we recommend continuous suppressive therapy during the remainder of pregnancy and for the first 2 weeks of the puerperium, because up to 60% of the patients will have a recurrence of pyelonephritis if left untreated. An alternative approach, frequent surveillance for recurrent infection with prompt treatment when significant bacteriuria is identified, has been claimed to be as effective as suppressive therapy.

2. **Perirenal abscess and renal abscess formation or carbuncle,** although infrequent complications of gestation, should be considered in the differential diagnosis of postpartum fever. It is important to recognize that a high incidence of positive urine cultures occurs in the postpartum period—perhaps 17% to 20% in the first few days after delivery, decreasing to 4% after the third postpartum day. These cases, which resolve spontaneously, may reflect a temporary breakdown in the normal host antibacterial mechanisms in the immediate postpartum period rather than true infection.

3. **Antibiotic use in pregnancy.** The first-choice antibiotic for symptomatic infections changes from decade to decade because of the rapid emergence of resistant strains, thus resulting in the use of drugs that have not yet withstood the test of time for safety in pregnancy. We continue to recommend starting treatment with cephalosporins, because a significant percentage of community-acquired *E. coli* infections are resistant to ampicillin. For routine cystitis, nitrofurantoin is often effective, and it is acceptable during pregnancy.

The physician should also be aware of problems specific to the use of antibiotics in obstetrics and anticipate the potential fetal toxicity of agents that cross the placental barrier. (Information concerning drug safety during pregnancy is listed in the *Physicians' Desk Reference*, which is updated annually.) In brief, sulfa drugs should not be used near term, because they may precipitate kernicterus in the newborn. The anti–folic acid activity of trimethoprim has been associated with anomalies such as cleft palate in animals, and this combination drug should also be avoided, at least before midpregnancy.

Aminoglycosides should also be prescribed sparingly, because streptomycin has been associated with fetal ototoxicity and nephrotoxicity. Fluoroquinolones cross the placenta and should be avoided if possible. Tetracyclines are contraindicated because they deposit in fetal bones and teeth and may cause severe reactions in the mother, including hepatic failure.

C. **Acute renal failure (ARF)**
1. **Incidence.** Before 1970, the incidence of ARF in pregnancy severe enough to require dialytic therapy was estimated at between 1 in 2,000 and 1 in 5,000 gestations, and it represented a considerable proportion of cases reported in large series. Since then, the number of patients with ARF from obstetric causes has declined markedly, and the incidence is now estimated to be less than 1 in 20,000 pregnancies. This trend, attributed to the liberalization of abortion laws and improvement of prenatal care, has not been shared by the poorer and less industrialized nations, in

which such patients compose up to 25% of referrals to dialysis centers and in which renal failure in pregnancy continues to be an important cause of maternal and fetal mortality.

The frequency distribution of ARF during gestation was bimodal, with one peak early in pregnancy (12 to 18 weeks) comprising most of the cases associated with septic abortion, and a second peak between gestational week 35 and the puerperium, primarily due to preeclampsia and bleeding complications, especially placental abruption.

2. **Causes.** ARF in pregnancy can be induced by any of the disorders leading to renal failure in the general population, such as acute tubular necrosis (ATN). Early in pregnancy, the most common problems are prerenal disease due to hyperemesis gravidarum, and ATN resulting from a septic abortion. Several different uncommon disorders can lead to ARF later in pregnancy. Mild to moderately severe preeclampsia is not usually associated with renal failure, because renal function is generally maintained in the normal or near-normal range for a nonpregnant woman. A variant of preeclampsia, the HELLP syndrome (*h*emolysis, *e*levated *l*iver enzymes, and *l*ow *p*latelet count; see section **VI.B**) may be associated with significant renal dysfunction, especially if not treated promptly.

a. **Thrombotic microangiopathy.** An important and difficult differential diagnosis is that of ARF in late pregnancy in association with microangiopathic hemolytic anemia and thrombocytopenia. Pregnancy is considered to be a risk factor for thrombotic thrombocytopenia purpura/hemolytic uremic syndrome (TTP/HUS). However, whether the pathogenesis of these disorders in pregnancy is similar to that in nonpregnant individuals is unclear. TTP/HUS is rare in pregnancy, and must be distinguished from the HELLP variant of preeclampsia, a much more common condition. The distinction of these syndromes is important for therapeutic and prognostic reasons, but considerable overlap exists in their clinical and laboratory features. Features that may be helpful in making the diagnosis include timing of onset and the pattern of laboratory abnormalities which in TTP may include decreased levels of a von Willebrand cleaving protease. Preeclampsia typically develops in the third trimester, with only a few cases developing in the postpartum period, usually within a few days of delivery. TTP usually occurs antepartum, with many cases developing in the second trimester, as well as the third. HUS is usually a postpartum disease. Symptoms may begin antepartum, but most cases are diagnosed postpartum.

Preeclampsia is much more common than TTP/HUS, and it is usually preceded by hypertension and proteinuria. Renal failure is unusual even with severe cases, unless significant bleeding or hemodynamic instability, or marked disseminated intravascular coagulation (DIC) occurs. In some cases, preeclampsia develops in the immediate postpartum period, and when thrombocytopenia is severe, it may be indistinguishable from HUS. However, preeclampsia spontaneously recovers, whereas HUS only infrequently improves.

In contrast to TTP/HUS, preeclampsia may be associated with mild DIC and prolongation of prothrombin and partial thromboplastin time. Another laboratory feature of preeclampsia/HELLP syndrome that is not usually associated with TTP/HUS is marked elevations in liver enzymes. The presence of fever is more consistent with a diagnosis of TTP than preeclampsia or HUS. The main distinctive features of HUS are its tendency to occur in the postpartum period and the severity of the associated renal failure. Treatment of preeclampsia/HELLP syndrome is delivery and supportive care. More aggressive treatment is rarely indicated. Treatment of TTP/HUS includes plasma infusion or exchange and other modalities used in nonpregnant patients with these disorders, although clinical trials of these modalities in pregnancy have not been performed.

b. Bilateral **renal cortical necrosis** may be induced by abruptio placenta or other clinical events complicated by severe obstetric hemorrhage (e.g., uterine rupture). Both primary DIC and severe renal ischemia have been proposed as the initiating events. Affected patients typically present with oliguria or anuria, hematuria, and flank pain. Ultrasonography or computed tomographic (CT) scanning may demonstrate hypoechoic or hypodense areas in the renal cortex. Most patients require dialysis, but 20% to 40% have partial recovery of renal function.

c. Acute pyelonephritis. Some pregnant women may develop ARF in association with pyelonephritis.

d. Acute fatty liver of pregnancy (fatty infiltration of hepatocytes without inflammation or necrosis) is a rare complication of pregnancy that is associated with significant azotemia. Women with this disorder often complain of anorexia and occasionally of abdominal pain in the third trimester. Clinical features suggesting preeclampsia, including hypertension and proteinuria, are not uncommon. Laboratory tests reveal elevations in liver enzymes, hypoglycemia, hypofibrinogenemia, and prolonged partial thromboplastin time. Delivery is indicated, and most patients improve shortly afterwards.

e. Urinary tract obstruction. Pregnancy is associated with dilation of the collecting system, which is not usually associated with renal dysfunction. Rarely, complications such as large uterine fibroids, which may enlarge in the setting of pregnancy, can lead to obstructive uropathy. Rarely, acute urinary tract obstruction in pregnancy is induced by a kidney stone. Diagnosis can usually be made by ultrasonography. Often the stones pass spontaneously, but occasionally cystoscopy is necessary for insertion of a stent to remove a fragment of stone and relieve obstruction, particularly if there is sepsis or a solitary kidney.

3. The **management** of ARF occurring in gestation or immediately postpartum is similar to that in nongravid subjects (see Chapter 11), but several points peculiar to pregnancy deserve emphasis. Because uterine hemorrhage near term may be concealed and blood loss underestimated, any overt blood loss should be replaced early. Gravidas should be slightly overtransfused to forestall the development of acute tubular or cortical necrosis. Both peritoneal dialysis and hemodialysis have been successfully used in patients with obstetric-related acute renal failure. Neither pelvic peritonitis nor the enlarged uterus is a contraindication to the former method. In fact, this form of treatment is more gradual than hemodialysis and thus less likely to precipitate labor. Because urea, creatinine, and other metabolites that accumulate in uremia traverse the placenta, dialysis should be undertaken early, with the aim of maintaining the blood urea nitrogen at approximately 50 mg per dL. In essence, the advantages of early dialysis in nongravid patients are even more important for the pregnant patient, making arguments for prophylactic dialysis quite compelling. Excessive fluid removal should be avoided, because it may contribute to hemodynamic compromise, reduction of uteroplacental perfusion, and premature labor. Some obstetricians and perinatologists recommend continuous fetal monitoring during hemodialysis treatments, starting at midpregnancy. Finally, the physician should be aware of potential dehydration in the neonate, because the newborn usually undergoes a brisk urea-induced diuresis.

D. Pregnancy in women with preexisting renal disease. The current approach to management of pregnancy in women with chronic renal disease (CRD) is primarily based on retrospective studies, and more definitive views must await prospective data from large series in which clinical, pathologic, and

Table 14-2. Summary of pregnancy in women with preexisting renal disease[a]

Disease	Comments
Chronic glomerulonephritis and focal glomerular sclerosis (FGS)	Increased incidence of high blood pressure occurs late in gestation, but usually no adverse effect results if renal function is preserved and hypertension is absent before gestation. Some disagree, believing that coagulation changes in pregnancy exacerbate disease, especially immunoglobulin A nephropathy, membranoproliferative glomerulonephritis, and FGS.
Systemic lupus erythematosus (SLE)	Controversial: prognosis is most favorable if disease is in remission 6 months or more before conception.
Periarteritis nodosa and scleroderma	Both fetal and maternal prognosis is poor. Therapeutic abortion should be considered.
Diabetic nephropathy	No adverse effect on the renal lesion. Increased frequency of infections. High incidence of heavy proteinuria and hypertension near term.
Chronic pyelonephritis (infectious tubulointerstitial disease)	Bacteriuria in pregnancy may lead to exacerbation.
Polycystic kidneys	Few problems when function is preserved and hypertension is absent. However, the incidence of preeclampsia is increased.
Urolithiasis	Ureteral dilation and stasis do not seem to affect natural history, but infections can be more frequent. Stents have been successfully placed during gestation.
Reflux nephropathy	Prognosis disputed. We believe such pregnancies have a good outcome, although urinary infection may be more common.
Previous urologic surgery	Urinary tract infection is common with urinary diversion, and renal function may undergo reversible decrease. Cesarean section might be necessary to avoid disruption of the continence mechanism if artificial sphincters or neourethras have been constructed.
After nephrectomy, solitary pelvic kidneys	Pregnancy is well tolerated. Might be associated with other malformations of the urogenital tract. Dystocia occurs rarely with a pelvic kidney.

[a]Generalizations are for women with only mild renal dysfunction (serum creatinine level <1.5 mg/dL) and without hypertension at conception.

functional observations are correlated. Nevertheless, several generalizations can be made and some guidelines presented regarding gestation in women with chronic kidney dysfunction (Table 14-2).

1. **Prognosis.** Counseling and managing women with CRD is based on the following general approach: Fertility and ability to sustain an uncomplicated pregnancy relate to the degree of functional impairment, and whether hypertension is present, and not to the underlying disorder.

   a. **Degree of impairment.** Patients are arbitrarily considered in three categories: preserved or mildly impaired renal function (serum creatinine less than or at 1.4 mg per dL), moderate renal insufficiency (creatinine 1.5 to 3.0 mg per dL), and severe renal insufficiency (creatinine higher than or equal to 3 mg per dL). In Table 14-3 are summarized the

Table 14-3. Pregnancy and renal disease: functional renal status and prospects[a]

| Prospects | Category | | |
	Mild Cr <1.5 mg/dL	Moderate Cr 1.5–3.0 mg/dL	Severe Cr >3.0 mg/dL
Pregnancy complications	25%	47%	86%
Successful obstetric outcome	96% (85%)	90% (59%)	47% (8%)
Long-term sequelae	<3% (9%)	25% (71%)	53% (92%)

Cr, serum creatinine.
[a]Estimates are based on 1,862 women with 2,799 pregnancies (1973–1992) and do not include collagen diseases. Numbers in parentheses refer to prospects when complication(s) develop before 28 weeks' gestation.
(From Davison JM, Lindheimer MD. Renal disorders. In: Creasy RK, Resnick RK, eds. *Maternal–fetal medicine,* 3rd ed. Philadelphia: WB Saunders, 1994. Reprinted with permission.)

maternal and fetal prognosis in each category, and Table 14-4 depicts the improvement in pregnancy outcomes that has occurred since the 1950s, reflecting advances in prenatal and neonatal care. We generally counsel avoidance of conception in women who have moderate or severe renal dysfunction, because up to 40% of pregnancies in the former category are complicated by either hectic hypertension or sudden declines in GFR, which may not reverse after delivery. An even higher incidence of serious maternal problems occurs when renal insufficiency is severe. This is especially true for women receiving dialytic therapy, in whom fewer than 50% of the gestations succeed, and problems of extreme prematurity plague many of those that do. Notably, although we base prognosis primarily on the degree of functional impairment, the underlying disease may also play a role. Thus, all authorities recommend against pregnancy in women with scleroderma and periarteritis nodosa, and some have reservations concerning patients who have lupus erythematosus, immunoglobulin A nephropathy, or focal glomerular sclerosis.

b. **Level of blood pressure (BP).** The BP level at time of gestation is an important prognostic index. In the absence of hypertension, the natural history of most established renal parenchymal disease is unaffected by gestation (although preeclampsia may occur more readily).

Table 14-4. Renal disease and pregnancy: improvements in perinatal mortality over four decades[a]

| Renal disease | Pregnancy outcome | Morbidity and mortality (%) | | | |
		1950s	1960s	1970s	1980s
Mild	Preterm delivery	8	10	19	25
(Cr <1.5 mg/dL)	Perinatal mortality	18	15	7	<5
Moderate	Preterm delivery	15	21	40	52
(Cr 1.5–3.0 mg/dL)	Perinatal mortality	58	45	23	10
Severe	Preterm delivery	100	100	100	100
(Cr >3.0 mg/dL)	Perinatal mortality	100	91	58	53

Cr, serum creatinine.
[a]Estimates are based on 2,952 women with 4,011 pregnancies (1954–1992) and do not include cases of lupus erythematosus.
(From Davison JM, Lindheimer MD. Renal disorders. In: Creasy RK, Resnick RK, eds. *Maternal–fetal medicine,* 3rd ed. Philadelphia: WB Saunders, 1994. Modified with permission.)

In contrast, when renal disease and hypertension coexist, the gestation is more likely to be complicated, either by severe increments in BP or by additional reductions in renal function. We permit women with well-controlled BP and only mild renal dysfunction to conceive or continue gestation, but these gravidas must be seen frequently and should understand that their gestation must be terminated if renal function deteriorates or if their BP becomes difficult to control.

E. **Proteinuria.** Urinary protein excretion, which increases in normal pregnancy, may increase markedly in pregnant women with underlying parenchymal renal disease. In one large series, one-third of the patients with preexisting renal disease developed nephrotic-range proteinuria during gestation. These increments do not necessarily reflect worsening of the underlying kidney disease.

1. **Renal hemodynamics.** Gravidas with kidney disorders who have only minimal renal dysfunction usually experience increments in GFR during gestation, even though levels do not reach those seen in normal pregnant women. Thus, a decrement in serum creatinine level early in pregnancy is a good prognostic sign. If serum creatinine levels before conception exceed 1.4 mg per dL, decrements during gestation are less common, and, as noted, the prognosis of such pregnancies is more guarded. Finally, Table 14-5 summarizes fetal and maternal outcomes of 906 pregnancies in women with various primary glomerular disorders. Of importance, the data are mainly retrospective, reflecting an important need for prospective observational studies.

F. **Glomerulonephritis.** Absence of gravidas in large epidemiologic surveys of poststreptococcal glomerulonephritis is remarkable and has led to speculations that pregnancy protects women from this disease. However, this form of immune complex nephritis does occur rarely in gestation, in which it may mimic preeclampsia. Its prognosis is favorable, because in those instances in which the occurrence of acute poststreptococcal glomerulonephritis during gestation was properly documented, renal function recovered rapidly and the pregnancy usually had a successful outcome.

The prognosis of chronic glomerulonephritis during pregnancy is difficult to evaluate because most reported cases are poorly documented, especially the prepregnancy level of renal function and BP. Still, it appears that if proteinuria or abnormal urinary sediment is the sole manifestation of the disease, pregnancy proceeds normally. Some authorities disagree, claiming that women with membranoproliferative glomerulonephritis (MPGN) and immunoglobulin A nephropathy are more prone to exacerbations during pregnancy, a view we do not share. Although C3 nephritic factor may pass from mother to fetus, the neonate appears unaffected, and maternal complement levels may actually rise during gestation.

Hereditary nephritis is an uncommon disorder that may first be manifested during pregnancy, when women with this disease develop frank nephrotic syndrome. A variety of hereditary nephritis accompanied by platelet abnormalities has been described. Pregnancy in these women has been successful from a renal standpoint, but their gestations have been complicated by bleeding problems.

G. **Collagen vascular disease**

1. **Lupus nephritis.** The effect of gestation in women with lupus erythematosus who have renal involvement is difficult to evaluate, in part because of the unpredictable course of the disease regardless of pregnancy. Activity of the disease in the 6 months before conception is often a useful prognostic guide (the longer the remission, the better the outlook). Although most pregnancies, in the presence of preserved function, proceed uneventfully or are accompanied by only transient functional declines; in approximately 10%, gestation appears to cause permanent renal damage and to accelerate the renal disease. Also, placental transmission of maternal autoantibodies is associated with an increased frequency of

spontaneous abortion in these women, and certain anticytoplasmic antibodies (especially SS-A/Ro) cause a neonatal lupus syndrome characterized by congenital heart block, transient cutaneous lesions, or both. Women with systemic lupus erythematosus (SLE) have a high incidence of detectable levels of antiphospholipid antibodies (anticardiolipin antibodies, lupus anticoagulant). High titers of these antibodies are associated with several complications of pregnancy, including spontaneous fetal loss, hypertensive syndromes indistinguishable from preeclampsia, and thrombotic events including deep vein thrombosis, pulmonary embolus, myocardial infarction, and strokes. Also, pregnant women with circulating antiphospholipid antibodies can manifest a rare form of rapid renal failure postpartum, associated with glomerular thrombi. Thus, women with SLE should be screened for antiphospholipid antibodies early in gestation. The therapeutic approach when gravidas manifest antiphospholipid antibodies is disputed, and many would not treat asymptomatic patients who manifest low titers. However, when titers are elevated [more than 40 GPL (immunoglobulin G antiphospholipid level)], most authorities prescribe aspirin (80 to 325 mg per day). Heparin in combination with aspirin is recommended for patients with a history of thrombotic events and may also be advisable when titers are higher than 80 GPL.

A flare of lupus nephritis may be difficult to distinguish from preeclampsia when a woman with a history of lupus develops worsening renal function, proteinuria, and hypertension. Elevation in liver enzymes and new onset severe hypertension is more consistent with preeclampsia. Hypocomplementemia, and severe nephritic syndrome without hypertension is more consistent with lupus nephritis. Often, a flare of nephritis in the third trimester appears to trigger "superimposed preeclampsia," and improvement in BP and proteinuria occurs only after delivery. However, in the presence of abnormal serologic testing, it is often reasonable to treat worsening proteinuria and azotemia with increased prednisone in the hope that it will improve, particularly if the fetus is immature. However, close maternal and fetal surveillance is of utmost importance, and delivery should be considered in the setting of obvious signs of HELLP syndrome, accelerating hypertension and/or azotemia, and other signs of worsening maternal condition.

Previously, patients with lupus nephropathy were believed to be prone to relapse in the immediate puerperium, and some physicians still start or increase steroid treatment during and after delivery. Such views of "stormy puerperium" are now disputed, and most authorities institute or change therapy only if signs of increased or *de novo* disease activity appear.

2. Pregnancy in patients with **periarteritis nodosa and scleroderma with renal involvement** appears to be disastrous, possibly due to the associated hypertension, which frequently becomes malignant in nature. Earlier case reports document poor fetal prognosis and maternal deaths particularly in the era before angiotensin converting enzyme (ACE) inhibitors. Although such a poor prognosis partly reflects the selectivity of a handful of case reports, prudence dictates that pregnancies of gravidas with these diseases be terminated at an early stage until more is known about their natural history during pregnancy.

H. **Diabetes mellitus** is among the more common medical disorders encountered in the prenatal clinic. Many of the patients are juvenile (type I, insulin-dependent) diabetics, who probably harbor early microscopical changes in their kidneys. Nevertheless, most gestations in diabetic patients with normal renal function succeed, especially if blood glucose levels are maintained close to the normal range during the prenatal period. These diabetic women, however, have an increased prevalence of bacteriuria and an increased susceptibility to symptomatic infection during pregnancy. With these exceptions, such women rarely have complications, although they seem to have a higher incidence of preeclampsia.

The effects of gestation in diabetic patients with overt nephropathy are similar to those in women with other forms of renal parenchymal disease. Patients with the mildest functional impairment have little trouble (although more than 50% experience third-trimester hypertension and increased proteinuria, the latter sometimes massive), whereas the presence of hypertension before conception imparts a poorer prognosis. Older reports of frequent deteriorations reflect experience from centers in which the gravidas were managed with stringent salt restriction and prophylactic diuretics. Without such restrictions, women with biopsy-proven diabetic nephropathy actually display increases in GFR during gestation.

I. **Nephrotic syndrome.** The most common cause of nephrotic-range proteinuria (more than 3.5 g per day) in late pregnancy is preeclampsia, a diagnosis that may be missed when diastolic pressures are between 85 and 95 mm Hg. The fetal prognosis in preeclampsia with heavy proteinuria is poorer than in other preeclamptic states, but maternal prognosis is similar. Most of the usual causes of nephrotic syndrome, including membranous nephropathy, proliferative or membranoproliferative glomerulonephritis, lipoid nephrosis (nil disease), diabetic nephropathy, amyloidosis, and focal segmental glomerulosclerosis have been described in gravidas. Many of these conditions do not respond to corticosteroids, and some may be aggravated by them, underscoring the importance of establishing a tissue diagnosis before starting therapy.

One should not confuse physiologic changes during gestation with the exacerbation of a disease causing the nephrotic syndrome; many women with a variety of non-nephrotic renal disorders develop heavy proteinuria when pregnant. Such increments in urinary protein may relate to the increased renal hemodynamics, alterations in the glomerular barrier, and possibly a rise in renal vein pressure. Other alterations in pregnancy that simulate symptoms accompanying nephrotic syndrome include decrements in serum albumin (approximately 0.5 to 1.0 g per dL), increments in the levels of cholesterol and other circulating lipids, and edema, which can occur at one time or another in up to 80% of normal gestations. Accordingly, an entity once termed *cyclic nephrotic syndrome of pregnancy* reflects instances of quiescent mild renal disease, which becomes more apparent during gestation.

Management of nephrotic pregnant patients includes dietary replenishment of urine protein losses (in rare instances, gestation has been sustained until an appropriate delivery date using albumin infusions). Although restriction of dietary protein has been recommended in certain forms of nephrotic syndrome in nonpregnant patients, and has led to decrements in the excretion of and increments in levels of circulating albumin, such therapy should not be attempted in gravid women, because it could be deleterious to fetal development. Diuretics should be avoided, if possible, because these women are already oligemic, and further intravascular volume depletion might impair uteroplacental perfusion. Also, because BP normally declines during pregnancy, diuretics might provoke more ready circulatory collapse or thromboembolic episodes. Exceptions to this, however, are certain nephrotics who also manifest salt-sensitive hypertension (mainly women with diabetic nephropathy). In such cases, modest salt restriction, combined with the judicious use of diuretics, may avoid termination in the early third trimester because of poorly controlled BP.

Prognosis in most nephrotic gravidas with preserved function is good, but some claim that fetal outcome is poorer if full-blown nephrotic syndrome is already present very early in gestation. In addition, hypoalbuminemia may be associated with small-for-date newborns. Focal segmental glomerulosclerosis is a disease of varied (and often unknown) etiology whose natural history during gestation remains disputed. Some claim pregnancy leads to irreversible functional loss and hypertension-sustained postpartum; others find the natural history of this entity in pregnancy similar to that of most other disorders.

J. Tubulointerstitial disease

1. **Chronic pyelonephritis.** Dilation and stasis in the urinary tract make chronic pyelonephritis in gravidas more prone to exacerbation. These women should have a high fluid intake and should be told to rest frequently on their sides. The prognosis of pregnant women with noninfectious interstitial nephritis seems similar to that of pregnant women with glomerular disease. Renal function deterioration may occur rapidly in this group of patients when they are inadvertently salt restricted during gestation.

2. **Reflux nephropathy.** Some authors believe that pregnancy adversely influences the course of reflux nephropathy. Others note that patients who do poorly have preexisting hypertension and moderate functional insufficiency. Obviously, the propensity for UTI in these patients demands close scrutiny during pregnancy, including frequent urine cultures and prompt treatment when signs of UTI appear.

3. **Adult dominant polycystic kidney disease** may remain undetected in gestation. Careful questioning of gravidas for a family history of renal problems and judicious use of ultrasonography may lead to its earlier detection. Patients with minimal functional impairment have few complications, but a greater propensity toward preeclampsia exists. They are also prone to UTIs, and it may therefore be prudent to culture their urines more frequently. Hypertension usually accompanies or antedates the onset of functional deterioration, and pregnancy in such gravidas is more hazardous.

   Some women with autosomal dominant polycystic kidney disease manifest cysts in their livers that may enlarge with repeated pregnancy as well as with oral contraceptive use. A high incidence of cerebral aneurysms also occurs in certain affected families. When aware of such family clustering, usually identified by a history of subarachnoid hemorrhages among relatives, the patient should undergo screening using magnetic resonance angiograph (MRA). If an aneurysm is detected, neurosurgical consultation should be obtained, and the obstetrician may wish to avoid natural labor. All these patients should undergo genetic counseling before pregnancy to ensure they are aware that 50% of their offspring are at risk. Finally, predicting the fetal outcome using molecular probes on cells cultured from the amniotic fluid is possible.

4. **Solitary and pelvic kidneys.** Women with solitary kidneys appear to tolerate gestation well. However, if the nephrectomy was performed for nephrolithiasis or chronic pyelonephritis, the remaining kidney is often infected. Patients with these conditions must be carefully scrutinized by frequent examination and culture of the urine throughout pregnancy and in the puerperium.

K. Pelvic kidneys are apparently associated with decreased fetal survival, often due to the presence of other malformations of the urogenital tract of the mother. In addition, dystocia may occur when the kidney is in the true pelvis.

L. Urolithiasis and hematuria. The prevalence of urolithiasis in gestation varies between 0.03% and 0.35% in the Western hemisphere. Many of the stones contain calcium, and some are infective in origin. The older literature tended to stress the dramatic complications that occur when calculi cause obstructive uropathy and infection supervenes, but more recent reports, including one survey of 148 gestations in 78 nonselected stone formers, suggest that pregnancy has little influence on the course of stone disease (although women with renal calculi may have an increased incidence of spontaneous abortions). It should be noted that most of the reported series focus on women whose calculi are mainly of the noninfective variety, and little is known of the natural history of the more serious infected struvite stones during gestation. In any event, UTI in the presence of nephrolithiasis requires prompt and prolonged treatment (3 to 5 weeks), followed by suppressive therapy through the immediate puerperium, because the calculus may represent a nidus of infection resistant to sterilization.

Experience with cystinuria in pregnancy is limited, but most women with this disease also do well in gestation. D-Penicillamine as used in these patients appears to have no apparent adverse effects on mother or fetus.

Renal calculi are among the most common causes of abdominal pain (of nonobstetric origin) requiring hospitalization during gestation, and, when complications suggest the need for surgical intervention, pregnancy should not be a deterrent to x-ray examination. If the stone obstructs the ureter, intervention with either uteteral stenting, percutaneous nephrostomy, or rarely, surgery, is indicated. Spontaneous gross or microscopical hematuria occasionally complicates an otherwise uneventful gestation. The differential diagnosis includes all causes of hematuria in nongravid patients (see Chapter 8), but frequently no etiology is demonstrable, and the bleeding subsides postpartum. It has been suggested that these events are due to the rupture of small veins around the dilatated renal pelvis. Hematuria may or may not occur in subsequent gestations. In any event, investigation of the hematuria can often be deferred until after delivery, and noninvasive techniques such as ultrasound and magnetic resonance imaging are helpful in arriving at such decisions.

IV. Renal transplantation

A. Fetal and maternal complications. Several thousand pregnancies have been reported in allograft recipients. As expected, prognosis is better when the transplanted kidney comes from a living donor. Most (more than 90%) gestations allowed to proceed beyond the first trimester succeed, but both maternal and fetal complications, due in part to the immunosuppressive therapy, can be anticipated; these include steroidinduced hyperglycemia, severe hypertension, UTI, septicemia, ectopic pregnancy, and uterine rupture. Fetal problems such as intrauterine growth retardation, congenital anomalies, prematurity, hypoadrenalism, hepatic insufficiency, thrombocytopenia, and serious infection have been reported.

B. Suggested criteria for pregnancy. The following relative criteria for transplant recipients wishing conception are suggested:

1. Good health and stable renal function for 1–2 years after transplantation
2. Stature compatible with good obstetric outcome
3. Absent or at most minimal proteinuria
4. No or easily managed hypertension
5. No evidence of pelvicalyceal distention on an excretory urogram performed before attempting pregnancy
6. Serum creatinine of 2 mg per dL or less, preferably less than 1.4 mg per dL
7. Drug therapy: prednisone, 15 mg per day or less; azathioprine, 2 mg per kg per day or less; cyclosporine, less than 5 mg per kg per day

   Several thousand woman have gone through pregnancy after renal transplantation, most of whom have received prednisone. Prednisone crosses the placenta in small amounts, and is not believed to adversely affect the fetus, although adrenal insufficiency and thymnic hypoplasia have been described. The well known impact of glucocorticoids on maternal BP and blood sugar are important issues during pregnancy. High doses of prednisone may be associated with premature rupture of membranes. Azathioprine has also been used extensively in pregnancy. Inactive metabolites appear in fetal blood, and high doses may lead to myelosuppression of the fetus. The National Transplantation Pregnancy Registry has reported on the experience with cyclosporine in pregnancy. This drug is associated with slightly lower birthweights, increased maternal hypertension and an increased frequency of preeclampsia, although the data have been collected retrospectively without a control population. Cyclosporine levels may decrease during pregnancy. No information on whether or not drug dosage should be increased is available. If renal function is normal, and the patient is more than 2 years post transplantation, it is probably not necessary to increase the cyclosporine dosage to maintain prepregnancy blood levels.

There is less experience with tacrolimus, although to date no serious concerns exist, and it appears similar to cyclosporine with respect to an association with premature delivery.

Although limited animal data regarding fetal effects of mycopheolate mofetil were a concern, no structural malformations have been noted among offspring exposed to this drug, although exposures are limited to less than 10 reported pregnancies. For this reason we do not recommend it during pregnancy. Limited experience exists with rapamycin, and this author is not aware of published reports of use during pregnancy.

V. Dialysis. Fertility is reduced in dialysis patients, and few women conceive once they have started dialysis. Most pregnancies occur during the first few years on dialysis. Although previously the outcomes of such pregnancies were poor, with only approximately 25% resulting in surviving infants, new information suggests that pregnancy in dialysis patients is successful as often as 30% to 50% of the time in pregnancies that reach the second trimester. Considerable problems exist in such pregnancies, however, and we do not encourage women on maintenance dialysis to conceive.

The National Registry for Pregnancy in Dialysis Patients has reported 318 pregnancies in women on dialysis. Prematurity is common, and approximately 85% of infants born to women who conceive after starting dialysis are born before 36 weeks' gestation. More than one-third of the infants reported by the registry weighed less than 1,500 g at birth, and growth restriction was common. Maternal complications are also common, including accelerated hypertension, and an increased maternal mortality rate. Management of pregnant women on dialysis should include attempts to minimize the uremic environment. In women with chronic renal disease, prophylactic dialysis should be considered when renal function is poor. In women already on dialysis, treatment time should be increased to five to seven dialysis sessions per week, with minimal heparinization and slow ultrafiltration to avoid dialysis hypotension and volume contraction. If peritoneal dialysis is used, decreasing exchange volumes and increasing exchange frequency is recommended. Adequate calorie and protein intake should be encouraged and supplemental vitamins prescribed. Antihypertensive therapy should be adjusted to be appropriate for pregnancy. Anemia should be corrected with iron, folic acid, and erythropoietin. Adequate calcium supplements should be administered but the dose of vitamin D may have to be decreased. And metabolic acidosis should be prevented. No evidence exists to support the superiority of one dialysis modality over another with respect to pregnancy outcome.

VI. Hypertensive disorders of pregnancy. Hypertension during gestation remains a major cause of morbidity and death in both mother and child.

A. Of the many **classifications** proposed for hypertension complicating pregnancy, that of the Committee on Terminology of the American College of Obstetricians and Gynecologists (1972) has been the most useful. The National High Blood Pressure Education Program in the United States endorsed this system in 1990 and again in 2000. The four categories of hypertensive disorders in pregnancy are:

1. Preeclampsia. Preeclampsia, characterized by hypertension, proteinuria, edema, and, at times, coagulation and liver function abnormalities, occurs in late pregnancy (after 20 weeks), primarily in nulliparas. Third-trimester hypertension is defined as a BP of 140/90 mm Hg or greater (Korotkoff V) sustained for 4 to 6 hours.

Attempts have been made to categorize this disease as severe (e.g., diastolic and systolic pressures of 110 and 160 mm Hg or greater, heavy proteinuria, oliguria, and neurologic symptoms) or mild. Because a seem-ingly mild preeclamptic patient (e.g., a teenage gravida with a systolic blood pressure of 140/85 mm Hg and trace proteinuria) may suddenly convulse (in which case the disease is called *eclampsia*, a complication as-sociated with maternal mortality), terms such as *mild* and *severe* may be misleading. Hypertension during late pregnancy in a nullipara, whether or not other signs are present, is sufficient reason to consider hospital-ization and treatment as if the patient were potentially preeclamptic.

2. **Chronic hypertension.** Most women in this category have essential hy-pertension, but in some the elevated BP is secondary to such conditions as renal artery stenosis, coarctation of the aorta, renal disease, primary al-dosteronism, and pheochromocytoma. Evidence of arteriolar disease and knowledge that hypertension was present before conception or early in gestation is helpful in establishing a diagnosis. Cocaine abuse may mas-querade as chronic hypertension in pregnancy. Pheochromocytoma has a catastrophic outcome during pregnancy; thus, measurement of urinary catecholamines or vanillylmandelic acid excretion should be considered in selected hypertensive gravidas not previously evaluated.

3. **Chronic hypertension with superimposed preeclampsia.** Hyperten-sive women are at increased risk for the development of superimposed preeclampsia, and, when this occurs, maternal and fetal morbidity and mortality are greater than when preeclampsia develops in a previously normotensive woman. Many of the maternal deaths attributable to hy-pertensive disease occur in previously hypertensive women with super-imposed preeclampsia

4. **Gestational hypertension,** which is high BP appearing first after mid-pregnancy, is distinguished from preeclampsia by the absence of pro-teinuria. This category is broad, and includes women who later develop diagnostic criteria for preeclampsia, as well as women with chronic hy-pertension in whom BP decreased in early pregnancy, masking the true diagnosis. Gestational hypertension that resolves postpartum, and which was not in retrospect preeclampsia, is more likely to occur in women who develop essential hypertension later in life.

5. The physician should be aware of two forms of hypertension that com-plicate the puerperium. One entity is called **_late postpartum eclampsia_** (hypertension and convulsions 48 hours to weeks after delivery). This disorder may be elicited by the administration of bromocriptine, a drug prescribed to suppress lactation. The second entity is **postpartum hyper-tension** in normotensive gravidas, presenting 2 weeks to 6 months after delivery, with normalization by the end of year 1. Its etiology is poorly understood.

B. **Pathophysiology of preeclampsia.** Preeclampsia is syndrome whose man-ifestations affect many organ systems, including brain, liver, kidney, blood vessels, and placenta. Thus, whereas the focus may be on hypertension and proteinuria, we must always be aware that such signs and symptoms may be minimal while other, life-threatening syndromes develop, including con-vulsions and liver failure, both often associated with thrombocytopenia, as well as signs of DIC.

The placenta may be critically involved in the genesis of preeclampsia, and failure of cytotrophoblastic invasion of the uterine spiral arteries is one of the earliest changes in this disorder. Thus, these vessels do not undergo the expected transformation into the dilated blood vessels characteristic of nor-mal placentation. This aberration may underlie the poor placental perfusion and growth retardation characteristic of preeclampsia. The reason for the failure of the trophoblast to invade the uterine spiral arteries is obscure. Re-cent research has focused on the abnormal modulation of cytotrophoblast ad-hesion molecules, integrins, and abnormal vascular endothelial growth fac-tor receptor-ligand interactions. The abnormal placentation leading to the maternal syndrome of preeclampsia is believed to occur early in pregnancy

(10 to 20 weeks gestation). Finally, recent evidence has implicated the production of antiangiogenic factors in the genesis of preeclampsia.

The mediators of hypertension in preeclampsia are not clearly understood. Evidence suggests that vasoconstriction results from a complex interplay of hormonal and vascular alterations. With respect to hormonal factors, the renin-angiotensin system is stimulated in normal pregnancy and relatively suppressed in women with preeclampsia. However, preeclamptic patients are more sensitive to the pressor effects of angiotensin II, and therefore this pressor peptide may play a role in their elevated BP. Aldosterone levels are also lower in preeclamptic women than in women with normal pregnancies, although still higher than nonpregnant levels.

Recent evidence suggests that alterations in vascular endothelial cell function are important features of the pathophysiology of preeclampsia. Endothelial cells produce a variety of substances important in modulating vascular tone and coagulation [e.g., nitric oxide (NO), prostacyclin, and endothelin]. Animal studies of gestational hypertension and limited clinical investigations suggest that decreased NO and prostacyclin, and increased endothelin, all sequelae of endothelial cell dysfunction, cause the vasoconstriction, platelet aggregation, and increased intravascular coagulation that then leads to the maternal clinical manifestations of preeclampsia. More recently soluble vascular endothelial growth factor variants have been postulated to modulate endothelial dysfunction.

The ability to excrete sodium may be impaired in preeclampsia, but the degree to which this occurs varies, as severe disease can occur in the absence of edema (the "dry preeclamptic" patient). Even when edema is marked, plasma volume is below that for normal pregnancy, and hemoconcentration is often present. This latter phenomenon may relate to the development of a "leaky" vasculature (thus, hypoalbuminemia in this disease may have three components: renal protein loss, liver dysfunction, and extravasation from the intravascular to the interstitial space). A decrement or suboptimal increase in intravascular volume also appears to precede the onset of overt hypertension.

Cardiac output is often decreased, and central venous and pulmonary capillary wedge pressures are normal or low. Thus, high BP is maintained by a marked increase in peripheral resistance. The alterations in cardiac output, combined with the decrements in intravascular volume, and the fact that placental perfusion is decreased in preeclampsia are major reasons that most authorities discourage use of diuretics in this disease.

In one variant of preeclampsia, HELLP, coagulation abnormalities and liver dysfunction predominate, whereas hypertension and proteinuria may be minimal. This syndrome is life threatening, because platelet counts may plunge far below 100 to 103 per mm^3, whereas transaminase and lactic acid dehydrogenase levels rise above 1,000 units per L and evidence of a marked microangiopathic hemolytic anemia appears on the peripheral blood smear, all in less than 24 hours. Early recognition of this HELLP variant and prompt termination of gestation are important; such action avoids substantial maternal morbidity.

The pathogenesis of the eclamptic convulsion is also poorly understood. Vasospasm, ischemia, and local hemorrhage may all play a role. The importance of hypertension per se in the genesis of the seizures is debated, because convulsions may be observed in women whose BP is only mildly elevated.

C. **Kidney function and morphology in preeclampsia**
   1. **GFR and RPF.** Both GFR and RPF decrease in preeclampsia. The decrements approximate 25% in most instances, so that the GFR of preeclamptic women often remains above pregravid values. However, in rare instances, large decreases in function may occur and, on occasion, lead to acute tubular or cortical necrosis.
   2. **Uric acid.** Changes occur in the renal handling of urate in preeclampsia. A decrease in the clearance of uric acid, accompanied by increments

A   **B**

Figure 14-2. A: Electron micrograph demonstrating complete capillary obliteration by a swollen endothelial cell. Note, however, that the basement membrane is normal and the epithelial foot processes are intact. **B:** Micrograph showing glomerulus from a preeclamptic kidney. Swollen endothelial and mesangial cells that display prominent vacuolization encroach on the capillary lumina. (Courtesy of B. H. Spargo, M.D.)

in blood levels of this solute, may occur weeks before any clinical signs of the disease appear. In pregnancy, serum urate levels above 4.5 mg per dL are suspect [to convert to SI units (μmol/L), multiply mg/dL by 59.48]. The level of hyperuricemia also correlates with the severity of the preeclamptic renal lesion, as well as with fetal outcome.

3. Increased **proteinuria,** which may be moderate or heavy, is a feature of preeclampsia, and the diagnosis is suspect in its absence. The magnitude of proteinuria does not appear to affect maternal prognosis, but protein excretion in the nephrotic range is associated with greater fetal loss.

4. **Calcium.** Studies have demonstrated that renal calcium handling is altered in preeclampsia, and that in contrast to normotensive gravidas, or those with chronic or transient hypertension, patients with preeclampsia demonstrate marked hypocalciuria. The basis for this abnormality is unknown.

5. Preeclampsia is accompanied by a characteristic histologic lesion: **glomerular capillary endotheliosis** (Fig. 14-2). In women diagnosed clinically as preeclamptic, this lesion is present in only about 85% of biopsies obtained from primiparas and in considerably fewer biopsies from multiparas. The remainder of patients have evidence of nephrosclerosis or another parenchymal disease. Some claim that preeclampsia is a cause of focal glomerular sclerosis, but others believe preeclampsia lesions to be completely reversible, with the presence of focal glomerular sclerosis reflecting preexisting nephrosclerosis or primary renal disease. Women with glomerular endotheliosis alone tend to have uneventful subsequent gestations, but when focal glomerular sclerosis or alterations in the renal vessels are present, hypertension is more likely to recur in later pregnancies.

D. Management of preeclampsia

1. **Hospitalization.** Ambulatory treatment is risky in the management of preeclampsia. Thus, suspicion of the disease is sufficient to consider hospitalization. Such an approach diminishes the frequency of convulsions and other consequences of diagnostic error. In general, fetal maturity is evaluated; if the gestation is near term, induction is the therapy of choice, whereas attempts to temporize are made if the pregnancy is at an earlier stage. Rest is an extremely important part of the therapeutic regimen, which must be prescribed rather than suggested. Termination of pregnancy should be considered when signs of impending eclampsia (e.g., hyperreflexia, headaches, epigastric pain) develop or persist; BP cannot be controlled; serum creatinine, urea nitrogen, and uric acid rise; laboratory evidence suggests DIC or abnormal liver function (increased transaminases); or specific obstetric tests suggest fetal jeopardy. When signs of impending convulsions (eclampsia) are present, parenteral magnesium sulfate is the drug of choice.

2. **Treatment of hypertension.** The approach to treatment of high BP in gravidas is disputed. As noted, morphologic examination of preeclamptic placentae demonstrates decreased trophoblastic invasion of the uterine spiral arteries, causing these vessels to be more constricted than normal. Thus, perfusion of the placenta is compromised. Therefore, aggressive reduction in maternal BP may decrease uteroplacental perfusion even further (i.e., poor autoregulation of uterine blood flow). Thus, large decrements in the mother's mean pressure should be avoided, especially in acute emergencies. Data on human pregnancy are limited, but they suggest that decrements in maternal pressure may indeed reduce placental perfusion. Others have argued that, based on evidence obtained from animal studies, uterine blood flow is autoregulated, and thus hypertension should be aggressively treated. Assuming that autoregulation of uterine blood flow exists, a critical but unanswered question is how quickly it takes place, because fetuses may be damaged by short periods of ischemia. In documented instances, precipitous decreases of pressure in response to diazoxide (even to diastolic levels above 85 mm Hg) were followed by immediate monitor signs of fetal distress. Thus, we prescribe the careful use of parenteral hydralazine or labetalol, in addition to close maternal scrutiny and fetal monitoring, when acute hypertension exceeds diastolic levels of 100 mm Hg or systolic levels of 150 mm Hg (Table 14-5). This approach is successful in most gravidas.

   Calcium channel blockers have also been used to treat acute hypertension associated with preeclampsia. However, these agents should be considered only after hydralazine or labetalol has been unsuccessful, because anecdotal reports exist of precipitous decreases in BP when calcium channel blockers have been used concomitantly with magnesium sulfate.

   Diazoxide can be used in rare resistant cases and should be administered only in small doses (30 mg at a time). Sodium nitroprusside should be avoided, because cyanide poisoning and fetal death have been observed in laboratory animals. ACE inhibitors and angiotensin receptor blockers (ARBs) should not be used in pregnancy.

3. **Treatment of the eclamptic convulsion.** Several large clinical trials have demonstrated that magnesium sulfate is superior to other anticonvulsants for prevention of recurrent eclamptic convulsions, and also, for primary prevention of eclampsia in women with preeclampsia. The usual protocol is to administer a loading dose of 4 g magnesium sulfate, infused over 15 minutes, followed by a sustaining infusion of 1 to 2 g per hour, aiming to achieve plasma levels of 2 to 4 μmol per L. Because the incidence of convulsion is highest in the immediate puerperium, it is common practice to begin magnesium sulfate immediately after delivery and continue it for 24 hours.

Table 14-5. Maternal and fetal outcomes (%) in 558 women with primary glomerulopathies

Renal lesion	Pregnancies	Spontaneous abortion	Perinatal loss	Preterm delivery	Reversible function	Progressive hypertension	Renal decrease	
							Reversible	Permanent
Focal glomerulosclerosis	85	3	23	32	13	5	32	10
Membranous glomerulopathy	110	12	4	35	3	2	22	3
Membranoproliferative	165	17	8	19	6	3	20	12
Immunoglobulin A nephropathy	268	5	15	21	12	2	25	12
Mesangial proliferative	278	5	12	9	2	3	36	7
Mean	906	8	13	19	8	3	27	9

(From Imbasciati E, Ponticelli C. Pregnancy and renal disease: predictors for fetal and maternal outcome [editorial]. *Am J Nephrol* 1991;11:353–362. Modified with permission.)

E. Prevention of preeclampsia. Many strategies to prevent preeclampsia have been attempted over the years, including sodium restriction, diuretics, high-protein diets, and antihypertensive medication—all have been unsuccessful. In the last decade, considerable resources have been allocated toward determining whether either low-dose aspirin or calcium supplementation are effective preventive strategies.

Several small studies conducted in the mid-1980s suggested that low-dose aspirin (50 to 150 mg per day), administered early in gestation may prevent preeclampsia. Since 1993, several large trials have now been completed, and most have not demonstrated a beneficial effect of aspirin for the prevention of preeclampsia. In a National Institutes of Health (NIH)–sponsored randomized placebo-controlled trial of 3,135 healthy nulliparous women, 4.6% of the aspirin group and 6.3% of the placebo group developed preeclampsia, a barely significant difference. There was a slight increase in placental abruption in the group taking aspirin. A larger trial conducted largely in the United Kingdom (the CLASP trial) of 9,309 women at slightly increased risk failed to demonstrate any decrease in the incidence of preeclampsia in the treated group. In this study, there was no increase in placental abruption in the aspirin-treated patients. Several subsequent large trials in Brazil, Barbados, Jamaica, and the United States, with a total of more than 13,000 women at moderate or high risk found no significant differences in the incidence of preeclampsia, fetal growth restriction, preterm births, or adverse outcomes between women receiving aspirin and controls. A summary of all large trials conducted suggests that aspirin treatment may prevent the occurrence of early onset preeclampsia in approximately 15% of women at risk and reduce fetal growth restriction by 18%. A recent systematic review of 14 trials including over 12,000 women showed a small but significant benefit of aspirin therapy in reducing perinatal death (OR .79) and preeclampsia (OR .86), and an increase of 215 g in mean birth weight. Aspirin therapy is safe and not associated with increased risk of bleeding or placental abruption.

It has been suggested that the women enrolled in the earlier trials were too "low risk" to detect a significant benefit of aspirin; however, a multicenter trial of women with high-risk pregnancies (chronic hypertension, diabetes, multiple gestation) did not demonstrate a reduced incidence of preeclampsia in the treated group. The present data therefore do not support the prophylactic use of low-dose aspirin in pregnant women at low or medium risk for preeclampsia, or in women with mild chronic hypertension. However, low-dose aspirin may be effective in a defined group of predominantly parous women at high risk, not only in preventing preeclampsia but in reducing its severity.

Another preventive strategy that has received considerable attention is calcium supplementation. Low calcium intake has been implicated in the pathogenesis of preeclampsia, and a trial of 1,094 nulliparous pregnant women, as well as a meta-analysis, suggested that calcium supplementation with 2 g of calcium carbonate daily can prevent preeclampsia. Again, a large NIH multicenter randomized clinical trial of 4,589 women failed to support these earlier findings. However, subsequent trials conducted outside the United States have continued to demonstrate a beneficial effect of calcium supplementation for the prevention of preeclampsia. A possible explanation for the discrepancy in these results is the dietary calcium intake in these populations. In the NIH trial, both the placebo and treated groups had a baseline calcium intake of greater than 1,000 g per day. In contrast, in those trials in which calcium has been beneficial, the calcium intake in the population was well below the recommended dietary allowance for pregnancy. Thus, calcium supplementation may be beneficial in women with low calcium intake but may not be necessary if calcium intake is adequate.

Most other approaches to prevention, including fish oil, diuretics, sodium restriction, and magnesium supplementation have not been successful.

Currently under investigation is the ability of antioxidants (e.g. vitamins C and E) to prevent preeclampsia. Nevertheless, although prevention of preeclampsia is usually not possible, avoidance of severe complications may be accomplished by early recognition of the disease before such complications develop. If early signs are detected, hospitalization should be strongly considered to permit close monitoring of the patient. If preeclampsia is detected early, bedrest and close monitoring of maternal and fetal condition may enable prolongation of pregnancy in some cases.

F. **The hypertensive patient without preeclampsia.** Increased risk is associated with pregnancy in women with chronic hypertension. Complications include superimposed preeclampsia, placental abruption, acute tubular and cortical necrosis, retardation of intrauterine growth, and midtrimester fetal death. Such events seem to correlate with the age of the gravida and the duration of her high BP. Thus, the majority of these complications occur in women over the age of 30 or with evidence of end-organ damage. Conversely, most women (approximately 85%) with essential hypertension have uncomplicated and successful gestations.

Women with chronic hypertension often have reductions in BP by midpregnancy, so that their BP may not exceed that observed in normotensive pregnant women. The failure of this decrement to occur, or increases in BP in early or midtrimester pregnancy, indicates a guarded prognosis for the gestation. Fetal outcome is poorer in hypertensive women with superimposed preeclampsia than in previously normotensive women with this complication, and the combination of chronic hypertension and preeclampsia seems responsible for most cases of cerebral hemorrhage in pregnancy. Patients with both conditions should be hospitalized and their hypertension controlled, but even with these precautions, most authorities consider delaying actions too risky and terminate the gestation.

1. **Antihypertensive therapy.** Guidelines for antihypertensive therapy during gestation are less clear than those for nonpregnant hypertensive women. For the latter, compelling data exist from large population studies to document the benefits of lowering BP with medication, even in women with only mild hypertension. During pregnancy, however, although maternal safety remains the primary concern, there is also a desire to minimize exposure of the fetus to drugs, given their unknown long-term effects on growth and development. A systematic review of clinical trials of hypertension found only 13 randomized clinical trials comparing antihypertensive therapy to either no treatment or placebo in women with chronic hypertension. The most commonly used drug, methyldopa, was given to just over 200 subjects. Six trials showed no reduction in perinatal mortality with antihypertensive treatment, whereas three reported a trend toward lower perinatal mortality with treatment. A debatable issue is whether lowering BP will prevent superimposed preeclampsia, but little or no convincing evidence supports this contention. Thus, it is permissible to tolerate higher BP levels during gestation that do no harm in the short term, while limiting use of antihypertensive drugs. In this respect, most pregnant women with chronic hypertension have only mild or very moderate elevations in BP and require little or no medication at all. However, "appropriate" or "tolerable" levels of BP for these patients during gestation seem to have been set empirically, and multicenter clinical trials are needed to support or reject such practices.

Whether mild degrees of hypertension during gestation should be treated is not generally agreed on. Although one group claimed that such therapy decreases the incidence of superimposed preeclampsia, most authorities would withhold treatment until diastolic levels are at least 15 mm Hg above borderline hypertension (defined in our clinics as 75 mm Hg

Table 14-6. Guidelines for treating severe hypertension near term or during labor

Regulation of blood pressure

The degree to which blood pressure should be decreased is disputed; we recommend maintaining diastolic levels between 90 and 110 mm Hg.

Drug therapy

Hydralazine administered intravenously is the drug of choice. Start with low doses (5 mg as an intravenous bolus), then administer 5 to 10 mg every 20 to 30 min to avoid precipitous decreases in pressure. Side effects include tachycardia and headache.

Labetalol, administered intravenously, is an effective and safe agent for preeclamptic hypertension. Start with 20 mg and repeat the dose every 20 min, up to 200 mg, until desired blood pressure is achieved. Side effects include headache.

Favorable results have been reported with *calcium channel blockers.* If *magnesium sulfate* is being infused, magnesium may potentiate the effects of calcium channel blockers, resulting in precipitous and severe hypotension.

Diazoxide should be used only in the rare instance that hydralazine, labetalol, or calcium channel blockers have been unsuccessful. Small doses (30 mg at a time) should be used. Side effects include arrest of labor and neonatal hypoglycemia.

Refrain from using *sodium nitroprusside,* because fetal cyanide poisoning has been reported in animals. However, maternal well-being should dictate the choice of therapy.

Prevention of convulsions

Parenteral *magnesium sulfate* is the drug of choice for preventing eclamptic convulsions. Therapy should be continued for 12 to 24 hr postpartum, because one-third of women with eclampsia have convulsions during this period.

---

in the second trimester and 85 mm Hg in late gestation). Very young gravidas, however, may require treatment at lower levels. Tables 14-6 and 14-7 summarize current knowledge on the use of antihypertensive drugs in pregnancy. Only since the mid-1980s have serious efforts been undertaken to determine the safety and efficacy of these medications in pregnant women, and only a handful of these efforts have involved controlled trials. Future endeavors should increase the availability of this information.

I recommend the guidelines of the National High Blood Pressure Education Program's Working Group Report on High Blood Pressure in Pregnancy, in which antihypertensive drug treatment is begun only when maternal BP reaches diastolic levels of 100 mm Hg or more. Exceptions, however, include parenchymal renal disease and evidence of target organ damage (e.g., retinopathy and cardiac hypertrophy), in which therapy is recommended once levels are 90 mm Hg or more.

The argument of whether to treat is debatable when fetal well-being is considered. Some evidence suggests fetal benefits when mild to moderate hypertension is treated with antihypertensive drugs during pregnancy.

In summary, the unknown but potential hazards of antihypertensive treatment during pregnancy are sufficient reasons for withholding drug treatment when mild hypertension (diastolic levels of 90 to 99 mm Hg) is present, particularly during the initial trimester. As noted, many of these patients experience a physiologic decrease in BP that on occasion reaches normotensive levels. Otherwise normal patients whose levels are 100 mm Hg or more, however, should be treated. Patients with evidence of renal disease or end-organ damage require the initiation of treatment at lower levels (less than 90 mm Hg).

Table 14-7. Antihypertensive drugs used to treat chronic hypertension in pregnancy

Alpha2 adrenergic receptor agonists
 Methyldopa is the most extensively used drug in this group. Its safety and efficacy
 are supported by evidence from randomized trials and a 7.5-year follow-up
 study of children born to mothers treated with methyldopa

Beta adrenergic receptor antagonists
 These drugs, especially *atenolol* and *metoprolol,* appear to be safe and efficacious
 in late pregnancy, but fetal growth retardation has been reported when
 treatment was started in early or midgestation. Fetal bradycardia can occur,
 and animal studies suggest that the fetus's ability to tolerate hypoxic stress may
 be compromised.

Alpha adrenergic receptor and beta adrenergic receptor antagonists
 Labetalol appears to be as effective as methyldopa, but no follow-up studies of
 children born to mothers given labetalol have been carried out, and concern
 about maternal hepatotoxicity still exists.

Arteriolar vasodilators
 Hydralazine is frequently used as adjunctive therapy with methyldopa and beta
 adrenergic receptor antagonists. Rarely, neonatal thrombocytopenia has been
 reported. Trials with *calcium channel blockers* look promising. The experience
 with *minoxidil* is limited, and this drug is not recommended.

Calcium channel blockers
 Small, uncontrolled studies suggest that these agents are safe and effective in
 pregnancy.

Angiotensin converting enzyme (ACE) inhibitors
 Captopril causes fetal death in diverse animal species, and several converting
 enzyme inhibitors have been associated with oligohydramnios and neonatal
 renal failure when administered to humans. Do not use in pregnancy.

Angiotensin II receptor blockers
 These drugs have not been used in pregnancy. In view of the deleterious effects of
 blocking angiotensin II generation with ACE inhibitors, angiotensin II receptor
 antagonists are also considered to be contraindicated in pregnancy.

Diuretics
 Many authorities discourage the use of diuretics, but others continue these
 medications if they were prescribed before conception or if a woman with
 chronic hypertension appears quite sensitive to salt.

(From Cunningham FG, Lindheimer MC. Hypertension in pregnancy [see comments]. *N Engl J Med*
1992;326:927–932. Reprinted with permission.)

Suggested readings

Armenti VT, Ahlswede KM, Ahlswede BA, et al. Variables affecting birthweight and
 graft survival in 197 pregnancies in cyclosporine-treated female kidney transplant
 recipients. *Transplantation* 1995;59:476–479.

August P, Lindheimer MD. Chronic hypertension in pregnancy. In: Lindheimer MD,
 Roberts JM, Cunningham FG, eds. *Chesley's hypertensive disorders in pregnancy,*
 2nd ed. Norwalk, CN: Appleton & Lange, 1999:605–633.

August P, Lindheimer MD. Pathophysiology of preeclampsia. In: Laragh JH, Brenner
 BM, eds. *Hypertension: pathophysiology, diagnosis, and management.* New York:
 Raven Press, 1995;2407–2426.

Burke JF. Variables affecting birthweight and graft survival in 197 pregnancies in cyclosporine-treated female kidney transplant recipients. *Transplantation*
 1995;59:476–479.

Cadnapaphornchai MA, Ohara M, Morris KG, Knotek M, Ragachev B, Ladtkow T,
 Carter EP, Schrier RW. Chronic NOS inhibition reverses systemic vasodilation

and glomerular hyperfiltration in pregnancy. *Am J Physiol Renal Physiol* 2001;280:F592–F598.

Chapman AB, Abraham WT, Zamudio S, Coffin C, et al. Temporal relationships between hormonal and hemodynamic changes in early human pregnancy. *Kid Int* 1998;54:2056–2063.

Conrad KP. Mechanisms of renal vasodilation in pregnancy. *J Soc gynec Invest* in press 2004.

Conrad KP and Lindheimer MK. Renal and cardiovascular alterations. In: Lindheimer MD, Roberts JM, and Cunningham FG, eds. *Chelsey's hypertensive disorders in pregnancy,* 2nd ed. Stamford, CT: Appleton & Lange, 1999:2263–2326.

Cunningham FC, Lucus MJ. Urinary tract infections complicating pregnancy. *Clin Obstet Gynaecol (Baillière)* 1994;8:363–383.

Davison JM. Pregnancy in renal allograft recipients: problems, prognosis, and practicalities. *Clin Obstet Gynaecol (Baillière)* 1994;8:511–535.

Davison JM, Dunlop M. Renal hemodynamics and tubular function in normal human pregnancy. *Kid Int* 1980;18:152.

Davison JM, Lindheimer MD; guest editors. New Developments in preeclampsia. *Seminars in Nephrol* in press 2004.

Hou S. Pregnancy in chronic renal insufficiency and end-stage renal disease. *Am J Kidney Dis* 1999;33:235–252.

Jones DC, Hayslett JP. Outcome of pregnancy in women with moderate or severe renal insufficiency. *N Engl J Med* 1996;335:226–232.

Jungers P, Chauveau D. Pregnancy in renal disease. *Kidney Int* 1997;52:871–885.

Lindheimer MD, Katz AI. Gestation in women with renal disease: prognosis and management. *Clin Obstet Gynaecol (Baillière)* 1994;8:397–414.

Lindheimer MD, Katz AI. Renal physiology and disease in pregnancy. In: Seldin DW, Giebisch G, eds. *The kidney: physiology and pathophysiology.* 3rd ed. Philadelphia: Lippincott Williams & Wilkins, 2000:1260–1265.

National High Blood Pressure Education Program Working Group Report on High Blood Pressure in Pregnancy. *Am J Obstet Gynecol* 2000;183:S1–S22.

Okundaye IB, Agrinko P, Hou S. A registry for pregnancy in dialysis patients. *Am J Kidney Dis* 1998;31:766–773.

Pertuisset N, Grünfeld J-P. Acute renal failure in pregnancy. *Clin Obstet Gynaecol (Baillière)* 1994;8:343–361.

Roberts JM, Redman CWG. Pre-eclampsia: more than pregnancy-induced hypertension. *Lancet* 1993;341:1447–1451.

Sibai BM. Drug therapy: treatment of hypertension in pregnant women. *N Engl J Med* 1996;335:257–265.

The Patient with Hypertension

Charles R. Nolan

I. **Definition and classification of hypertension.** The definition of hypertension is somewhat arbitrary, because blood pressure (BP) is not distributed bimodally in the population. Instead, the distribution of BP readings in the population is unimodal, and an arbitrary level of BP must be defined as the threshold above which hypertension can be diagnosed. The correlation between the levels of systolic BP and diastolic BP and cardiovascular risk has long been recognized. It has become clear that in patients over age 50, systolic BP of more than 140 mm Hg is a much more important cardiovascular risk disease risk factor than is diastolic BP. Increasing BP clearly has an adverse effect on mortality over the entire range of recorded pressures, even those generally considered to be in the normal range. Lifespan and health are progressively reduced as BP rises. The goal of identifying and treating high BP is to reduce the risk of cardiovascular disease and associated morbidity and mortality. In this regard, classifying hypertension in adults is useful in identifying high-risk individuals and providing guidelines for follow-up and treatment of hypertension. The seventh report of the Joint National Committee on Prevention, Detection, Evaluation, and Treatment of High Blood Pressure (JNC 7) has established criteria for the diagnosis and classification of BP in adult patients (Table 15-1). The optimal BP in an individual who is not acutely ill is lower than 120/80 mm Hg. Individuals with a systolic BP of 120 to 139 mm Hg or a diastolic BP of 80 to 89 mm Hg should be considered as prehypertensive; these patients require health-promoting lifestyle modifications to prevent cardiovascular disease. Patients with prehypertension are at twice the risk of developing hypertension as those with lower values. Although normotensive by definition, these prehypertensive patients should be rechecked annually to exclude the development of hypertension. Hypertension is arbitrarily defined as a systolic BP of 140 mm Hg or greater or a diastolic BP of 90 mm Hg or greater, or by virtue of the patient taking antihypertensive medications. The stage of hypertension (stage 1 or 2) is determined by the levels of both systolic BP and diastolic BP (Table 15-1). This classification should be based on the average of two or more blood pressure readings at each of two or more visits after the initial BP screening. When systolic BP and diastolic BP fall into different categories, the higher category should be selected to classify the individual's BP.

II. **Epidemiology of hypertension.** The prevalence of hypertension ranges from 20% to 30% of the entire adult population of the United States. Hypertension affects approximately 50 million individuals in the United States and approximately 1 billion individuals worldwide. The prevalence increases with advancing age, so that approximately one-third of patients in their fifth decade meet the criteria for hypertension. Data from the Framingham Heart Study indicate that even individuals who are normotensive at 55 years of age have a 90% lifetime risk for developing hypertension. As the mean age in the general population increases, the prevalence of hypertension will no doubt increase further unless effective preventative measures are implemented. Many hypertensive patients have a positive family history of parental hypertension. The mode of inheritance is complex and probably polygenic in most instances. Black men and women have a twofold higher prevalence of hypertension (30%) than white men and women (15%) in a sampling of almost 18,000 American

Table 15-1. Classification of blood pressure for adults [a]

BP classification[b]	Systolic BP (mm Hg)[c]		Diastolic BP (mm Hg)[c]
Normal	< 120	and	< 80
Prehypertension	120–139	or	80–89
Stage 1 hypertension	140–159	or	90–99
Stage 2 hypertension	≥ 160	or	≥ 100

[a]Adults aged 18 years and older.
[b]Classification should be based on the mean of two or more properly measured seated blood pressure readings obtained on each of two or more office visits.
[c]When systolic and diastolic BP fall into different categories, classify based on the higher category.
(Adapted with permission from Chobanian AV, Bakris GL, Black HR, et al. The seventh report of the Joint National Committee on prevention, detection, evaluation and treatment of high blood pressure. The JNC 7 Report. *JAMA* 2003;289:2560–2572.)

adults aged 48 to 75 years in the National Health and Nutrition Examination Survey (NHANES). Prevalence appears to be equal in men and women in most surveys. Obese individuals have significantly more hypertension than nonobese individuals. In childhood, obesity is a major cause of hypertension. Proof of the significant relationship between body weight and blood pressure is found in the observation that BP falls with weight reduction. The intake of dietary salt (sodium chloride) has significant effects on BP, especially in patients with other factors predisposing to the development of hypertension, such as advancing age, obesity, adult onset diabetes, positive family history of hypertension, black race, or underlying renal disease. Numerous epidemiologic studies have shown that the dietary intake of salt correlates with the average BP in a population. Northern Japanese fisherman who ingest 450 mEq of sodium daily have a 40% prevalence of hypertension. In contrast, indigenous Alaskan populations and the Yanomamo Indians in Brazil and Venezuela, who have dietary intakes of 1 mEq of sodium daily, do not develop hypertension at any age. Intersalt, an international epidemiologic study, examined the relation between dietary sodium intake (based on 24-hour urinary sodium excretion) and BP in more than 10,000 individuals aged 20 to 59 years from 52 countries around the world. The results demonstrate a significant correlation between median systolic BP and diastolic BP and dietary sodium intake. These observations can be explained based on the role of abnormal renal sodium handling in the pathogenesis of hypertension, which is discussed in section **IV**. The therapeutic implications of these observations include dietary sodium restriction as part of nonpharmacologic therapy and the recommendation of thiazide diuretics as first-line drug therapy for the treatment of hypertension in most patients. Despite the known cardiovascular risks of untreated hypertension and the widespread availability of effective pharmacologic treatment, the identification and effective control of hypertension remains a significant public health problem in the United States. From the 1976–1980 NHANES survey (NHANES II) to the 1991–1994 survey (NHANES III, phase 2), the percentage of hypertensive Americans who are aware that they have high BP increased from 51% to 68%. Among persons with hypertension, the prevalence of treatment increased from 31% to 54% during the same period. The number of persons with high BP controlled to below 140/90 mm Hg increased from 10% in NHANES II to 27% in NHANES III. Alarmingly, data computed for 1999–2000 reveal that more than 65% of patients with hypertension still have inadequate control of their BP. The continued high prevalence of hypertension and hypertension-related complications such as stroke, cardiovascular complications, heart failure, and end-stage renal disease (ESRD) represent a major public health challenge.

III. Cardiovascular disease risk. The relationship of blood pressure to cardiovascular risk is continuous and independent of other cardiovascular risk factors.

Table 15-2. Cardiovascular risk factors and target-organ damage

Major Risk Factors
  Hypertension[a]
  Cigarette smoking
  Obesity (BMI)[b] > 30)[a]
  Physical inactivity
  Dyslipidemia[a]
  Diabetes mellitus[a]
  Microalbuminuria or estimated GFR[c] < 60 mL/min
  Age (> 55 years for men, > 65 years for women)
  Family history of premature cardiovascular disease (men < 55 years or
    women < 65 years)

Target-Organ Damage
  Heart
    Left ventricular hypertrophy
    Angina or prior myocardial infarction
    Prior coronary revascularization
    Heart failure
  Brain
    Prior stroke or transient ischemic attack
  Chronic kidney disease
  Peripheral arterial disease
  Retinopathy (see Table 14-8)

[a] Components of the metabolic syndrome associated with insulin resistance and hyperinsulinemia.
[b] BMI indicates body mass index calculated as weight in kilograms divided by the square of height in meters.
[c] GFR indicates glomerular filtration rate.
(Adapted with permission from Chobanian AV, Bakris GL, Black HR, et al. The seventh report of the Joint National Committee on prevention, detection, evaluation and treatment of high blood pressure. The JNC 7 Report. *JAMA* 2003;289:2560–2572.)

Beginning at 115/75 mm Hg and across the entire BP range, each increment of 20/10 mm Hg doubles the risk of cardiovascular disease. The overall risk of cardiovascular morbidity and mortality in patients with hypertension is determined not only by the stage of hypertension, but also by the presence of other risk factors, such as smoking, hyperlipidemia, and diabetes, and by the existence of target-organ damage (Table 15-2). The major target organs affected by hypertension are the heart, peripheral vasculature, central nervous system, the kidney, and the eye. Most of the consequences of hypertension are the result of progressive vascular injury. Hypertension accelerates atherosclerotic vascular disease and aggravates the deleterious effects of diabetes, smoking, and hyperlipidemia on the aorta and its major branches. Atherosclerotic disease results in significant morbidity from myocardial infarction (MI), atherothrombotic cerebral infarction, peripheral vascular disease with claudication, and renal disease due to ischemia or cholesterol embolization. Hypertensive renal disease may result from hypertension-induced vasculitis in the setting of malignant hypertension or more insidious renal injury from long-standing essential hypertension with hypertensive nephrosclerosis. Hypertension is also an important cofactor in the progression of other renal diseases, especially diabetic nephropathy. Hypertension may also cause cerebrovascular disease in the form of lacunar infarction or intracerebral hemorrhage. Left ventricular hypertrophy (LVH) and congestive heart failure (CHF), often due to isolated diastolic dysfunction, are the result of the heightened peripheral vascular resistance (afterload) imposed by systemic hypertension. In clinical trials, antihypertensive therapy has been associated with significant reductions in the incidence of stroke (35% to 40%), MI (20% to 25%), and heart failure (50%). It has been estimated that in patients with stage 1 hypertension (systolic BP

140 to 159 mm Hg and/or diastolic BP 90 to 99 mm Hg) and additional cardio-vascular risk factors, achieving a sustained 12 mm Hg reduction in systolic BP for 10 years will prevent 1 death for every 11 patients treated. In the setting of pre-existing cardiovascular disease or target-organ damage, treatment of 9 patients would prevent 1 death.

IV. **Pathogenesis of hypertension.** Experiments with isolated, perfused kidneys demonstrate that the magnitude of urinary sodium excretion is a direct function of the renal arterial perfusion pressure. The level of perfusion pressure may alter sodium excretion by changing the peritubular hydrostatic pressure. Thus, an increase in perfusion pressure should increase peritubular hydro-static pressure with a resultant decrease in sodium reabsorption. Micropuncture studies in the rat have shown an inverse relationship between renal perfusion pressure and proximal sodium reabsorption. It has been argued that if this pressure natriuresis mechanism was operating in a normal fashion, in the presence of hypertension, profound volume depletion would result. The fact that this does not occur suggests that in every hypertensive state, a shift in the pressure natriuresis curve must occur so that a higher perfusion pressure is required to achieve any given level of natriuresis. In this regard, Guyton and colleagues have postulated that this shift in the pressure natriuresis curve is the fundamental underlying pathophysiologic abnormality that leads to essential hypertension and virtually all secondary forms of hypertension (Fig. 15-1). If a primary renal defect in natriuresis does exist in hypertension, then, to avert disaster due to persistent positive sodium balance with inexorable fluid accumulation, compensatory mechanisms must be invoked that restore sodium balance. These compensatory processes restore sodium balance and normal extracellular fluid (ECF) volume but, in the process, cause systemic hypertension.

Guyton's hypothesis states that the most important and fundamental mechanism in determining the long-term control of BP is the renal fluid-volume feedback mechanism. In simple terms, through this basic mechanism, the kidneys regulate arterial pressure by altering renal excretion of sodium and water, thereby controlling circulatory volume and cardiac output. Changes in BP, in turn, directly influence the renal excretion of sodium and water, thus providing a negative feedback mechanism for the control of ECF volume, cardiac output, and BP. The hypothesis is that derangements in this renal fluid-volume pressure control mechanism are the fundamental cause of virtually all hypertensive states (Fig. 15-1). In every hypertensive state, an underlying abnormality exists in the intrinsic natriuretic capacity of the kidney, so that the daily salt intake cannot be excreted normally, and the development of hypertension is necessary to induce a pressure natriuresis that allows the kidney to excrete the daily salt intake. Normal sodium balance and ECF volume are maintained, but at the expense of systemic hypertension. The underlying cause for the abnormality in the natriuretic capacity depends on the etiology of hypertension. In essential hypertension, some underlying abnormality increases renal avidity for sodium. In patients with obesity and insulin resistance (metabolic syndrome), hyperinsulinemia increases proximal tubular sodium reabsorption. Increased angiotensin II levels and sympathetic nervous system activity also enhance sodium reabsorption. Mineralocorticoids enhance distal tubular sodium reabsorption. Renal parenchymal disease causes nephron loss, resulting in a natriuretic defect. Abnormalities in renal endothelin or nitric oxide (NO) levels may also impair natriuresis. To date, each of the genetic causes of hypertension that have been elucidated has been shown to relate to an abnormality of renal sodium handling. For example, Liddle's syndrome results from enhanced distal tubular sodium reabsorption due to an abnormality in sodium channels in the distal nephron. Cross-transplant experiments in hypertensive and normotensive rat strains validate the importance of the kidney in the pathogenesis of hypertension, because the presence or absence of hypertension depends on the donor source of the kidney. Guyton's hypothesis states that this decreased natriuretic capacity of the kidney initially leads to renal

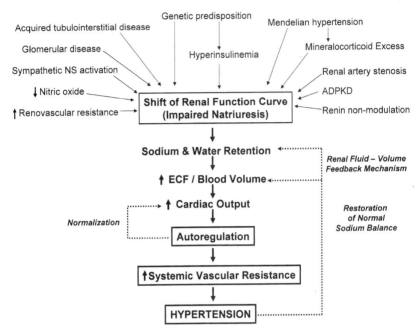

Figure 15-1. Abnormal renal sodium handling in the pathogenesis of hypertension (Guyton's hypothesis). In the setting of essential hypertension, primary renal disease, mineralocorticoid excess, or insulin resistance with hyperinsulinemia, a defect in the intrinsic natriuretic capacity of the kidney is present that prevents sodium balance from being maintained at a normal level of BP. Initially, this impairment in natriuresis leads to increases in extracellular fluid (ECF) volume and cardiac output. This hemodynamic state is short lived, however. Circulatory autoregulation occurs to maintain normal perfusion of the tissues, resulting in an increase in the systemic vascular resistance (SVR). The increase in SVR leads to systemic hypertension. With pressure-induced natriuresis, the renal fluid–volume feedback mechanism returns sodium balance, ECF volume, and cardiac output to normal. Systemic hypertension can be conceptualized as an essentially protective mechanism that prevents life-threatening fluid overload in the setting of reduced renal natriuretic capacity. Normal salt balance and fluid volume are maintained, but at the expense of systemic hypertension. (AII, angiotensin II.) (Adapted with permission from Nolan CR, Schrier RW. The kidney in hypertension. In: Schrier RW, ed. *Renal and electrolyte disorders*, 6th ed. Philadelphia: Lippincott Williams & Wilkins, 2003.)

salt and water retention, ECF volume expansion, and increased cardiac output with hypertension. This phase of volume expansion and high cardiac output is short lived. In the setting of high cardiac output, autoregulatory vasoconstriction of each vascular bed matches the blood flow to the metabolic requirements of the tissues. This phenomenon of circulatory autoregulation leads to an increase in systemic vascular resistance (SVR). Thus, hypertension that was initially caused by high cardiac output becomes high-SVR hypertension.

The development of hypertension represents a protective mechanism, because it induces the kidney to undergo a pressure natriuresis and diuresis, thereby restoring normal salt balance and returning ECF volume to normal. This mechanism explains why an underlying problem with sodium excretion, as in salt-sensitive hypertension, is manifest as high-SVR hypertension without evidence of overt fluid overload. Support for this hypothesis is found in animal models of mineralocorticoid-induced hypertension. To substantiate the role of direct pressure–induced natriuresis in the regulation of sodium balance in mineralocorticoid hypertension, Hall and colleagues compared the systemic BP and natriuretic effect of aldosterone infusion in a dog model in which the renal perfusion pressure was either allowed to increase or mechanically servocontrolled to maintain renal artery pressure at normal levels. In the intact animal, continuous aldosterone infusion caused a transient period of sodium and water retention with a mild increase in BP. This sodium retention lasted only a few days, however, and was followed by an escape from the sodium-retaining effects of aldosterone and a restoration of normal sodium balance. In contrast, when the renal perfusion pressure was servocontrolled during aldosterone infusion, no aldosterone escape occurred, and a relentless increase in sodium and water retention occurred, accompanied by severe hypertension, edema, ascites, and pulmonary edema. When the servocontrol device was removed and the renal perfusion pressure was allowed to rise to the systemic level, a prompt natriuresis and diuresis ensued, with the restoration of sodium balance and a fall in BP. These observations highlight the pivotal role of BP in the regulation of renal sodium and water excretion. Moreover, the observation that abnormal renal sodium handling is central in the pathogenesis of all forms of hypertension provides a sound pathophysiologic rationale for the JNC 7 recommendation regarding thiazide-type diuretics as first-line antihypertensive therapy in most patients.

V. **Diagnostic evaluation of hypertension.** Detection of hypertension begins with proper measurement of BP at each health care encounter. Repeated BP measurements are used to determine whether initial elevations persist and require prompt attention or have returned to normal values and require only periodic surveillance. BP measurement should be standardized as follows: After at least 5 minutes of rest, the patient should be seated in a chair with the back supported and one arm bared and supported at heart level. The patient should refrain from smoking or ingesting caffeine for 30 minutes before the examination. For an appropriately sized cuff, the bladder should encircle at least 80% of the arm. Many patients require a large adult cuff. Measurements should ideally be taken with a mercury sphygmomanometer. Alternatively, a recently calibrated aneroid manometer or a validated electronic device can be used. The first appearance of sound (phase 1) is used to define systolic BP. The disappearance of sound (phase 5) is used to define diastolic BP. The BP should be confirmed in the contralateral arm. Measurement of BP outside of the physician's office may provide some valuable information with regard to the diagnosis and treatment of hypertension. Self-measurement is useful in distinguishing sustained hypertension from "white-coat hypertension," a condition in which the patient's pressure is consistently elevated in the clinician's office but normal at other times. Self-measurement may also be used to assess the response to antihypertensive medications and as a tool to improve patient adherence to treatment. Ambulatory monitoring is useful for the evaluation of suspected white-coat hypertension, patients with apparent drug resistance, hypotensive symptoms with antihypertensive medications, and episodic hypertension. However, ambulatory BP measurement is not appropriate for the routine evaluation of patients with suspected hypertension. In elderly patients, the possibility of **pseudohypertension** should always be considered in the diagnostic evaluation of possible hypertension. Pseudohypertension is a condition in which the indirect measurement of arterial pressure using a cuff sphygmomanometer is artificially high in comparison to direct intra-arterial pressure measurement. Failure to recognize pseudohypertension can result in unwarranted and sometimes frankly dangerous treatment. Pseudohypertension can result from Monckeberg's medial calcification (a clinically benign form of arterial calcification) or advanced atherosclerosis with widespread calcification of intimal plaques. In these entities, stiffening of the arterial wall may prevent its collapse by externally applied pressure, resulting

Table 15-3. Identifiable causes of hypertension

Metabolic syndrome (obesity, insulin resistance, impaired glucose tolerance,
  dyslipidemia, hypertension)
Obstructive sleep apnea
Drug-induced hypertension (see Table 14-7)
Chronic kidney disease
Primary hyperaldosteronism
Renovascular disease
Chronic steroid use or Cushing syndrome
Pheochromocytoma
Coarctation of the aorta
Thyroid or parathyroid disease

(Adapted with permission from Chobanian AV, Bakris GL, Black HR, et al. The seventh report of the
Joint National Committee on Prevention, Detection, Evaluation and Treatment of High Blood Pressure.
The JNC 7 Report. *JAMA* 2003;289:2560–2572.)

in artificially high indirect BP readings affecting both systolic and diastolic measurements. The presence of a positive Osler's maneuver, in which the radial or brachial artery remains palpable despite being made pulseless by proximal inflation of a cuff above systolic pressure, is an important physical examination finding that should suggest the diagnosis. Roentgenograms of the extremities frequently reveal calcified vessels. The diagnosis can only be made definitely by a direct measurement of intra-arterial pressure. Patients with pseudohypertension are often elderly and therefore may have a critical limitation of blood flow to the brain or heart, such that inappropriate BP treatment may precipitate life-threatening ischemic events.

The initial history and physical examination of patients with documented hypertension should be designed to assess lifestyle, identify other cardiovascular risk factors, and identify the presence of target-organ damage that may affect prognosis and impact treatment decisions (Table 15-2). Although the vast majority of hypertensive patients have essential (primary) hypertension without a clearly definable etiology, the initial evaluation is also designed to screen for identifiable causes of secondary hypertension (Table 15-3). A medical history should include information about prior BP measurements, to assess the duration of hypertension, and details about adverse effects from any prior antihypertensive therapy. History or symptoms of coronary heart disease, CHF, cerebrovascular disease, peripheral vascular disease, or renal disease should be carefully evaluated. Symptoms suggesting unusual secondary causes of hypertension should be queried, such as weakness (hyperaldosteronism) or episodic anxiety, headache, diaphoresis, and palpitations (pheochromocytoma). Information regarding other risk factors, such as diabetes, tobacco use, hyperlipidemia, physical activity, and any recent weight gain, should be obtained. Dietary assessment regarding the intake of salt, alcohol, and saturated fat is also important. Detailed information should be sought regarding all prescription and over-the-counter medication use, including herbal remedies and illicit drugs, some of which may raise BP or interfere with the effectiveness of antihypertensive therapy. For example, nonsteroidal anti-inflammatory drugs (NSAIDs) impair the response to virtually all antihypertensive agents and increase the risk of hyperkalemia or renal insufficiency with ACE inhibitor therapy. Stimulants such as cocaine, ephedra, amphetamines, and anabolic steroids can raise BP. A family history of hypertension, diabetes, premature cardiovascular disease, or renal disease should be sought. A psychosocial history is important to identify family situation, working conditions, employment status, educational level, and sexual dysfunction that may influence adherence to antihypertensive treatment.

Physical examination should include the measurement of height, weight, and calculation of body mass index (weight in kg divided by the square of height in meters). Funduscopic examination is important to identify striate hemorrhages, cotton-wool spots, and papilledema, the characteristic findings of hypertensive neuroretinopathy, which are indicative of the presence of malignant hypertension. Documentation of the presence of arteriosclerotic retinopathy (e.g., arteriolar narrowing, arteriovenous crossing changes, changes in light reflexes) is less important, given its lack of prognostic significance with regard to the potential long-term cardiovascular complications of hypertension. Examination of the neck for carotid bruits, distended neck veins, and thyromegaly is important. Cardiac examination should include investigation for abnormalities of rate or rhythm, murmurs, and third or fourth heart sounds. The lungs should be examined for rales and evidence of bronchospasm. Abdominal examination should include auscultation for bruits (an epigastric bruit present in both systole and diastole suggests renal artery stenosis), abdominal or flank masses (polycystic kidney disease), or increased aortic pulsation (abdominal aortic aneurysm). Peripheral pulses should be examined for quality and bruits. The lower extremities should be examined for edema. A neurologic screening examination is used to identify prior cerebrovascular events. Routine laboratory tests are recommended before the initiation of antihypertensive therapy to identify other risk factors and screen for the presence of target-organ damage. These routine tests include blood chemistry (sodium, potassium, creatinine, fasting glucose), lipid profile (total cholesterol, low-density lipoprotein (LDL) and high-density lipoprotein (HDL) cholesterol), and a complete blood cell count. Creatinine clearance should be estimated using either the Cockcroft-Gault or the Modification of Diet in Renal Disease (MDRD) study forumulae. A urinalysis is used to identify proteinuria or hematuria that would suggest the presence of underlying primary renal disease. A 12-lead electrocardiogram (ECG) is used to identify left atrial enlargement, LVH, or prior MI. Optional tests, depending on the clinical situation, include 24-hour creatinine clearance, 24-hour urine protein or urine protein to creatinine ratio, serum uric acid, glycosylated hemoglobin, and thyroid function tests. A limited ECG to identify the presence of LVH may be useful in selected patients to determine the clinical significance of labile hypertension. The majority of patients with hypertension have primary (essential) hypertension in which no clearly definable underlying etiology is apparent.

A. In contrast, a wide variety of uncommon conditions can lead to so-called **secondary hypertension,** some of which are potentially amenable to surgical correction (Table 15-3). Secondary causes of hypertension include underlying chronic kidney disease (CKD), primary hyperaldosteronism, pheochromocytoma, renovascular hypertension due to fibromuscular dysplasia or atherosclerotic renal artery stenosis, coarctation of the aorta, and Cushing's syndrome. Secondary causes of hypertension amenable to surgical intervention are so unusual that extensive diagnostic testing is not warranted. More extensive laboratory and radiographic testing for identifiable causes of hypertension is not indicated unless adequate control of BP cannot be achieved with a multidrug antihypertensive regimen that includes a diuretic. The initial history, physical examination, and routine laboratory tests are usually all that is required to evaluate for the possibility of secondary hypertension. A normal estimated creatinine clearance and urinalysis are usually sufficient to exclude underlying renal disease as a secondary cause of hypertension. Examination for abdominal or flank masses is used to screen for polycystic kidney disease, which can be confirmed by ultrasound examination. Because most patients with primary hyperaldosteronism have unprovoked hypokalemia while not on diuretic therapy, a measurement of serum potassium is a suitable screening test, and routine measurement of aldosterone levels is not necessary. Assessment for any delay or diminution of pulses in the lower extremities, or a discrepancy between arm and leg BP can be used to screen for coarctation of the aorta. A careful assessment for a history of episodic hypertension, associated with headache, palpitations, diaphoresis, and pallor, is all that is usually required to screen for pheochromocytoma. The routine measurement of serum or urine catecholamines is not warranted. Likewise, evaluation for truncal obesity and abdominal purple striae is all that is usually required to screen for Cushing's syndrome; therefore, routine measurement of serum cortisol or cortisol suppression testing is unnecessary. Several tests are notably absent from the recommended list of routine screening tests for secondary hypertension. Hypertensive intravenous pyelography, renal scanning, captopril renography, and arterial digital subtraction angiography all lack sufficient specificity to be of any value as routine screening tests for renovascular hypertension. In this regard, the prevalence of renovascular hypertension in the general hypertensive population is so low that the predictive value of a positive test from any of these procedures is abysmal when used as a general screening test.

VI. Treatment of hypertension

A. Goals of treatment. The goal of treating hypertension is the reduction of cardiovascular and renal morbidity and mortality. Because systolic BP correlates best with target-organ damage and mortality, the primary focus should be on achieving the systolic BP goal. The goal of treatment is a systolic BP less than 140 mm Hg and a diastolic BP less than 90 mm Hg. In hypertensive patients with diabetes or underlying chronic kidney disease, a BP goal of less than 130/80 mm Hg is recommended.

B. Nonpharmacologic treatment. Lifestyle modification is recommended in the management of all individuals with hypertension, even in those who require antihypertensive drug treatment. All patients should be encouraged to adopt the lifestyle modificationis outlined in Table 15-4, especially if they have additional cardiovascular risk factors such as hyperlipidemia or diabetes. Modest weight reduction of as little as 4 kg (10 lbs) significantly reduces BP. Anorectic agents should be avoided because they may contain stimulants that raise BP. Obstructive sleep apnea (OSA) is now recognized as an important treatable cause of hypertension. Clues to the presence of OSA include morbid obesity, daytime hypersomnolence, headache, snoring, or fitful sleep. The diagnosis can be confirmed with a sleep study to document apneic episodes. Appropriate treatment with a continuous positive airway pressure (CPAP) device may result in a significant reduction in BP. Dietary sodium intake in the form of sodium chloride (NaCl; table salt) has a strong epidemiologic link to hypertension. Meta-analysis of clinical trials indicates that the limitation of dietary sodium intake to 75 to 100 mEq per day lowers BP over a period of several weeks to a few years. The restriction of sodium intake has been shown to reduce the need for antihypertensive medication, reduce diuretic-induced renal potassium wasting, lead to regression of LVH, and prevent renal stones through a reduction in renal calcium excretion. Average American dietary sodium intake is in excess of 150 mEq per day, most of which (75%) is derived from processed foods. Moderation of sodium intake to a level of less than 100 mEq per day (2.4 g of sodium or 6 g of sodium chloride) is recommended for the nonpharmacologic treatment of hypertension.

Excessive intake of ethanol is an important risk factor for high BP, and it can lead to resistant hypertension. Ethanol intake should be limited to not more than 30 mL (1 oz) per day in men and 15 mL (0.5 oz) per day in women and lighter-weight men. This type of moderate ethanol intake may be associated with a reduction in risk of coronary heart disease.

Regular aerobic exercise can enhance weight loss and reduce the risk for cardiovascular disease and all-cause mortality.

Inadequate potassium intake may increase BP, whereas high dietary potassium intake may improve BP control in patients with hypertension. An intake of 90 mEq per day in the form of fresh fruits and vegetables should be recommended.

Table 15-4. Lifestyle modifications to manage hypertension

Modification	Recommendation	Approximate SBP reduction
Weight loss	Maintain normal weight (BMI[a] 18.5–24.9)	5–20 mm Hg/10 kg
Dietary sodium restriction	Limit dietary sodium intake to less than 100 mEq/day (2.4 gm sodium or 6 gm sodium chloride)	2–8 mm Hg
Adopt DASH diet	Consume diet rich in fruits, vegetables, and low-fat dairy products with a reduced content of saturated and total fat	8–14 mm Hg
Increase physical activity	Engage in regular aerobic physical activity such as brisk walking (at least 30 minutes per day, most days of the week)	4–9 mm Hg
Moderate alcohol consumption	Limit consumption to no more than two drinks per day (1 oz or 30 mL ethanol per day; e.g., 24 oz beer, 10 oz wine, 3 oz 80-proof whiskey) in most men, and no more than one drink per day in women and lighter-weight men	2–4 mm Hg

[a]BMI indicates body mass index calculated as weight in kilograms divided by the square of height in meters.
(Adapted with permission from Chobanian AV, Bakris GL, Black HR, et al. The seventh report of the Joint National Committee on Prevention, Detection, Evaluation and Treatment of High Blood Pressure. The JNC 7 Report. *JAMA* 2003;289:2560–2572.)

An increase in dietary calcium may lower blood pressure in some patients with hypertension, but the effect is negligible. Nonetheless, adequate calcium intake is recommended for general health and osteoporosis prophylaxis.

Smoking cessation and reductions in dietary fat and cholesterol are also recommended to reduce overall cardiovascular risk. Although caffeine may acutely raise BP, tolerance to this effect develops quickly. Most epidemiologic studies have found no direct relationship between caffeine intake and BP.

C. **Pharmacologic treatment of hypertension.** The decision to treat hypertension with medications after the failure of lifestyle modifications to adequately control BP or initially, as an adjunct to lifestyle modifications, is based on the severity (stage) of hypertension and an assessment of the risk of cardiovascular morbidity, given the presence of other cardiovascular risk factors and pre-existing target organ damage or cardiovascular disease (see Table 15-2). Reducing BP with drugs clearly decreases cardiovascular morbidity and mortality regardless of age, gender, race, stage of hypertension, or socioeconomic status. Benefit has been demonstrated for stroke, coronary events, heart failure, progression of primary renal disease, prevention of progression to malignant hypertension, and all-cause mortality. Numerous clinical trials have demonstrated that lowering BP with several classes of drugs, including thiazide-type diuretics, angiotensin-converting enzyme (ACE) inhibitors, angiotensin-receptor blockers (ARBs), beta-blockers, and

Table 15-5. Results of the antihypertensive lipid-lowering to prevent heart attack trial

	6-Year Incidence (%)		
Outcome	Chlorthalidone	Amlodipine	Lisinopril
Primary outcome			
Coronary heart disease[a]	11.5	11.3	11.4
Secondary outcomes			
All-cause mortality	17.3	16.8	17.2
Stroke	5.6	5.4	6.3[b]
Combined coronary heart disease[c]	19.9	19.9	20.8
Combined cardiovascular disease[d]	30.9	32.0	33.3[b]
Angina	12.1	12.6	13.6[b]
Coronary revascularization	9.2	10.0	10.2[b]
Heart failure	7.7	10.2[b]	8.7[b]
End-stage renal disease	1.8	2.1	2.0
Cancer	9.7	10.0	9.9

[a]Fatal coronary heart disease or nonfatal myocardial infarction.
[b]$p \leq 0.05$.
[c]Combined coronary heart disease death, nonfatal myocardial infarction, coronary revascularization, and hospitalized angina.
[d]Combined coronary heart disease death, nonfatal myocardial infarction, coronary revascularization, angina, heart failure, and peripheral arterial disease.
(Adapted with permission from The ALLHAT Officers and Coordinators for the ALLHAT Collaborative Research Group. Major outcomes in high-risk hypertensive patients randomized to angiotensin-converting enzyme inhibitor or calcium channel blocker vs. diuretic. The Antihypertensive and Lipid-Lowering Treatment to Prevent Heart Attack Trial (ALLHAT). *JAMA* 2002;288:2981–2997.)

calcium channel blockers (CCBs), reduces all the complications of hypertension. Thiazide-type diuretics have been the treatment regimen employed in most large-scale outcome trials. In these trials, including the recently published Antihypertensive and Lipid-Lowering Treatment to Prevent Heart Attack Trial (ALLHAT), thiazide diuretics are unsurpassed in antihypertensive efficacy and for prevention of the cardiovascular complications of hypertension. In ALLHAT, stage 1 or 2 hypertensive patients older than age 55, with at least one other cardiovascular risk factor, received first-line treatment with chlorthalidone (thiazide-type diuretic), doxazocin (selective alpha-blocker), amlodipine (CCB), or lisinopril (ACE inhibitor). In this study, 47% of patients were women, 35% were black, 19% were Hispanic, 36% were diabetic, and the mean body mass index (BMI) was nearly 30. The doxazocin arm was terminated prematurely because of an excess of CHF. After a mean follow-up of 4.9 years, neither the primary clinical outcome (fatal coronary heart disease or nonfatal MI), nor the secondary outcomes of all-cause mortality, combined coronary heart disease, peripheral arterial disease, cancer, or ESRD had occurred more often in the clorthalidone group than in the amlodipine or lisinopril groups. Furthermore, event rates were signficantly lower in the chlorthalidone group than in one or both of the other groups for some of the secondary outcomes (Table 15-5). As expected, patients in the chlorthalidone group developed higher cholesterol levels, lower serum potassium levels, and higher fasting blood glucose levels than patients in other groups. The mean cholesterol was 216 mg per dL at baseline, falling at 4 years to 197 mg per dL in the chlorthalidone group, to 196 mg per dL in the amlodipine group (p = 0.009 versus chlorthalidone), and to 195 mg per dL in the lisinopril group (p < 0.001 versus chlorthalidone). At 4 years, 8.5% of the chlorthalidone group had developed hypokalemia (serum potassium less than 3.5 mEq per L), compared with 1.9% in the amlodipine group (p < 0.001) and 0.8% in the lisinopril group (p < 0.001). The incidence of new-onset diabetes (fasting blood glucose greater than 126 mg per dL) was 11.6% with chlorthalidone, compared with 9.8% in the amlodipine group (p = 0.04) and 8.1% in the lisinopril group (p < 0.001). Nonetheless, the presence of these metabolic abnormalities did not translate into more cardiovascular events or deaths in the chlorthalidone group. The public health implications of ALLHAT are enormous. The *2002 Drug Topics Red Book* indicates that generic chlorthalidone costs $15.95 for 100 tablets, compared with $97.96 for Prinavil (lisinopril) 10 mg, $102.76 for Zestril (lisinopril) 10 mg, and $145.13 for Norvasc (amlodipine) 5 mg. Using the less expensive generic diuretic to treat the more than 50 million hypertensive patients in the United States could lead to a cost savings of billions of dollars annually. Based on the results of the ALLHAT and other trials, the JNC 7 report has recommended that thiazide-type diuretics should be used as initial therapy for most patients with hypertension, either alone or in combination with one of the other classes of drugs (ACE inhibitors, ARBs, beta-blockers, or CCBs). An algorithm outlining the approach to treatment of hypertension is shown in Fig. 15-2. Diuretic therapy potentiates the antihypertensive effect of most other antihypertensive drugs. For this reason, the drug treatment algorithm outlined in JNC 7 recommends the addition of diuretic as a second-step agent if BP is inadequately controlled with any other drug chosen as a first-line agent. The mechanism of action of thiazide diuretics is to block sodium reabsorption by inhibiting the thiazide-sensitive NaCl cotransporter in the distal tubule. The sustained antihypertensive effect of thiazides however, is mediated through a reduction in systemic vascular resistance rather than through chronic volume depletion and a reduction of cardiac output, as one might predict. In fact, thiazides do not cause a large, sustained decrease in intravascular volume or sodium balance when used for the treatment of hypertension. Within a few days to weeks of the initiation of therapy with thiazide diuretics, salt balance returns toward normal, and total-body sodium and intravascular volume returns toward pretreatment levels. This seeming paradox can be understood in the context of Guyton's hypothesis regarding the pathogenesis of hypertension, whereby the development of systemic hypertension is conceptualized as an essential protective mechanism to maintain normal fluid volume in various disease states in which an underlying renal impairment exists with regard to excreting the daily sodium load at a normal BP (Fig. 15-2). In this context, diuretics lower BP by addressing the primary renal defect in salt excretion, so that systemic hypertension (high SVR) is no longer a prerequisite for maintaining sodium balance. It should be noted that in ALLHAT and most clinical trials, achievement of the desired BP goal often requires treatment with two or more antihypertensive agents. Addition of a second drug from a different class should be implemented when use of a single drug in optimal doses fails to adequately control BP. When the BP is more than 20 mm Hg systolic or 10 mm Hg diastolic above goal, treatment may be initiated with two drugs (usually including a thizide-type diuretic), either as separate prescriptions or in fixed-dose combinations.

D. Treatment of hypertension in special populations. The presence of certain comorbidities or target-organ damage in the individual hypertensive patient may provide a compelling indication for treatment with a certain class of antihypertensive agent, based on favorable outcome data from clinical trials (Table 15-6). In hypertensive patients with diabetes mellitus, thiazide diuretics, beta-blockers, ACE inhibitors, ARBs, and CCBs have been shown to reduce cardiovascular disease and the incidence of stroke. In patients with evidence of diabetic nephropathy, ACE inhibitor- or ARB-based treatment regimens have been shown to retard the progression of nephropathy, reduce urine albumin excretion, and slow progression from

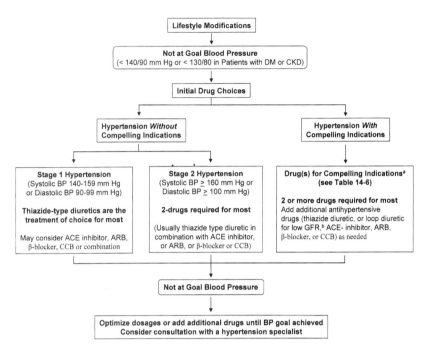

Figure 15-2. Algorithm for treatment of hypertension. [a]Compelling indications are special high-risk conditions for which clinical trials demonstrate benefit of specific classes of antihypertensive drugs: treatment of hypertension in the setting of diabetes, chronic kidney disease, heart failure, high coronary disease risk, post-MI, and for recurrent stroke prevention. [b]In the setting of advanced chronic kidney disease with GFR less than 30 mL per minute or in patients with fluid overload unresponsive to thiazide diuretics, more potent loop diuretic therapy may be requried. (BP, blood pressure; DM, diabetes mellitus; CKD, chronic kidney disease; ACE, angiotensin-converting enzyme; ARB, angiotensin-receptor blocker; and CCB, calcium channel blocker.) (Adapted with permission from Chobanian AV, Bakris GL, Black HR, et al. The seventh report of the Joint National Committee on Prevention, Detection, Evaluation and Treatment of High Blood Pressure. The JNC 7 Report. *JAMA* 2003;289:2560–2572.)

microalbuminuria to overt proteinuria. Chronic kidney disease (CKD) is present in patients with estimated glomerular filtration rate less than 60 mL per minute or if albuminuria (greater than 300 mg per day or 200 mg albumin per gram creatinine on spot urine specimen) is present. ACE inhibitors and ARBs have been shown to slow the progression of both diabetic and nondiabetic CKD. Thus, these agents should be included as part of the multidrug regimen often required for adequate BP control in CKD. Potent loop diuretics are usually needed in combination with other classes of drugs when the estimated GFR falls below 30 mL per minute. LVH is an independent risk factor for subsequent cardiovascular disease. Regression of LVH occurs with aggressive BP management using all classes of drugs except the direct-acting vasodilators such as hydralazine and minoxidil. Ischemic heart disease is a common form of target-organ damage in hypertension. In patients with hypertension and stable angina pectoris, the treatment regimen should include a beta-blocker or, alternatively, a long-acting CCB.

Table 15-6. Clinical trial and guideline basis for compelling indications for treatment with individual drug classes

High-risk condition with compelling Indication	Diuretic	Beta-blocker	ACE inhibitor	ARB	CCB	Aldosterone antagonist	Clinical trial basis[a]
Diabetes mellitus	•	•	•	•	•		ALLHAT, UKPDS, NKF Guideline, ADA Guideline
Chronic kidney disease			•	•			Captopril Trial, RENAAL, IDNT, REIN, AASK, NKF Guideline
Heart failure	•	•	•	•		•	ACC/AHA Heart Failure Guideline, MERIT-HF, COPERNICUS, CIBIS, SOLVD, AIRE, TRACE, ValHEFT, RALES
High coronary disease risk	•	•	•		•		ALLHAT, HOPE, ANBP2, Life, CONVINCE
Post-myocardial infarction		•	•			•	ACC/AHA Post-MI Guideline, BHAT, SAVE, Capricorn, EPHESUS
Recurrent stroke prevention	•		•				PROGRESS

[a]Compelling indications for certain classes of antihypertensive drugs are based on proven benefit from outcome studies or existing clinical practice guidelines. The compelling indication must be managed in parallel with blood pressure. Patients with these high-risk conditions usually require combination treatment with two to three additional antihypertensive drugs from different classes in order to achieve the recommended blood pressure treatment goal. AASK, African American Study of Kidney Disease and Hypertension; ACC/AHA, American College of Cardiology/American Heart Association; ACE, angiotensin-converting enzyme; AIRE, Acute Infarction Ramipril Efficacy; ALLHAT, Antihypertensive and Lipid-Lowering to Prevent Heart Attack Trial; ANBP2, Second Australian National Blood Pressure Study; ARB, angiotensin-receptor blocker; BHAT, Beta-Blocker Heart Attack Trial; CCB, calcium channel blocker; CIBIS, Cardiac Insufficiency Bisoprolol Study; CONVINCE, Controlled Onset Verapamil Investigation of Cardiovascular Endpoints; COPERNICUS, Carvedilol Prospective Randomized Cumulative Survival Study; EPHESUS, Eplerenone Post-Acute Myocardial Infarction Heart Failure Efficacy and Survival Study; HOPE, Heart Outcomes Prevention Evaluation Study; INDT, Irbesartan Diabetic Nephropathy Trial; LIFE, Losartan Intervention for Endpoint Reduction in Hypertension Study; MERIT-HT, Metoprolol CR/SL Randomized Intervention Trial in Congestive Heart Failure; NKF, National Kidney Foundation; PROGRESS, Perindopril Protection against Recurrent Stroke Study; RALES, Randomized Aldactone Evaluation Study; EEIN, Ramipril Efficacy in Nephropathy Study; RENAAL, Reduction of Endpoints in Non-Insulin Dependent Diabetes Mellitus with the Angiotensin II Antagonist Losartan Study; SAVE, Survival and Ventricular Enlargement Study; SOLVD, Studies of Left Ventricular Dysfunction; TRACE, Trandolapril Cardiac Evaluation Study; USPDS, United Kingdom Prospective Diabetes Study; ValHEFT, Valsartan Heart Failure Trial. (Adapted from Chobanian AV, Bakris GL, Black HR, et al. The seventh report of the Joint National Committee on Prevention, Detection, Evaluation and Treatment of High Blood Pressure. The JNC 7 Report. *JAMA* 2003;289:2560–2572.)

In patients with acute coronary syndromes (unstable angina or acute MI), hypertension should be treated initially with beta-blockers and ACE inhibitors, with the addition of other agents such as thiazide diuretics as needed for BP control. In the chronic BP management of post-MI patients, beta-blockers, ACE inhibitors, and aldosterone receptor antagonists have proven to be of highest benefit. In patients with ischemic heart disease, low-dose aspirin therapy and intensive lipid lowering therapy are also indicated. Heart failure represents another special hypertensive patient population; it can occur in the setting of either systolic or diastolic dysfunction. In asymptomatic patients with LV dysfunction, ACE inhibitors and beta-blockers are recommended. In patients with symptomatic heart failure or end-stage heart disease, ACE inhibitors, beta-blockers, ARBs, and aldosterone receptor blockers (spironolactone or eplerenone) are recommended, along with potent loop diuretics as needed for fluid overload. Treatment of hypertension in patients with cerebrovascular disease requires special consideration. Lowering of BP during the acute phase of an ischemic stroke may worsen ischemia and extend the infarct. However, treatment of chronic hypertension following a cerebrovascular accident with ACE inhibitors and thiazide-type diuretics may reduce the rate of recurrent stroke. The treatment of elderly patients with predominant systolic hypertension should follow the same treatment algorithm. In the Systolic Hypertension in the Elderly Program (SHEP) trial, a double-blind placebo-controlled trial of low-dose chlorthalidone in patients over age 60 with isolated systolic hypertension (systolic BP greater than 160 mm Hg with diastolic BP less than 90 mm Hg), the relative risks of stroke, left ventricular failure, nonfatal MI or fatal coronary heart disease, and the requirement for coronary artery bypass grafting were all significantly reduced in the active treatment group. Because of the risks of orthostatic hypotension and falls, selective alpha-blockers should be avoided in the treatment of older individuals with hypertension.

E. Treatment of the patient with resistant hypertension. Resistant hypertension is defined as a failure to reach BP less than 140/90 mm Hg in an adherent patient treated with a three-drug regimen including a diuretic. Truly resistant hypertension should prompt an investigation for underlying potentially treatable forms of secondary hypertension (Table 15-3). Table 15-7 outlines other causes of resistant hypertension. Consultation with a hypertension specialist should be considered if the BP goal cannot be achieved.

VII. Benign versus malignant hypertension. The classification of hypertension as benign or malignant is based on funduscopic examination. The finding of hypertensive neuroretinopathy (HNR) is the clinical sine qua non for the diagnosis of malignant hypertension (Fig. 15-3). In the absence of HNR, malignant hypertension cannot be diagnosed, regardless of the severity of the hypertension. Hypertensive neuroretinopathy is defined by the presence of striate hemorrhages and cotton-wool spots with or without papilledema (Table 15-8). The clinical importance of the finding of HNR is that it signifies the presence of a systemic hypertensive vasculopathy with fibrinoid necrosis and obliterative arteriopathy that, left untreated, will lead to ESRD or death within 1 year. Fortunately, malignant hypertension is a relatively rare disorder, occurring in less than 1% of hypertensive patients. The term **"benign hypertension"** is clearly a misnomer, because although the clinical course is less dramatic and precipitous than that seen in patients with malignant hypertension, the eventual cerebrovascular and cardiovascular complications are quite devastating, and they represent a major cause of morbidity and mortality in the general population. Benign hypertension is defined based on the absence of hypertensive neuroretinopathy. Retinal arteriosclerosis and arteriosclerotic retinopathy (see Table 15-8), which are the characteristic funduscopic findings in benign hypertension, are of little clinical utility, because they may be found in elderly normotensive individuals. These findings have no predictive value with regard to the risk of cardiovascular or cerebrovascular complications.

Table 15-7. Causes of resistant hypertension

Improper blood pressure measurement (use of inadequately sized BP cuff in
   obese patients)
Pseudohypertension in elderly individuals
White coat (office) hypertension
Volume overload or pseudotolerance
   Excess dietary sodium intake
   Fluid retention from underlying renal disease
   Inadequate diuretic therapy (failure to use loop diuretic with advanced CKD)
Noncompliance
   Patient nonadherence with therapy due to ignorance, cost, or side-effects
   Physician noncompliance (inadequate drug dosage or failure to include diuretic
      in regimen)
Drug-induced
   Nonsteroidal anti-inflammatory agents (NSAIDs) or cyclooxygenase 2 (Cox 2)
      inhibitors
   Cocaine, amphetamines, or other illicit drugs
   Sympathomimetics (decongestants or anoretic agents)
   Oral contraceptives
   Adrenal steroids
   Erythropoietin
   Licorice
   Over-the-counter dietary supplements (ephedra, ma huang, bitter orange)
Excessive alcohol consumption
Identifiable secondary causes of hypertension (see Table 15-3)

   A. Definition of hypertensive crises. The vast majority of hypertensive
      patients are asymptomatic for many years until complications due to
      atherosclerosis, cerebrovascular disease, or CHF supervene. In a minority
      of patients, this "benign" course is punctuated by a hypertensive crisis. A
      hypertensive crisis is defined as the turning point in the course of an illness
      at which acute management of the elevated BP plays a decisive role in the
      eventual outcome. The haste with which the BP must be controlled varies
      with the type of hypertensive crisis. However, the crucial role of hyper-
      tension in the disease process must be identified and a plan for managing
      the BP successfully implemented if the patient's outcome is to be optimal.
      The absolute level of the BP is clearly not the most important factor in de-
      termining the existence of a hypertensive crisis. For example, in children,
      pregnant women, and other previously normotensive individuals in whom
      mild to moderate hypertension develops suddenly, a hypertensive crisis can
      occur at a BP level that is normally well tolerated by adults with chronic
      hypertension. Furthermore, in adults with mild to moderate hypertension,
      a crisis can occur with the onset of acute end-organ dysfunction involving
      the heart or brain. Table 15-9 outlines the spectrum of hypertensive crises.
   B. Malignant hypertension is a clinical syndrome characterized by a marked
      elevation of BP with widespread acute arteriolar injury (hypertensive vas-
      culopathy). Funduscopy reveals HNR with flame-shaped hemorrhages,
      cotton-wool spots (soft exudates), and sometimes papilledema (Fig. 15-3).
      Regardless of the severity of BP elevation, in the absence of HNR, malig-
      nant hypertension cannot be diagnosed. HNR is thus an extremely impor-
      tant clinical finding, indicating the presence of a hypertension-induced ar-
      teriolitis that may involve the kidneys, heart, and central nervous system.
      With malignant hypertension, a rapid and relentless progression to ESRD
      occurs if effective BP control is not implemented. Mortality can result from

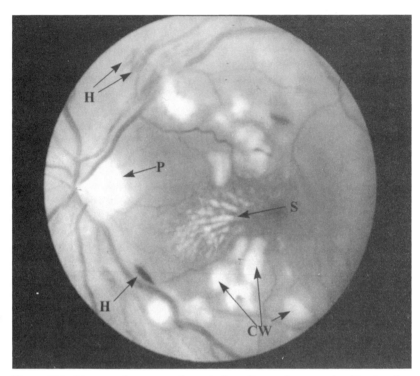

Figure 15-3. Hypertensive neuroretinopathy in malignant hypertension. Fundus photograph in a 30-year-old man with malignant hypertension demonstrates all the characteristic features of hypertensive neuroretinopathy, including striate hemorrhages (H), cotton-wool spots (CW), papilledema (P), and a star figure at the macula (S).

acute hypertensive heart failure, intracerebral hemorrhage, hypertensive encephalopathy, or complications of uremia. Malignant hypertension represents a hypertensive crisis; adequate control of BP clearly prevents these morbid complications.

C. **Hypertensive crises due to nonmalignant hypertension with acute complications.** Even in patients with benign hypertension, in whom HNR is absent, a hypertensive crisis may be diagnosed based on the presence of concomitant acute end-organ dysfunction (Table 15-9). Hypertensive crises due to nonmalignant hypertension with acute complications include hypertension accompanied by hypertensive encephalopathy, acute hypertensive heart failure, acute aortic dissection, intracerebral hemorrhage, subarachnoid hemorrhage, severe head trauma, acute MI or unstable angina, and active bleeding. Poorly controlled hypertension in a patient requiring surgery increases the risk of intraoperative cerebral or myocardial ischemia and postoperative acute renal failure. Severe postoperative hypertension, including post–coronary artery bypass hypertension and post–carotid endarterectomy hypertension, increases the risk of postoperative bleeding, hypertensive encephalopathy, pulmonary edema, and myocardial ischemia. The various catecholamine-excess states can cause a hypertensive crisis with hypertensive encephalopathy or acute hypertensive heart failure. Preeclampsia and eclampsia represent hypertensive crises that are unique

Table 15-8. Classification of hypertensive retinopathy

Retinal arteriosclerosis and arteriosclerotic retinopathy (characteristic of benign hypertension)
Arteriolar narrowing (focal or diffuse)
Arteriovenous crossing changes
Broadening of the arteriolar light reflex
Copper or silver wiring changes
Perivasculitis
Solitary round retinal hemorrhages
Hard exudates
Central or branch venous occlusion

Hypertensive neuroretinopathy (sine qua non of malignant hypertension)
Generalized arteriolar narrowing
Striate (flame-shaped hemorrhages)[a]
Cotton-wool spots (soft exudates)[a]
Bilateral papilledema[a]
Star figure at the macula

[a]These features distinguish retinal arteriosclerosis (benign hypertension) from hypertensive neuroretinopathy (malignant hypertension). (Adapted with permission from Nolan CR. Malignant hypertension and other hypertensive crises. In: RW Schrier, (ed.) *Diseases of the kidney and urinary tract,* 7th ed. Boston: Lippincott Williams & Wilkins, 2000;1513–1592.)

Table 15-9. Spectrum of hypertensive crises

Malignant hypertension (*hypertensive neuroretinopathy present*)
Hypertensive encephalopathy (*occurs with either malignant or severe benign hypertension*)
Nonmalignant ("benign") hypertensin with acute complications (*acute end-organ dysfunction in the absence of hypertensive neuroretinopathy*)
 Acute hypertensive heart failure (pulmonary edema due to acute diastolic dysfunction)
 Acute coronary syndromes
  Acute myocardial infarction
  Unstable angina
 Acute aortic dissection
 Central nervous system catastrophe
  Hypertensive encephalopathy
  Intracerebral hemorrhage
  Subarachnoid hemorrhage
  Severe head trauma
 Catecholamine excess states
  Pheochromocytoma crisis
  Monoamine oxidase inhibitor–tyramine interactions
  Antihypertensive drug withdrawal syndromes
  Phenylpropanolamine overdose
 Preeclampsia and eclampsia
 Active bleeding (including postoperative bleeding)
 Poorly controlled hypertension in patients requiring emergency surgery
 Severe postoperative hypertension
  Postcoronary artery bypass hypertension
  Postcarotid endarterectomy hypertension
 Scleroderma renal crisis
 Autonomic hyperreflexia in quadriplegic patients

(Adapted from Nolan CR. Malignant hypertension and other hypertensive crises. In: Schrier RW, ed. *Diseases of the kidney and urinary tract,* 7th ed. Boston: Lippincott Williams & Wilkins, 2001.)

to pregnancy. Scleroderma renal crisis is a hypertensive crisis in which failure to adequately control BP with a regimen that includes an ACE inhibitor results in rapid irreversible loss of renal function. Hypertensive crises can also occur in quadriplegic patients due to autonomic hyperreflexia induced by bowel or bladder distention. The sudden onset of hypertension in this setting can lead to hypertensive encephalopathy or acute pulmonary edema.

D. **Treatment of malignant hypertension.** Malignant hypertension must be treated expeditiously to prevent complications such as hypertensive encephalopathy, acute hypertensive heart failure, and renal failure. The traditional approach to patients with malignant hypertension has been the initiation of potent parenteral agents. In general, parenteral therapy should be used in patients with evidence of acute end-organ dysfunction (hypertensive encephalopathy or pulmonary edema) or those unable to tolerate oral medications. Nitroprusside is the treatment of choice for patients requiring parenteral therapy. In general, reducing the mean arterial pressure by 20% or to a level of 160 to 170/100 to 110 mm Hg is safe. The use of a short-acting agent such as nitroprusside has obvious advantages, because BP can quickly be stabilized at a higher level if complications develop during rapid BP reduction. If no evidence of vital organ hypoperfusion is apparent during the initial reduction, the diastolic BP can gradually be lowered to 90 mm Hg over a period of 12 to 36 hours. Oral antihypertensive agents should be initiated as soon as possible to minimize the duration of parenteral therapy. The nitroprusside infusion can be weaned as the oral agents become effective. The cornerstone of initial oral therapy should be arteriolar vasodilators such as hydralazine or minoxidil. Beta-blockers are required to control reflex tachycardia, and a diuretic must be initiated within a few days to prevent salt and water retention in response to vasodilatator therapy when the patient's dietary salt intake increases. Diuretics may not be necessary as a part of initial parenteral therapy, because patients with malignant hypertension often present with volume depletion due to pressure-induced natriuresis. Although many patients with malignant hypertension definitely require initial parenteral therapy, some patients may not yet have evidence of cerebral or cardiac dysfunction or rapidly deteriorating renal function and therefore do not require instantaneous control of BP. These patients can often be managed with an intensive oral regimen, often with a beta-blocker and minoxidil, designed to bring the BP under control within 12 to 24 hours. After the immediate crisis has resolved and the hypertension has been controlled with initial parenteral therapy, oral therapy, or both, lifelong surveillance of BP is mandatory. If control lapses, malignant hypertension can recur even after years of successful antihypertensive therapy. Triple therapy with a diuretic, a beta-blocker, and a vasodilator is often required to maintain satisfactory long-term BP control.

E. **Treatment of other hypertensive crises.** Sodium nitroprusside is the drug of choice for the management of virtually all hypertensive crises outlined in Table 15-9, including malignant hypertension, hypertensive encephalopathy, acute hypertensive heart failure, intracerebral hemorrhage, perioperative hypertension, catecholamine-related hypertensive crises, and acute aortic dissection (in combination with beta-blockers). Intravenous nitroglycerin may also be useful in patients with concomitant myocardial ischemia, because it dilatates intracoronary collaterals.

Sodium nitroprusside is a potent intravenous hypotensive agent with an immediate onset and brief duration of action. The site of action is the vascular smooth muscle. It has no direct action on the myocardium, although it may indirectly affect cardiac performance through alterations in systemic hemodynamics. Nitroprusside is an iron-coordination complex with five cyanide moieties and a nitroso group. The nitroso group combines with cysteine to form nitrosocysteine, a potent activator of guanylate cyclase that causes cyclic guanosine monophosphate (cGMP) accumulation and the relaxation of vascular smooth muscle. Nitroprusside causes vasodilation of both arteriolar resistance vessels and venous capacitance vessels. Its hypotensive action is a result of a decrease in SVR. The combined decrease in preload and afterload reduces myocardial wall tension and myocardial oxygen demand. The net effect of nitroprusside on cardiac output and heart rate depends on the intrinsic state of the myocardium. In patients with left ventricular systolic dysfunction and elevated left ventricular end-diastolic pressure, it causes an increase in stroke volume and cardiac output as a result of afterload reduction. Heart rate may actually decrease in response to improved cardiac performance. In contrast, in the absence of left ventricular dysfunction, venodilation and preload reduction can result in a reflex increase in sympathetic tone and heart rate. For this reason, nitroprusside must be used in conjunction with a beta-blocker in acute aortic dissection.

The hypotensive action of nitroprusside appears within seconds and is immediately reversible when the infusion is stopped. The cGMP in vascular smooth muscle is rapidly degraded by cGMP-specific phosphodiesterases. Nitroprusside is rapidly metabolized, with a half-life of 3 to 4 minutes. Cyanide is formed, as a short-lived intermediate product, by direct combination with sulfhydryl groups in red blood cells and tissues. The cyanide groups are rapidly converted to thiocyanate by the liver, in a reaction in which thiosulfate acts as a sulfur donor. Thiocyanate is excreted by the kidney, with a half-life of 1 week in patients with normal renal function. Thiocyanate accumulation and toxicity can occur when a high dose or prolonged infusion is required, especially in patients with renal insufficiency. When these risk factors are present, thiocyanate levels should be monitored and the infusion stopped if the level is over 10 mg per dL. Thiocyanate toxicity is rare in patients with normal renal function requiring less than 3 μg per kg per minute for less than 72 hours. Cyanide poisoning is a very rare complication, unless hepatic clearance of cyanide is impaired by severe liver disease, or massive doses of nitroprusside (more than 10 μg per kg per minute) are used to induce deliberate hypotension during surgery. Once the hypertensive crisis has resolved and the BP is adequately controlled, oral antihypertensive therapy should be initiated. The nitroprusside infusion is weaned as the oral antihypertensive agents become effective.

F. **Treatment of severe uncomplicated hypertension in the acute care setting.** The benefits of acute reduction in blood pressure in the setting of true hypertensive crisis are obvious (Fig. 15-4). Fortunately, true hypertensive crises are relatively rare events that never affect the vast majority of hypertensive patients. Much more common than true hypertensive crisis is the patient who presents with markedly elevated BP (greater than 180/100 mm Hg) in the absence of HNR (malignant hypertension) or acute end-organ damage that would signify a true crisis. This entity, known as severe uncomplicated hypertension, is very common in the emergency department or other acute-care settings. Of patients with severe uncomplicated hypertension, 60% are entirely asymptomatic and present for prescription refills or routine blood pressure checks, or are found to have elevated pressure during routine physical examinations. The other 40% present with nonspecific findings such as headache, dizziness, or weakness in the absence of evidence of acute end-organ dysfunction.

In the past, this entity was referred to as *urgent hypertension*, reflecting the erroneous notion that an acute reduction of BP over a few hours before discharge from the acute care facility was essential to minimize the risk of short-term complications from severe hypertension. Commonly used treatment regimens included oral clonidine loading or sublingual nifedipine. However, the practice of acute BP reduction in severe uncomplicated hypertension is no longer considered the standard of care. The Veterans Administration Cooperative Study of patients with severe hypertension included 70 placebo-treated patients who had an average diastolic BP of 121 mm Hg at entry. Among these untreated patients, 27 experienced morbid events at a mean of 11 (plus or minus 2) months of follow-up. However, the earliest

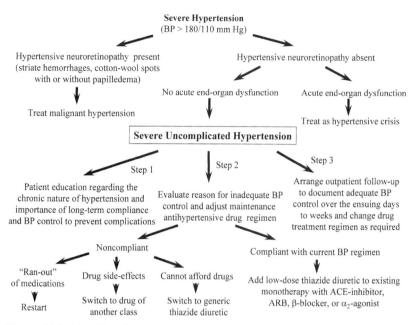

Figure 15-4. Algorithm for treatment of severe uncomplicated hypertension. ACE, angiotensin-converting enzyme; BP, blood pressure; CCB, calcium channel blocker. (Adapted with permission from Nolan CR. Hypertensive crises. In: Schrier RW, ed. *Atlas of diseases of the kidney*, vol. 3. Philadelphia: Current Medicine, 1999.)

morbid event occurred after 2 months. These data suggest that in patients with severe uncomplicated hypertension in which severe hypertension is not accompanied by evidence of malignant hypertension or acute end-organ dysfunction, eventual complications due to stroke, MI, or heart failure tend to occur over a time frame of months to years rather than hours to days. Although the long-term control of BP can clearly prevent these eventual complications, a hypertensive crisis cannot be diagnosed, because no evidence indicates that the acute reduction of BP results in an improvement in short- or long-term prognosis. Although the acute reduction of BP in patients with severe uncomplicated hypertension using sublingual nifedipine or oral clonidine loading was once the de facto standard of care, this practice was often an emotional response on the part of the treating physician to the dramatic elevation of BP, or it was motivated by the fear of medicolegal repercussions in the unlikely event of a hypertensive complication occurring within hours to days. Observing and documenting the dramatic fall in BP is a satisfying therapeutic maneuver, but no scientific basis for this approach exists. No literature supports the notion that some goal level of BP reduction must be achieved before the patient with severe uncomplicated hypertension leaves the acute care setting. In fact, the acute reduction of BP is often counterproductive, because it can produce untoward side effects that render the patient less likely to comply with long-term drug therapy. Instead, the acute therapeutic intervention should focus on tailoring an effective, well-tolerated maintenance antihypertensive regimen, with patient education regarding the chronic nature of the disease process and the importance of long-term compliance and medical follow-up. If the patient has simply run out of medicines, reinstitution of the previously effective drug regimen should suffice. If the patient is thought to be compliant with an existing drug regimen, a sensible change in the regimen, such as an increase in a suboptimal dosage of an existing drug or the addition of a drug of another class, is appropriate. In this regard, the addition of a low dose of a thiazide diuretic as a second-step agent to existing monotherapy with ACE inhibitor, ARB, CCB, beta-blocker, or central alpha-agonist is often remarkably effective. Another essential goal of the acute intervention should be to arrange suitable outpatient follow-up within a few days. A gradual reduction of BP to normotensive levels over a few days to a week should be accomplished in conjunction with frequent outpatient visits to modify the drug regimen and reinforce the importance of lifelong compliance with therapy. Although less dramatic than the acute reduction of BP in the acute care setting, this type of approach to the treatment of chronic hypertension is more likely to prevent long-term hypertensive complications and recurrent episodes of severe uncomplicated hypertension.

Suggested readings

Acute Infarction Ramipril Efficacy (AIRE) Study Investigators. Effects of ramipril on mortality and morbidity of survivors of acute myocardial infarction with clinical evidence of heart failure. *Lancet* 1993;342:821–828.

ALLHAT Collaborative Research Group. Major cardiovascular events in hypertensive patients randomized to doxazosin vs. chlorthalidone: the antihypertensive and lipid-lowering to prevent heart attack trial (ALLHAT). *JAMA* 2000;238:1967–1975.

ALLHAT Officers and Coordinators for the ALLHAT Collaborative Research Group. Major outcomes in high-risk hypertensive patients randomized to angiotensin-converting enzyme inhibitor, calcium channel blocker vs. diuretic. *JAMA* 2002;288:2981–2997.

American Diabetes Association. Treatment of hypertension in adults with diabetes. *Diabetes Care* 2003;26(Suppl 1):S80–S82.

β-blocker Heart Attack Trial Research Group. A randomized trial of propranolol in patients with acute myocardial infarction, I: mortality results (BHAT). *JAMA* 1982;247:1707–1714.

Black HR, Elliott JW, Grandits G, et al. Principal results of the Controlled Onset Verapamil Investigation of Cardiovasculaar End Points (CONVINCE) trial. *JAMA* 2003;289:2073–2082.

Braunwald E, Antgman EM, Beasley JW, et al. AHA 2002 guideline update for the management of patients with unstable angina and non-ST-segment elevation myocardial infarction (ACC/AHA Post MI Guideline). *J Am Coll Cardiol* 2002;40:1366–1374.

Brenner BM, Copper ME de Zeeuq D, et al. Effects of losartan on renal and cardiovascular outcomes in patients with type 2 diabetes and nephropathy (RENAAL). *N Engl J Med* 2001;345:861–869.

Capricorn Investigators. Effect of varvedilol on outcome after myocardial infarction in patients with left-ventricular dysfunction: The CAPRICORN randomized trial. *Lancet* 2001;357:1358–1390.

Chobanian AV, Bakris GL, Black HR, et al. The seventh report of the Joint National Committee on Prevention, Detection, Evaluation, and Treatment of Hypertension. The JNC 7 report. *JAMA* 2003;289:2560–2572.

CIBIS Investigators and Committees. A randomized trial of beta-blockade in heart failure: the Cardiac Insufficiency Bisprolol Study (CIBIS). *Circulation* 1994;90:1765–1773.

Cohn J, Tognoni G. A randomized trial of the angiotensin receptor blocker valsartan in chronic heart failure (ValHEFT). *N Engl J Med* 2001;345:1667–1675.

Dahlof B, Devereux RB, Kjeldsen SE, et al. Cardiovascular morbidity and mortality in the Losartan Intervention for Endpoint Reduction in Hypertension Study (LIFE). *Lancet* 2002;359:995–1003.

GISEN (Cruppo Italiano di Studi Epidemiologici in Nefrologia) Group. Randomized placebo-controlled trial of effect of ramipril on decline in glomerular filtration rate and risk of terminal renal failure in proteinuric, non-diabetic nephropathy (REIN). *Lancet* 1997;349:1857–1863.

Guyton AC, Manning RD, Norman RA, et al. Current concepts and perspectives of renal volume regulation in relationship to hypertension. *J Hypertens* 1986;4(Suppl 4):S49–S56.

Hager WD, Davis BR, Riba A, et al., for the Survival and Ventricular Enlargement (SAVE) Investigators. Absence of a deleterious effect of calcium channel blockers in patients with left ventricular dysfunction after myocardial infarction: the SAVE Study Experience. *Am Heart J* 1998;135:406–423.

Hall JE, Granger JP, Smith MJ, et al. Role of renal hemodynamics and arterial pressure in aldosterone "escape." *Hypertension* 1984;6(Suppl 1):I183–I192.

Heart Outcomes Prevention Evaluation Study Investigators. Effects of an angiotensin-converting-enzyme inhibitor, ramipril on cardiovascular events in high-risk patients (HOPE). *N Engl J Med* 2000;342:145–153.

Hunt SA, Baker DW, Chin MH, et al. ACC/AHA guidelines for the evaluation and management of chronic heart failure in the adult. *J Am Coll Cardiol* 2001;38:2101–2113.

Intersalt Cooperative Research Group. Intersalt: an international study of electrolyte excretion and blood pressure. Results for 24 hour urinary sodium and potassium excretion. *Br Med J* 1988;297:319–330.

Kober L, Torp-Pedersen C, Carlsen JE, et al., for Trandolapril Cardiac Evaluation (TRACE) Study Group. A clinical trial of the angiotensin-converting enzyme inhibitor trandolapril in patients with left ventricular dysfunction after myocardial infarction. *N Engl J Med* 1995;333:1670–1676.

Lewis EJ, Hunsicker LG, Bain RP, et al. The effect of angiotensin-converting enzyme inhibitor on diabetic nephropathy: the Collaborative Study Group (Captopril Trial). *N Engl J Med* 1993;329:1456–1462.

Lewis EJ, Hunsicker LG, Clarke WR, et al. Renoprotective effect of the angiotensin-receptor antagonist irbesartan in patients with nephropathy due to type 2 diabetes (INDT). *N Engl J Med* 2001;345:851–860.

Lifton RP, Gharavi AG, Geller DS. Molecular mechanisms of human hypertension. *Cell* 2001;104:545–556.

National Kidney Foundation Guideline. K/DOQI clinical practice guidelines for chronic kidney disease: Kidney Disease Outcome Quality Initiative. *Am J Kidney Dis* 2002;39(suppl 2):S1–S246.

Nolan CR. Hypertensive crises. In: RW Schrier, ed. *Atlas of diseases of the kidney,* Vol. 3. Philadelphia: Current Medicine, 1999.

Nolan CR. Malignant hypertension and other hypertensive crises. In: RW Schrier, ed. *Diseases of the kidney and urinary tract,* 7th ed. Boston: Lippincott Williams & Wilkins, 2001:1513–1592.

Nolan CR, Schrier RW. The kidney in hypertension. In: RW Schrier, ed. *Renal and electrolyte disorders,* 6th ed. Philadelphia: Lippincott Williams & Wilkins, 2003.

Packer M, Coats AJ, Fowler MB, et al. Effect of carvedolo on survival in severe chronic heart failure (COPERNICUS). *N Engl J Med* 2001;344:1651–1658.

Pitt B, Remme W, Zannad F, et al. Eplerenone, a selective aldosterone blocker, in patients with left ventricular dysfunction after myocardial infarction (EPHESUS). *N Engl J Med* 2003;348:1309–1321.

Pitt B, Zannad F, Remme WJ, et al., for Randomized Aldactone Evaluation Study Investigators. The effect of spironolactone on morbidity and mortality in patients with severe heart failure (RALES). *N Engl J Med* 1999;341:709–717.

PROGRESS Collaborative Study Group. Randomised trial of perindopril-based blood pressure lowering regimen among 6105 individuals with previous stroke or transient ischaemic attack. *Lancet* 2001;358:1033–1041.

Pstay BM, Smith NL, Siscovick DS, et al. Health outcomes associated with antihypertensive therapies used as first-line agents. *JAMA* 1997;277:739–745.

SHEP Cooperative Research Group. Prevention of stroke by antihypertensive treatment in older persons with isolated systolic hypertension. Final results of the Systolic Hypertension in the Elderly Program (SHEP). *JAMA* 1991;265:3255–3264.

SOLVD Investigators. Effect of enalapril on survival in patients with reduced ventricular ejection fractions and congestive heart failure. *N Engl J Med* 1991;325:293–302.

Tepper D. Frontiers in congestive heart failure: effect of metoprolol CR/XL in chronic heart failure (MERIT-HF). *Congest Heart Fail* 1999;5:184–185.

UK Prospective Diabetes Study Group. Efficacy of atenolol and captopril in reducing risk of macrovascular and microvascular complications in type 2 diabetes: UKPDS 39. *BMJ* 1998;317:713–720.

Wing LMH, Reid CM, Ryan P, et al., for Second Australian National Blood Pressure Study Group. A comparison of outcomes with angiotensin-converting-enzyme inhibitors and diuretics for hypertension in the elderly (ANBP2). *N Engl J Med* 2003;348:583–592.

Wright JT Jr., Agadoa L, Contreras G, et al. Successful blood pressure control in African American Study of Kidney Disease and Hypertension (AASK). *Arch Intern Med* 2002;162:1636–1643.

Practical Guidelines for Drug Dosing in Patients with Renal Impairment

George R. Aronoff

Uremia influences every organ system and every aspect of drug disposition. The physiologic changes associated with renal disease have pronounced effects on the pharmacology of many drugs. This chapter provides a rational schema for drug dosing in patients with decreased renal function and for those requiring renal replacement therapy.

Figure 16-1 outlines an approach to drug dosing in patients with renal disease. When possible, a specific diagnosis should be established before drug therapy is initiated. The use of fewer drugs and the recognition of potential drug interactions decreases adverse drug effects and the potential for drug interactions.

I. **History and physical examination.** Clinical evaluation always begins with a careful history and physical examination. Are the history of previous drug allergy or toxicity and the use of concurrent medications or recreational drugs are particularly important for this purpose. Physical assessment should include an estimate of the extracellular fluid (ECF) volume. Edema or ascites increases the distribution volume of many drugs, whereas dehydration contracts this volume. Measurements of body weight and height are needed to tailor the dosage regimen. For obese patients, an average of the calculated ideal body weight and the measured body weight is useful for estimating drug doses. Evidence of the impaired function of other excretory organs should be sought. Stigmata of liver disease are clues that the drug dose may need to be altered.

II. **Measurement of renal function.** The rate of elimination of drugs excreted by the kidneys is proportional to the glomerular filtration rate (GFR). The serum creatinine or creatinine clearance rate is needed to determine renal function before prescribing any drug. The Cockcroft-Gault equation is useful for this purpose:

$$\text{Clcr} = \frac{(140 - \text{age}) \times (\text{IBW})}{72 \times \text{Scr}} \times (0.85 \text{ if female})$$

where:
Clcr = Creatinine clearance (mL/min).
Scr = Serum creatinine (mg/dL).
IBW (in kg) = Ideal body weight (men) = 50 kg + 2.3 kg per inch over 5 feet.
= Ideal body weight (women) = 45.5 kg + 2.3 kg per inch over 5 feet.
For obese men and women the equation is modified:

$$\text{Clcr} = \frac{(137 - \text{age}) \times [(0.285 \times \text{wgt}) + (12.1 \times \text{hgt}^2)]}{51 \times \text{Scr}}$$
(obese men)

$$\text{Clcr} = \frac{(146 - \text{age}) \times [(0.287 \times \text{wgt}) + (9.74 \times \text{hgt}^2)]}{60 \times \text{Scr}}$$
(obese women)

where:
wgt = patient's weight in kg.
hgt = patient's height in cm.
In cases of changing renal function, the serum creatinine no longer reflects the true clearance rate. In these cases, a timed urine collection is needed to

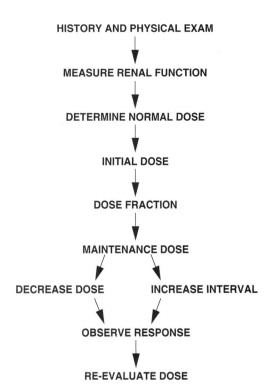

HISTORY AND PHYSICAL EXAM

MEASURE RENAL FUNCTION

DETERMINE NORMAL DOSE

INITIAL DOSE

DOSE FRACTION

MAINTENANCE DOSE

DECREASE DOSE   INCREASE INTERVAL

OBSERVE RESPONSE

RE-EVALUATE DOSE

Figure 16-1. A schema for drug dosing in patients with impaired renal function.

estimate renal function. The midpoint serum creatinine is useful to calculate the creatinine clearance for the collection period. If the patient is oliguric, the creatinine clearance is less than 5 mL per minute.

The serum creatinine reflects muscle mass as well as GFR. Serum creatinine measurements within the "normal" range are frequently used to establish "normal" renal function. This erroneous assumption may cause serious overdose and resultant toxic drug accumulation in elderly or debilitated patients with decreased muscle mass.

III. **Calculation of the initial dose.** The purpose of the initial dose is to achieve therapeutic plasma drug concentrations rapidly. A loading dose should be considered when the half-life of a drug is particularly long in patients with impaired renal function and the clinical situation requires rapidly achieved therapeutic levels. When the physical examination suggests that the ECF volume is normal, the loading dose of a drug given to a patient with renal insufficiency is the same as the initial dose given to a patient with normal renal function. Initial doses for most drugs requiring loading are already known. However, the loading dose may be calculated using the following formula:

Loading Dose = Vd (L/kg) × Wt (kg) × Cp (mg/L)

where:
Vd = volume of distribution of the drug.
Wt = patient's ideal body weight.
Cp = desired plasma drug level.

If the patient has edema or ascites, a larger loading dose may be required. Conversely, dehydrated or debilitated patients should receive smaller initial drug doses.

IV. **Calculation of the maintenance dose.** Several methods can be used to decide subsequent doses. The following relationship is useful for calculating the fraction of the normal dose recommended for a patient with renal insufficiency:

Dose Fraction = F[(Clcr/120) − 1)] + 1

where:

F = fraction of the drug excreted unchanged in the urine.

Clcr = creatinine clearance.

When F is not known, the ratio of the drug's half-life in patients with normal renal function ($T_{1/2}$ normal) to that measured in patients with renal failure ($T_{1/2}$ renal failure) may be substituted as below:

$$\text{Dose Fraction} = \frac{T_{1/2}\ \text{normal}}{T_{1/2}\ \text{renal failure}}[(\text{Clcr}/120) - 1] + 1$$

Table 16-1 lists commonly used drugs that require substantial dose alteration when used in patients with renal failure and suggestions for dose adjustment and for dialysis.

A. **Use of the table.** Prolonging the dose interval is often a convenient and cost-effective method for altering the drug dose in patients with renal impairment. This recommendation is indicated in the table by "I" in the Method column. This method is particularly useful for drugs with wide therapeutic ranges and long plasma half-lives. Extended parenteral therapy can be completed without prolonged hospitalization when the dose interval can safely be lengthened to allow for home therapy. If the range between the therapeutic and toxic levels is too narrow, either potentially toxic or subtherapeutic plasma concentrations may result.

To maintain the same dose interval as in patients with normal renal function, one may decrease the amount of each individual dose given to renal impaired patients. This recommendation is indicated in the table by "D" in the Method column. This method is effective for drugs with narrow therapeutic ranges and short plasma half-lives in patients with renal insufficiency.

In practice, a combination of the methods is often effective and convenient. The combination method uses a modification of both the dose and dose interval. For drugs with particularly long half-lives in patients with impaired renal function, give the total daily dose as a single dose each day, or divide the total daily dose in half and give twice daily.

The decision to extend the dosing interval beyond a 24-hour period should be based on the necessity to maintain therapeutic peak or trough drug levels. When the peak level is most important, prolong the dose interval. However, when the minimum trough level must be maintained, modification of the individual dose or a combination of the dose and interval methods may be preferred.

V. **Drug dosing in dialysis patients.** Drug removal by hemodialysis (HD) is most effective for drugs that weigh less than 500 Daltons, are less than 90% protein bound, and those that have small volumes of distribution. Table 16-1 also lists commonly used drugs removed by HD or peritoneal dialysis (PD). For many drugs, alter the dosage schedule such that the dose can be given at the end of the HD treatment, thus eliminating the need for a reloading dose. For example, give aminoglycosides to chronic HD patients as a post-dialysis dose.

Continuous renal replacement therapies (CRRT), such as continuous venovenous hemofiltration (CVVH) and sustained, low-efficiency dialysis (SLED)

Table 16-1. Drug dosing recommendations for patients with renal failure and on dialysis

Drug	Dose method	GFR >50 (mL/min)	GFR 10–50 (mL/min)	GFR <10 (mL/min)	Supplemental dose after hemodialysis	CAPD	CRRT
Acarbose	D	50–100%	Avoid	Avoid	Unknown	Unknown	Avoid
Acebutolol	D	100%	50%	30% to 50%	None	None	Dose for GFR 10–50
Acetazolamide	I	q6h	q12h	Avoid	No data	No data	Avoid
Acetohexamide	I	Avoid	Avoid	Avoid	Unknown	None	Avoid
Acetohydroxamic acid	D	100%	100%	Avoid	Unknown	Unknown	Unknown
Acetominophen	I	q4h	q6h	q8h	None	None	Dose for GFR 10–50
Acetylsalicylic acid	I	q4h	q4–6h	Avoid	Dose after dialysis	None	Dose for GFR 10–50
Acrivastine	D	Unknown	Unknown	Unknown	Unknown	Unknown	Unknown
Acyclovir	D,I	5 mg/kg q8h	5 mg/kg q12–24h	2.5 mg/kg q24h	Dose after dialysis	Dose for GFR <10	3.5 mg/kg d
Adenosine	D	100%	100%	100%	None	None	Dose for GFR 10–50
Albuterol	D	100%	75%	50%	Unknown	Unknown	Dose for GFR 10–50
Alcuronium	D	Avoid	Avoid	Avoid	Unknown	Unknown	Avoid
Alfentanil	D	100%	100%	100%	Not applicable	Not applicable	NA
Allopurinol	D	75%	50%	25%	1/2 dose	Unknown	Dose for GFR 10–50
Alprazolam	D	100%	100%	100%	None	Unknown	NA
Altretamine	D	Unknown	Unknown	Unknown	No data	No data	Unknown
Amantadine	I	q24–48h	q48–72h	q7d	None	None	Dose for GFR 10–50
Amikacin	D,I	60% to 90% q12h	30% to 70% q12–18h	20% to 30% q24–48h	2/3 normal dose	15–20 mg/L d	Dose for GFR 10–50
Amiloride	D	100%	50%	Avoid	Not applicable	Not applicable	Not applicable
Amiodarone	D	100%	100%	100%	None	None	Dose for GFR 10–50
Amitriptyline	D	100%	100%	100%	None	Unknown	NA

(continued)

Table 16-1. (Continued)

Drug	Dose method	GFR >50 (mL/min)	GFR 10–50 (mL/min)	GFR <10 (mL/min)	Supplemental dose after hemodialysis	CAPD	CRRT
Amlodipine	D	100%	100%	100%	None	None	Dose for GFR 10–50
Amoxapine	D	100%	100%	100%	Unknown	Unknown	NA
Amoxicillin	I	q8h	q8–12h	q24h	Dose after dialysis	250 mg q12h	Not applicable
Amphotericin	I	q24h	q24h	q24–36h	None	Dose for GFR <10	Dose for GFR 10–50
Amphotericin B colloidal	I	q24h	q24h	q24–36h	None	Dose for GFR <10	Dose for GFR 10–50
Amphotericin B lipid	I	q24h	q24h	q24–36h	None	Dose for GFR <10	Dose for GFR 10–50
Ampicillin	I	q6h	q6–12h	q12–24h	Dose after dialysis	250 mg q12h	Dose for GFR 10–50
Amrinone	D	100%	100%	50% to 75%	No data	No data	Dose for GFR 10–50
Anistreplase	D	100%	100%	100%	Unknown	Unknown	Dose for GFR 10–50
Astemizole	D	100%	100%	100%	Unknown	Unknown	NA
Atenolol	D,I	100% q24h	50% q48h	30% to 50% q96h	25–50 mg	None	Dose for GFR 10–50
Atovaquone	—	100%	100%	100%	None	None	Dose for GFR 10–50
Atracurium	D	100%	100%	100%	Unknown	Unknown	Dose for GFR 10–50
Auranofin	D	50%	Avoid	Avoid	None	None	None
Azathioprine	D	100%	75%	50%	Yes	Unknown	Dose for GFR 10–50
Azithromycin	D	100%	100%	100%	None	None	None
Azlocillin	I	q4–6h	q6–8h	q8h	Dose after dialysis	Dose for GFR <10	Dose for GFR 10–50
Aztreonam	D	100%	50% to 75%	25%	0.5 g after dialysis	Dose for GFR <10	Dose for GFR 10–50
Benazepril	D	100%	50% to 75%	25% to 50%	None	None	Dose for GFR 10–50
Bepridil	—	Unknown	Unknown	Unknown	None	None	No data
Betamethasone	D	100%	100%	100%	Unknown	Unknown	Dose for GFR 10–50
Betaxolol	D	100%	100%	50%	None	None	Dose for GFR 10–50
Bezafibrate	D	70%	50%	25%	Unknown	Unknown	Dose for GFR 10–50
Bisoprolol	D	100%	75%	50%	Unknown	Unknown	Dose for GFR 10–50

Drug	Method	Dose for normal renal function	GFR >50	GFR 10–50	GFR <10	Supplement for hemodialysis	Supplement for CAPD
Bleomycin	D	100%	75%	50%	None	Unknown	Dose for GFR 10–50
Bopindolol	D	100%	100%	100%	None	None	Dose for GFR 10–50
Bretylium	D	100%	25% to 50%	25%	None	None	Dose for GFR 10–50
Bromocriptine	D	100%	100%	100%	Unknown	Unknown	Unknown
Brompheniramine	D	100%	100%	100%	Unknown	Unknown	NA
Budesonide	D	100%	100%	100%	None	None	Dose for GFR 10–50
Bumetanide	D	100%	100%	100%	None	Unknown	Not applicable
Bupropion	D	100%	100%	100%	None	None	NA
Buspirone	D	100%	100%	100%	None	Unknown	NA
Busulfan	D	100%	100%	100%	Unknown	Unknown	Dose for GFR 10–50
Butorphanol	D	100%	75%	50%	Unknown	Unknown	NA
Capreomycin	I	q24h	q24h	q48h	None	Give dose after HD only	Dose for GFR 10–50
Captopril	D,I	100% q8–12h	75% q12–18h	50% q24h	25–30%	None	Dose for GFR 10–50
Carbamazepine	D	100%	100%	100%	None	None	None
Carbidopa	D	100%	100%	100%	Unknown	Unknown	Unknown
Carboplatin	D	100%	50%	25%	1/2 dose	Unknown	Dose for GFR 10–50
Carmustine	D	Unknown	Unknown	Unknown	Unknown	Unknown	Unknown
Carteolol	D	100%	50%	25%	None	None	Dose for GFR 10–50
Carvedilol	D	100%	100%	100%	None	None	Dose for GFR 10–50
Cefaclor	D	100%	50% to 100%	50%	250 mg q8–12h	250 mg after dialysis	Not applicable
Cefadroxil	I	q12h	q12–24h	q24–48h	0.5 g/d	0.5–1.0 g after dialysis	Not applicable
Cefamandole	I	q6h	q6–8h	q12h	0.5–1.0 g q12h	0.5–1.0 g after dialysis	Dose for GFR 10–50
Cefazolin	I	q8h	q12h	q24–48h	0.5 g q12h	0.5–1.0 g after dialysis	Dose for GFR 10–50
Cefepime	I	q12h	q16–24h	q24–48h	Dose for GFR <10	1.0 g after dialysis	Not recommended

(continued)

Table 16-1. (Continued)

Drug	Dose method	GFR >50 (mL/min)	GFR 10–50 (mL/min)	GFR <10 (mL/min)	Supplemental dose after hemodialysis	CAPD	CRRT
Cefixime	D	100%	75%	50%	300 mg after dialysis	200 mg/d	Not recommended
Cefmenoxime	D,I	1.0 g q8h	0.75 g q8h	0.75 g q12h	0.75 g after dialysis	0.75 g q12h	Dose for GFR 10–50
Cefmetazole	I	q16h	q24h	q48h	Dose after dialysis	Dose for GFR <10	Dose for GFR 10–50
Cefonicid	D,I	0.5 g/d	0.1g to 0.5 g/d	0.1 g/d	None	None	None
Cefoperazone	D	100%	100%	100%	1 g after dialysis	None	None
Ceforanide	I	q12h	q12–24h	q24–48h	0.5–1.0 g after dialysis	None	1.0 g/d
Cefotaxime	I	q6h	q8–12h	q24h	1 g after dialysis	1 g/d	1 g q12h
Cefotetan	D	100%	50%	25%	1 g after dialysis	1 g/d	750 mg q12h
Cefoxitin	I	q8h	q8–12h	q24–48h	1 g after dialysis	1 g/d	Dose for GFR 10–50
Cefpodoxime	I	q12h	q16h	q24–48h	200 mg after dialysis	Dose for GFR <10	Not applicable
Cefprozil	D,I	250 mg q12h	250 mg q12–16h	250 mg q24h	250 mg after dialysis	Dose for GFR <10	Dose for GFR <10
Ceftazidime	I	q8–12h	q24–48h	q48h	1 g after dialysis	0.5 g/d	Dose for GFR 10–50
Ceftibutin	D	100%	50%	25%	300 mg after dialysis	Dose for GFR <10	Dose for GFR 10–50
Ceftizoxime	I	q8–12h	q12–24h	q24h	1 g after dialysis	0.5–1.0 g/d	Dose for GFR 10–50
Ceftriaxone	D	100%	100%	100%	Dose after dialysis	750 mg q12h	Dose for GFR 10–50
Cefuroxime axetil	D	100%	100%	100%	Dose after dialysis	Dose for GFR <10	Not applicable
Cefuroxime sodium	I	q8h	q8–12h	q12h	Dose after dialysis	Dose for GFR <10	1 g q12h
Celiprolol	D	100%	100%	75%	Unknown	None	Dose for GFR 10–50
Cephalexin	I	q8h	q12h	q12h	Dose after dialysis	Dose for GFR <10	Not applicable
Cephalothin	I	q6h	q6–8h	q12h	Dose after dialysis	1 g q12h	1 g q8h
Cephapirin	I	q6h	q6–8h	q12h	Dose after dialysis	1 g q12h	1 g q8h

Cephradine	D	100%	50%	25%	None	Unknown	Not applicable
Cetirizine	D	100%	100%	30%	None	Unknown	NA
Chloral hydrate	D	100%	Avoid	Avoid	Unknown	Unknown	NA
Chlorambucil	D	Unknown	Unknown	Unknown	None	None	Unknown
Chloramphenicol	D	100%	100%	100%	None	Unknown	None
Chlorazepate	D	100%	100%	100%	Unknown	Unknown	NA
Chlordiazepoxide	D	100%	100%	50%	None	None	Dose for GFR 10–50
Chloroquine	D	100%	100%	50%	None	Unknown	None
Chlorpheniramine	D	100%	100%	100%	None	None	NA
Chlorpromazine	D	100%	100%	100%	None	None	Dose for GFR 10–50
Chlorpropamide	D	50%	Avoid	Avoid	Unknown	Not applicable	Avoid
Chlorthalidone	I	q24h	q24h	Avoid	Not applicable	None	Not applicable
Cholestyramine	D	100%	100%	100%	None	None	Dose for GFR 10–50
Cibenzoline	D,I	100% q12h	100% q12h	66% q24h	None	None	Dose for GFR 10–50
Cidofovir	D	50% to 100%	avoid	avoid	No data	No data	Avoid
Cilastin	D	100%	50%	Avoid	Avoid	Avoid	Avoid
Cilazapril	D,I	75% q24h	50% q24–48h	10% to 25% q72h	None	None	Dose for GFR 10–50
Cimetidine	D	100%	50%	25%	None	None	Dose for GFR 10–50
Cinoxacin	D	100%	50%	Avoid	Avoid	Avoid	Avoid
Ciprofloxacin	D	100%	50% to 75%	50%	250 mg q12h	250 mg q8h	200 mg iv q12h
Cisapride	D	100%	100%	50%	Unknown	Unknown	50–100%
Cisplatin	D	100%	75%	50%	Yes	Unknown	Dose for GFR 10–50
Cladribine	D	Unknown	Unknown	Unknown	Unknown	Unknown	Unknown
Clarithromycin	D	100%	75%	50% to 75%	Dose after dialysis	None	None
Clavulanic acid	D	100%	100%	50% to 75%	Dose after dialysis	Dose after dialysis	Dose for GFR <10
Clindamycin	D	100%	100%	100%	None	None	None
Clodronate	D	Unknown	Unknown	Avoid	Unknown	Unknown	Unknown

(continued)

Table 16-1. (Continued)

Drug	Dose method	GFR >50 (mL/min)	GFR 10–50 (mL/min)	GFR <10 (mL/min)	Supplemental dose after hemodialysis	CAPD	CRRT
Clofazamine	—	100%	100%	100%	None	None	No data
Clofibrate	I	q6–12h	q12–18h	Avoid	None	Unknown	Dose for GFR 10–50
Clomipramine	D	Unknown	Unknown	Unknown	Unknown	Unknown	NA
Clonazepam	D	100%	100%	100%	None	Unknown	NA
Clonidine	D	100%	100%	100%	None	None	Dose for GFR 10–50
Codeine	D	100%	75%	50%	Unknown	Unknown	Dose for GFR 10–50
Colchicine	D	100%	100%	50%	None	Unknown	Dose for GFR 10–50
Colestipol	D	100%	100%	100%	None	None	Dose for GFR 10–50
Cortisone	D	100%	100%	100%	None	Unknown	Dose for GFR 10–50
Cyclophosphamide	D	100%	100%	75%	1/2 dose	Unknown	Dose for GFR 10–50
Cycloserine	I	q12h	q12–24h	q24h	None	None	Dose for GFR 10–50
Cyclosporine	D	100%	100%	100%	None	None	100%
Cytarabine	D	100%	100%	100%	Unknown	Unknown	Dose for GFR 10–50
Dapsone	—	100%	No data	No data	None	Dose for GFR <10	No data
Daunorubicin	D	100%	100%	100%	Unknown	Unknown	Unknown
Delavirdine	—	100%	100%	100%	None	No data	Dose for GFR 10–50
Desferoxamine	D	100%	100%	100%	Unknown	Unknown	Dose for GFR 10–50
Desipramine	D	100%	100%	100%	None	None	NA
Dexamethasone	D	100%	100%	100%	Unknown	Unknown	Dose for GFR 10–50
Diazepam	D	100%	100%	100%	None	Unknown	100%
Diazoxide	D	100%	100%	100%	None	None	Dose for GFR 10–50
Diclofenac	D	100%	100%	100%	None	None	Dose for GFR 10–50
Dicloxacillin	D	100%	100%	100%	None	None	Not applicable
Didanosine	I	q12h	q24h	q24–48h	Dose after dialysis	Dose for GFR <10	Dose for GFR <10
Diflunisal	D	100%	50%	50%	None	None	Dose for GFR 10–50
Digitoxin	D	100%	100%	50% to 75%	None	None	Dose for GFR 10–50

274

Digoxin	D,I	100% q24h	25% to 75% q36h	10% to 25% q48h	None	None	Dose for GFR 10–50
Dilevalol	D	100%	100%	100%	None	None	Unknown
Diltiazem	D	100%	100%	100%	None	None	Dose for GFR 10–50
Diphenhydramine	D	100%	100%	100%	None	None	None
Dipyridamole	D	100%	100%	100%	Unknown	Unknown	NA
Dirithromycin	—	100%	100%	100%	None	None	Dose for GFR 10–50
Disopyramide	I	q8h	q12–24h	q24–40h	None	None	Dose for GFR 10–50
Dobutamine	D	100%	100%	100%	No data	No data	Dose for GFR 10–50
Doxacurium	D	100%	50%	50%	Unknown	Unknown	Dose for GFR 10–50
Doxazosin	D	100%	100%	100%	None	None	Dose for GFR 10–50
Doxepin	D	100%	100%	100%	None	None	Dose for GFR 10–50
Doxorubicin	D	100%	100%	100%	None	Unknown	Dose for GFR 10–50
Doxycycline	D	100%	100%	100%	None	None	Dose for GFR 10–50
Dyphylline	D	75%	50%	25%	1/3 dose	Unknown	Dose for GFR 10–50
Enalapril	D	100%	75% to 100%	50%	20–25%	None	Dose for GFR 10–50
Epirubicin	D	100%	100%	100%	None	Unknown	Dose for GFR 10–50
Erbastine	D	100%	50%	50%	Unknown	Unknown	Dose for GFR 10–50
Erythromycin	D	100%	100%	50% to 75%	None	None	None
Estazolam	D	100%	100%	100%	Unknown	Unknown	NA
Ethacrynic acid	I	q8–12h	q8–12h	Avoid	None	None	Not applicable
Ethambutol	I	q24h	q24–36h	q48h	Dose after dialysis	Dose for GFR <10	Dose for GFR 10–50
Ethchlorvynol	D	100%	Avoid	Avoid	None	None	NA
Ethionamide	D	100%	100%	50%	None	None	None
Ethosuximide	D	100%	100%	100%	None	Unknown	Unknown
Etodolac	D	100%	100%	100%	None	None	None
Etomidate	D	100%	100%	100%	Unknown	Unknown	Dose for GFR 10–50
Etoposide	D	100%	75%	50%	None	Unknown	Dose for GFR 10–50
Famciclovir	I	100%	q12–48h	50% q48h	Dose after dialysis	No data	Dose for GFR 10–50

(continued)

Table 16-1. (Continued)

Drug	Dose method	GFR >50 (mL/min)	GFR 10–50 (mL/min)	GFR <10 (mL/min)	Supplemental dose after hemodialysis	CAPD	CRRT
Famotidine	D	50%	25%	10%	None	None	Dose for GFR 10–50
Fazadinium	D	100%	100%	100%	Unknown	Unknown	Dose for GFR 10–50
Felodipine	D	100%	100%	100%	None	None	Dose for GFR 10–50
Fenoprofen	D	100%	100%	100%	None	None	Dose for GFR 10–50
Fentanyl	D	100%	75%	50%	Not applicable	Not applicable	NA
Fexofenadine	I	q12h	q12–24h	q24h	Unknown	Unknown	Dose for GFR 10–50
Flecainide	D	100%	100%	50% to 75%	None	None	Dose for GFR 10–50
Fleroxacin	D	100%	50% to 75%	50%	400 mg after dialysis	400 mg/d	Not applicable
Fluconazole	D	100%	100%	100%	200 mg after dialysis	Dose for GFR <10	Dose for GFR 10–50
Flucytosine	I	q12h	q16h	q24h	Dose after dialysis	0.5–1.0 g/d	Dose for GFR 10–50
Fludarabine	D	100%	75%	50%	Unknown	Unknown	Dose for GFR 10–50
Flumazenil	D	100%	100%	100%	None	Unknown	NA
Flunarizine	D	100%	100%	100%	None	None	None
Fluorouracil	D	100%	100%	100%	Yes	Unknown	Dose for GFR 10–50
Fluoxetine	D	100%	100%	100%	Unknown	Unknown	NA
Flurazepam	D	100%	100%	100%	None	Unknown	NA
Flurbiprofen	D	100%	100%	100%	None	None	Dose for GFR 10–50
Flutamide	D	100%	100%	100%	Unknown	Unknown	Unknown
Fluvastatin	D	100%	100%	100%	Unknown	Unknown	Dose for GFR 10–50
Fluvoxamine	D	100%	100%	100%	None	Unknown	NA
Foscarnet	D	28 mg/kg	15 mg/kg	6 mg/kg	Dose after dialysis	Dose for GFR <10	Dose for GFR 10–50
Fosinopril	D	100%	100%	75% to 100%	None	None	Dose for GFR 10–50
Furosemide	D	100%	100%	100%	None	None	Not applicable

Drug							
Gabapentin	D,I	400 mg tid	300 q12–24h	300 mg qd	300 mg load, then 200–300	—	Dose for GFR 10–50
Gallamine	D	75%	Avoid	Avoid	Not applicable	Not applicable	Dose for GFR 10–50
Ganciclovir	I	q12h	q24–48h	q48–96h	Dose after dialysis	Dose for GFR <10	2.5 mg/kg d
Gemfibrozil	D	100%	100%	100%	None	Unknown	Dose for GFR 10–50
Gentamicin	D,I	60% to 90% q8–12h	30% to 70% q12h	20% to 30% q24–48h	2/3 normal dose	3–4 mg/L d	Dose for GFR 10–50
Glibornuride	D	Unknown	Unknown	Unknown	Unknown	Unknown	Avoid
Gliclazide	D	Unknown	Unknown	Unknown	Unknown	Unknown	Avoid
Glipizide	D	100%	100%	100%	Unknown	Unknown	Avoid
Glyburide	D	Unknown	Avoid	Avoid	None	None	Avoid
Gold sodium thiomalate	D	50%	Avoid	Avoid	None	None	Avoid
Griseofulvin	D	100%	100%	100%	None	None	None
Guanabenz	D	100%	100%	100%	Unknown	Unknown	Dose for GFR 10–50
Guanadrel	I	q12h	q12–24h	q24–48h	Unknown	Unknown	Dose for GFR 10–50
Guanethidine	I	q24h	q24h	q24–36h	Unknown	Unknown	Avoid
Guanfacine	D	100%	100%	100%	None	None	Dose for GFR 10–50
Haloperidol	D	100%	100%	100%	None	None	Dose for GFR 10–50
Heparin	D	100%	100%	100%	None	None	Dose for GFR 10–50
Hexobarbital	D	100%	100%	100%	None	Unknown	NA
Hydralazine	I	q8h	q8h	q8–16h	None	None	Dose for GFR 10–50
Hydrocortisone	D	100%	100%	100%	Unknown	Unknown	Dose for GFR 10–50
Hydroxyurea	D	100%	50%	20%	Unknown	Unknown	Dose for GFR 10–50
Hydroxyzine	D	100%	Unknown	Unknown	100%	100%	100%
Ibuprofen	D	100%	100%	100%	None	None	Dose for GFR 10–50
Idarubicin	—	Unknown	Unknown	Unknown	Unknown	Unknown	Unknown
Ifosfamide	D	100%	100%	75%	Unknown	Unknown	Dose for GFR 10–50
Iloprost	D	100%	100%	50%	Unknown	Unknown	Dose for GFR 10–50
Imipenem	D	100%	50%	25%	Dose after dialysis	Dose for GFR <10	Dose for GFR 10–50

(continued)

Table 16-1. (Continued)

Drug	Dose method	GFR >50 (mL/min)	GFR 10–50 (mL/min)	GFR <10 (mL/min)	Supplemental dose after hemodialysis	CAPD	CRRT
Imipramine	D	100%	100%	100%	None	None	NA
Indapamide	D	100%	100%	Avoid	None	None	Not applicable
Indinavir	—	100%	100%	100%	None	Dose for GFR <10	No data
Indobufen	D	100%	50%	25%	Unknown	Unknown	NA
Indomethacin	D	100%	100%	100%	None	None	Dose for GFR 10–50
Insulin	D	100%	75%	50%	None	None	Dose for GFR 10–50
Ipratropium	D	100%	100%	100%	None	None	Dose for GFR 10–50
Isoniazid	D	100%	100%	50%	Dose after dialysis	Dose for GFR <10	Dose for GFR <10
Isosorbide	D	100%	100%	100%	10–20 mg	None	Dose for GFR 10–50
Isradipine	D	100%	100%	100%	None	None	Dose for GFR 10–50
Itraconazole	D	100%	100%	50%	100 mg q12–24h	100 mg q12–24h	100 mg q12–24h
Kanamycin	D,I	60% to 90% q8–12h	30% to 70% q12h	20% to 30% q24–48h	2/3 normal dose	15–20 mg/L d	Dose for GFR 10–50
Ketamine	D	100%	100%	100%	Unknown	Unknown	Dose for GFR 10–50
Ketanserin	D	100%	100%	100%	None	None	Dose for GFR 10–50
Ketoconazole	D	100%	100%	100%	None	None	None
Ketoprofen	D	100%	100%	100%	None	None	Dose for GFR 10–50
Ketorolac	D	100%	50%	50%	None	None	Dose for GFR 10–50
Labetolol	D	100%	100%	100%	None	None	Dose for GFR 10–50
Lamivudine	D,I	100%	50–150 mg qd	25 mg qd	Dose after dialysis	Dose for GFR <10	Dose for GFR 10–50
Lamotrigine	D	100%	100%	100%	Unknown	Unknown	Dose for GFR 10–50
Lansoprazole	D	100%	100%	100%	Unknown	Unknown	Unknown
Levodopa	D	100%	100%	100%	Unknown	Unknown	Dose for GFR 10–50
Levofloxacin	D	100%	50%	25–50%	Dose for GFR <10	Dose for GFR <10	Dose for GFR 10–50
Lidocaine	D	100%	100%	100%	None	None	Dose for GFR 10–50
Lincomycin	I	q6h	q6–12h	q12–24h	None	None	Not applicable

Drug							
Lisinopril	D	100%	50% to 75%	25% to 50%	20%	None	Dose for GFR 10–50
Lispro Insulin	D	100%	75%	50%	None	None	None
Lithium carbonate	D	100%	50% to 75%	25% to 50%	Dose after dialysis	None	Dose for GFR 10–50
Lomefloxacin	D	100%	50% to 75%	50%	Dose for GFR <10	None	Not applicable
Loracarbef	I	q12h	q24h	q 3–5d	Dose after dialysis	Dose for GFR <10	Dose for GFR 10–50
Lorazepam	D	100%	100%	100%	None	Unknown	Dose for GFR 10–50
Losartan	D	100%	100%	100%	Unknown	Unknown	Dose for GFR 10–50
Lovastatin	D	100%	100%	100%	Unknown	Unknown	Dose for GFR 10–50
Low-molecular-weight heparin	D	100%	100%	50%	Unknown	Unknown	Dose for GFR 10–50
Maprotiline	D	100%	100%	100%	Unknown	Unknown	NA
Meclofenamic acid	D	100%	100%	100%	None	None	Dose for GFR 10–50
Mefenamic acid	D	100%	100%	100%	None	None	Dose for GFR 10–50
Mefloquine	—	100%	100%	100%	None	None	Dose for GFR 10–50
Melphalan	D	100%	75%	50%	Unknown	Unknown	Dose for GFR 10–50
Meperidine	D	100%	75%	50%	Avoid	None	Avoid
Meprobamate	I	q6h	q9–12h	q12–18h	None	Unknown	NA
Meropenem	D,I	500 mg q6h	250 – 500 mg q12h	250 – 500 mg q24h	Dose after dialysis	Dose for GFR <10	Dose for GFR 10–50
Metaproterenol	D	100%	100%	100%	Unknown	Unknown	Dose for GFR 10–50
Metformin	D	50%	25%	Avoid	Unknown	Unknown	Avoid
Methadone	D	100%	100%	50% to 75%	None	None	NA
Methenamine mandelate	D	100%	Avoid	Avoid	Not applicable	Not applicable	Not applicable
Methicillin	I	q4–6h	q6–8h	q8–12h	None	None	Dose for GFR 10–50
Methimazole	D	100%	100%	100%	Unknown	Unknown	Dose for GFR 10–50
Methotrexate	D	100%	50%	Avoid	Yes	None	Dose for GFR 10–50
Methyldopa	I	q8h	q8–12h	q12–24h	250 mg	Unknown	Dose for GFR 10–50
Methylprednisolone	D	100%	100%	100%	Yes	Unknown	Dose for GFR 10–50
Metoclopramide	D	100%	75%	50%	None	Unknown	50–75%

(continued)

Table 16-1. (Continued)

Drug	Dose method	GFR >50 (mL/min)	GFR 10–50 (mL/min)	GFR <10 (mL/min)	Supplemental dose after hemodialysis	CAPD	CRRT
Metocurine	D	75%	50%	50%	Unknown	Unknown	Dose for GFR 10–50
Metolazone	D	100%	100%	100%	None	None	Not applicable
Metoprolol	D	100%	100%	100%	50 mg	None	Dose for GFR 10–50
Metronidazole	D	100%	100%	50%	Dose after dialysis	Dose for GFR <10	Dose for GFR 10–50
Mexiletine	D	100%	100%	50% to 75%	None	None	None
Mezlocillin	I	q4–6h	q6–8h	q8h	None	None	Dose for GFR 10–50
Miconazole	D	100%	100%	100%	None	None	None
Midazolam	D	100%	100%	50%	Not applicable	Not applicable	NA
Midodrine	—	5–10 mg q8h	5–10 mg q8h	Unknown	5 mg q8h	No data	Dose for GFR 10–50
Miglitol	D	50%	Avoid	Avoid	Unknown	Unknown	Avoid
Milrinone	D	100%	100%	50% to 75%	No data	No data	Dose for GFR 10–50
Minocycline	D	100%	100%	100%	None	None	Dose for GFR 10–50
Minoxidil	D	100%	100%	100%	None	None	Dose for GFR 10–50
Mitomycin C	D	100%	100%	75%	Unknown	Unknown	Unknown
Mitoxantrone	D	100%	100%	100%	Unknown	Unknown	Dose for GFR 10–50
Mivacurium	D	100%	50%	50%	Unknown	Unknown	Unknown
Moricizine	D	100%	100%	100%	None	None	Dose for GFR 10–50
Morphine	D	100%	75%	50%	None	None	Dose for GFR 10–50
Moxalactam	I	q8–12h	q12–24h	q24–48h	Dose after dialysis	Dose for GFR <10	Dose for GFR 10–50
Nabumetone	D	100%	100%	100%	None	None	Dose for GFR 10–50
N–Acetylcysteine	D	100%	100%	75%	Unknown	Unknown	100%
Nadolol	D	100%	50%	25%	40 mg	None	Dose for GFR 10–50
Nafcillin	D	100%	100%	100%	None	None	Dose for GFR 10–50
Nalidixic acid	D	100%	Avoid	Avoid	Avoid	Avoid	Not applicable
Naloxone	D	100%	100%	100%	Not applicable	Not applicable	Dose for GFR 10–50
Naproxen	D	100%	100%	100%	None	None	Dose for GFR 10–50
Nefazodone	D	100%	100%	100%	Unknown	Unknown	NA

Nelfinavir	—	No data	No data	No data	No data	No data	No data
Neostigmine	D	100%	50%	25%	Unknown	Unknown	Dose for GFR 10–50
Netlimicin	D,I	50% to 90% q8–12h	20% to 60% q12h	10% to 20% q24–48h	2/3 normal dose	3–4 mg/L d	Dose for GFR 10–50
Nevirapine	D	100%	100%	100%	None	Dose for GFR <10	Dose for GFR 10–50
Nicardipine	D	100%	100%	100%	None	Unknown	Dose for GFR 10–50
Nicotinic acid	D	100%	50%	25%	Unknown	Unknown	Dose for GFR 10–50
Nifedipine	D	100%	100%	100%	None	None	Dose for GFR 10–50
Nimodipine	D	100%	100%	100%	None	None	Dose for GFR 10–50
Nisoldipine	D	100%	100%	100%	None	None	Dose for GFR 10–50
Nitrazepam	D	100%	100%	100%	Unknown	Unknown	NA
Nitrofurantoin	D	Avoid	Avoid	Avoid	Not applicable	Not applicable	Not applicable
Nitroglycerine	D	100%	100%	100%	No data	No data	Dose for GFR 10–50
Nitroprusside	D	100%	100%	100%	None	None	Dose for GFR 10–50
Nitrosoureas	D	100%	75%	25% to 50%	None	Unknown	Unknown
Nizatidine	D	75%	50%	25%	Unknown	Unknown	Dose for GFR 10–50
Norfloxacin	I	q12h	q12–24h	Avoid	Not applicable	Not applicable	Not applicable
Nortriptyline	D	100%	100%	100%	None	None	NA
Ofloxacin	D	100%	50%	25% to 50%	100 mg bid	Dose for GFR <10	300 mg/d
Omeprazole	D	100%	100%	100%	Unknown	Unknown	Unknown
Ondansetron	D	100%	100%	100%	Unknown	Unknown	Dose for GFR 10–50
Orphenadrine	D	100%	100%	100%	Unknown	Unknown	NA
Ouabain	I	q12–24h	q24–36h	q36–48h	None	None	Dose for GFR 10–50
Oxaproxin	D	100%	100%	100%	None	None	Dose for GFR 10–50
Oxatomide	D	100%	100%	100%	None	None	NA
Oxazepam	D	100%	100%	100%	None	Unknown	Dose for GFR 10–50
Oxcarbazepine	D	100%	100%	100%	Unknown	Unknown	Unknown
Paclitaxel	D	100%	100%	100%	Unknown	Unknown	Dose for GFR 10–50
Pancuronium	D	50%	50%	Avoid	Unknown	Unknown	Dose for GFR 10–50
Paroxetine	D	100%	50% to 75%	50%	Unknown	Unknown	NA

(continued)

Table 16-1. (Continued)

Drug	Dose method	GFR >50 (mL/min)	GFR 10–50 (mL/min)	GFR <10 (mL/min)	Supplemental dose after hemodialysis	CAPD	CRRT
PAS	D	100%	50% to 75%	50%	Dose after dialysis	Dose for GFR <10	Dose for GFR <10
Penbutolol	D	100%	100%	100%	None	None	Dose for GFR 10–50
Penicillamine	D	100%	Avoid	Avoid	1/3 dose	Unknown	Dose for GFR 10–50
Penicillin G	D	100%	75%	20% to 50%	Dose after dialysis	Dose for GFR <10	Dose for GFR 10–50
Penicillin VK	D	100%	100%	100%	Dose after dialysis	Dose for GFR <10	Dose for GFR 10–50
Pentamidine	I	q24h	q24–36h	q48h	None	None	Not applicable
Pentazocine	D	100%	75%	50%	None	Unknown	None
Pentobarbital	D	100%	100%	100%	None	Unknown	Dose for GFR 10–50
Pentopril	D	100%	50% to 75%	50%	Unknown	Unknown	Dose for GFR 10–50
Pentoxifylline	D	100%	100%	100%	Unknown	Unknown	100%
Perfloxacin	D	100%	100%	100%	None	None	Dose for GFR 10–50
Perindopril	D	100%	75%	50%	25–50%	Unknown	Dose for GFR 10–50
Phenelzine	D	100%	100%	100%	Unknown	Unknown	NA
Phenobarbital	I	q8–12h	q8–12h	q12–16h	Dose after dialysis	1/2 normal dose	Dose for GFR 10–50
Phenylbutazone	D	100%	100%	100%	None	None	Dose for GFR 10–50
Phenytoin	D	100%	100%	100%	None	None	None
Pindolol	D	100%	100%	100%	None	None	Dose for GFR 10–50
Pipecuronium	I	q4–6h	50%	25%	Unknown	Unknown	Dose for GFR 10–50
Piperacillin	I	q4–6h	q6–8h	q8h	Dose after dialysis	Dose for GFR <10	Dose for GFR 10–50
Piretanide	D	100%	100%	100%	None	None	Not applicable
Piroxicam	D	100%	100%	100%	None	None	Dose for GFR 10–50
Plicamycin	D	100%	75%	50%	Unknown	Unknown	Unknown
Pravastatin	D	100%	100%	100%	Unknown	Unknown	Dose for GFR 10–50
Prazepam	D	100%	100%	100%	Unknown	Unknown	NA
Prazosin	D	100%	100%	100%	None	None	Dose for GFR 10–50

Drug						
Prednisolone	D	100%	100%	Yes	Unknown	Dose for GFR 10–50
Prednisone	D	100%	100%	None	Unknown	Dose for GFR 10–50
Primaquine	—	100%	100%	None	None	Dose for GFR 10–50
Primidone	I	q8h	q12–24h	1/3 dose	Unknown	Unknown
Probenecid	D	100%	Avoid	Avoid	Unknown	Avoid
Probucol	D	100%	100%	Unknown	Unknown	Dose for GFR 10–50
Procainamide	I	q4h	q6–12h	200 mg	None	Dose for GFR 10–50
Promethazine	D	100%	100%	Unknown	Unknown	Dose for GFR 10–50
Propafenone	D	100%	100%	None	None	Dose for GFR 10–50
Propofol	D	100%	100%	Unknown	Unknown	Dose for GFR 10–50
Propoxyphene	D	100%	Avoid	None	None	NA
Propranolol	D	100%	100%	None	None	Dose for GFR 10–50
Propylthiouracil	D	100%	100%	Unknown	Unknown	Dose for GFR 10–50
Protryptyline	D	100%	100%	None	None	NA
Pyrazinimide	D	Avoid	Avoid	Avoid	Avoid	Avoid
Pyridostigmine	D	50%	20%	Unknown	Unknown	Dose for GFR 10–50
Pyrimethamine	D	100%	100%	None	None	None
Quazepam	D	Unknown	Unknown	Unknown	Unknown	NA
Quinapril	D	100%	75% to 100%	75%	25%	None	Dose for GFR 10–50
Quinidine	D	100%	100%	75%	100–200 mg	None	None
Quinine	I	q8h	q8–12h	q24h	Dose after dialysis	Dose for GFR <10	Dose for GFR 10–50
Ramipril	D	100%	50% to 75%	25% to 50%	20%	None	Dose for GFR 10–50
Ranitidine	D	75%	50%	25%	1/2 dose	None	Dose for GFR 10–50
Reserpine	D	100%	100%	Avoid	None	None	Dose for GFR 10–50
Ribavirin	D	100%	100%	50%	Dose after dialysis	Dose for GFR <10	Dose for GFR <10
Rifabutin	—	100%	100%	100%	None	None	Dose for GFR 10–50

(continued)

Table 16-1. (*Continued*)

Drug	Dose method	GFR >50 (mL/min)	GFR 10–50 (mL/min)	GFR <10 (mL/min)	Supplemental dose after hemodialysis	CAPD	CRRT
Rifampin	D	100%	50% to 100%	50 to 100%	None	Dose for GFR <10	Dose for GFR <10
Ritonavir	—	100%	100%	100%	None	Dose for GFR <10	Dose for GFR 10–50
Saquinavir	—	100%	100%	100%	None	Dose for GFR <10	Dose for GFR 10–50
Secobarbital	D	100%	100%	100%	None	None	NA
Sertraline	D	100%	100%	100%	Unknown	Unknown	NA
Simvastatin	D	100%	100%	100%	Unknown	Unknown	Dose for GFR 10–50
Sodium valproate	D	100%	100%	100%	None	None	None
Sotalol	D	100%	30%	15% to 30%	80 mg	None	Dose for GFR 10–50
Sparfloxacin	D,I	100%	50% to 75%	50% q48h	Dose for GFR <10	No data	Dose for GFR 10–50
Spectinomycin	D	100%	100%	100%	None	None	None
Spironolactone	I	q6–12h	q12–24h	Avoid	Not applicable	Not applicable	Avoid
Stavudine	D,I	100%	50% q12–24h	50% q24h	Dose after dialysis	No data	Dose for GFR 10–50
Streptokinase	D	100%	100%	100%	Not applicable	Not applicable	Dose for GFR 10–50
Streptomycin	I	q24h	q24–72h	q72–96h	1/2 normal dose	20–40 mg/L d	Dose for GFR 10–50
Streptozotocin	D	100%	75%	50%	Unknown	Unknown	Unknown
Succinylcholine	D	100%	100%	100%	Unknown	Unknown	Dose for GFR 10–50
Sufentanil	D	100%	100%	100%	Unknown	Unknown	Dose for GFR 10–50
Sulbactam	I	q6–8h	q12–24h	q24–48h	Dose after dialysis	0.75–1.5 g/d	750 mg q12h
Sulfamethoxazole	I	q12h	q18h	q24h	1 g after dialysis	1 g/d	Dose for GFR 10–50
Sulfinpyrazone	D	100%	100%	Avoid	None	None	Dose for GFR 10–50
Sulfisoxazole	I	q6h	q8–12h	q12–24h	2 g after dialysis	3 g/d	Not applicable
Sulindac	D	100%	100%	100%	None	None	Dose for GFR 10–50
Sulotroban	D	50%	30%	10%	Unknown	Unknown	Unknown
Tamoxifen	D	100%	100%	100%	Unknown	Unknown	Dose for GFR 10–50
Tazobactam	D	100%	75%	50%	1/3 dose	Dose for GFR <10	Dose for GFR 10–50

Drug		Dose for GFR >50	Dose for GFR 10–50	Dose for GFR <10	Hemodialysis	Peritoneal dialysis	CVVH
Teicoplanin	I	q24h	q48h	q72h	None	Dose for GFR <10	Dose for GFR 10–50
Temazepam	D	100%	100%	100%	None	None	NA
Teniposide	D	100%	100%	100%	None	None	Dose for GFR 10–50
Terazosin	D	100%	100%	100%	Unknown	Unknown	Dose for GFR 10–50
Terbutaline	D	100%	50%	Avoid	Unknown	Unknown	Dose for GFR 10–50
Terfenadine	D	100%	100%	100%	None	None	NA
Tetracycline	I	q8–12h	q12–24h	q24h	None	None	Dose for GFR 10–50
Theophylline	D	100%	100%	100%	1/2 dose	Unknown	Dose for GFR 10–50
Thiazides	D	100%	100%	Avoid	Not applicable	Not applicable	Not applicable
Thiopental	D	100%	100%	75%	Not applicable	Not applicable	NA
Ticarcillin	D,I	1–2 g q4h	1–2 g q8h	1–2 g q12h	3 g after dialysis	Dose for GFR <10	Dose for GFR 10–50
Ticlopidine	D	100%	100%	100%	Unknown	Unknown	Dose for GFR 10–50
Timolol	D	100%	100%	100%	None	None	Dose for GFR 10–50
Tobramycin	D,I	60% to 90% q8–12h	30% to 70% q12h	20% to 30% q24–48h	2/3 normal dose	3–4 mg/L d	Dose for GFR 10–50
Tocainide	D	100%	100%	50%	200 mg	None	Dose for GFR 10–50
Tolazamide	D	100%	100%	100%	Unknown	Unknown	Avoid
Tolbutamide	D	100%	100%	100%	None	None	Avoid
Tolmetin	D	100%	100%	100%	None	None	Dose for GFR 10–50
Topiramate	D	100%	50%	25%	Unknown	Unknown	Dose for GFR 10–50
Topotecan	D	75%	50%	25%	Unknown	Unknown	Dose for GFR 10–50
Torsemide	D	100%	100%	10%	None	None	NA
Tranexamic acid	D	50%	25%	10%	Unknown	Unknown	Unknown
Tranylcypromine	D	Unknown	Unknown	Unknown	Unknown	Unknown	NA
Trazodone	D	100%	100%	Unknown	Unknown	Unknown	NA
Triamcinolone	D	100%	100%	100%	Not applicable	Not applicable	Dose for GFR 10–50
Triamterene	I	q12h	q12h	Avoid	None	None	Avoid
Triazolam	D	100%	100%	100%	Unknown	Unknown	NA
Trihexyphenidyl	D	Unknown	Unknown	Unknown	Unknown	Unknown	Unknown
Trimethadione	I	q8h	q8–12h	q12–24h	Unknown	Unknown	Dose for GFR 10–50

(continued)

Table 16-1. (*Continued*)

Drug	Dose method	GFR >50 (mL/min)	GFR 10–50 (mL/min)	GFR <10 (mL/min)	Supplemental dose after hemodialysis	CAPD	CRRT
Trimethoprim	I	q12h	q18h	q24h	Dose after dialysis	q24h	q18h
Trimetrexate	D	100%	50–100%	Avoid	No data	No data	No data
Trimipramine	D	100%	100%	100%	None	None	NA
Tripelennamine	D	Unknown	Unknown	Unknown	Unknown	Unknown	NA
Triprolidine	D	Unknown	Unknown	Unknown	Unknown	Unknown	NA
Tubocurarine	D	75%	50%	Avoid	Unknown	Unknown	Dose for GFR 10–50
Urokinase	D	Unknown	Unknown	Unknown	Unknown	Unknown	Dose for GFR 10–50
Vancomycin	D,I	500 mg q6–12h	500 mg q24–48h	500 mg q48–96h	Dose for GFR <10	Dose for GFR <10	Dose for GFR 10–50
Vecuronium	D	100%	100%	100%	Unknown	Unknown	Dose for GFR 10–50
Venlafaxine	D	75%	50%	50%	None	Unknown	NA
Verapamil	D	100%	100%	100%	None	None	Dose for GFR 10–50
Vidarabine	D	100%	100%	75%	Infuse after dialysis	Dose for GFR <10	Dose for GFR 10–50
Vigabatrin	D	100%	50%	25%	Unknown	Unknown	Dose for GFR 10–50
Vinblastine	D	100%	100%	100%	Unknown	Unknown	Dose for GFR 10–50
Vincristine	D	100%	100%	100%	Unknown	Unknown	Dose for GFR 10–50
Vinorelbine	D	100%	100%	100%	Unknown	Unknown	Dose for GFR 10–50
Warfarin	D	100%	100%	100%	None	None	None
Zafirlukast	D	100%	100%	100%	Unknown	Unknown	Dose for GFR 10–50
Zalcitabine	I	100%	q12h	q24h	Dose after dialysis	No data	Dose for GFR 10–50
Zidovudine (AZT)	D,I	200 mg q8h	200 mg q8h	100 mg q8h	Dose for GFR <10	Dose for GFR <10	100 mg q8h
Zileuton	—	100%	100%	100%	None	Unknown	Dose for GFR 10–50

are frequently used to maintain fluid and electrolyte homeostasis and remove waste products in critically ill patients. The rate and extent of drug removal by CRRT depends less on the drug's molecular weight and more on the membrane characteristics, blood flow rate, the amount of hemofiltration by convection and the addition of dialysate to the extracorporeal circuit. During hemofiltration, a filtration rate of 10 to 30 mL per minute is achieved. The addition of diffusion by continuous dialysis adds 15 to 20 mL per minute. Therefore, continuous dialysis and continuous hemofiltration together may provide a drug clearance of 10 to 50 mL per minute. The serum creatinine, as an estimate of creatinine clearance, can be used as an estimate of drug clearance during CRRT for drugs that are not highly protein bound and have relatively small volumes of distribution. Underestimating drug removal in these circumstances risks ineffective therapy.

VI. **Adverse drug reactions** occur more frequently in patients with impaired renal function. Untoward effects may be the result of direct toxicity or the additive effects of the drug or its metabolites. The lack of efficacy of the drug in patients with compromised renal function, or increased drug-induced metabolic load also causes adverse drug effects. The acute onset of any unexplained symptoms should alert clinicians of a possible adverse drug effect.

VII. **Therapeutic drug monitoring.** The measurement of plasma drug concentrations may be helpful in assessing a particular drug dosing regimen when efficacy or toxicity corresponds to drug levels. These measurements are most important for drugs with a narrow therapeutic range or for drugs whose pharmacologic effects are not easily measured.

Measure serum levels following the administration of an appropriate loading dose. If no loading dose is administered, give three or four doses of the drug before measuring serum levels to ensure that steady-state serum concentrations have been established. For some drugs, both maximum and minimum concentrations are relevant. Peak levels are most meaningful when measured after rapid drug distribution has occurred. For example, measure aminoglycoside peak concentrations 30 minutes after the end of the infusion; minimum concentrations are usually measured just before administration of the next scheduled dose. Included in Table 16-1 are recommendations for drug level monitoring. Appropriate pharmacokinetic application of drug level measurements can improve patient care and decrease cost.

Patients with renal disease are heterogeneous, and their responses to drug therapy are variable. Dosage nomograms, drug tables, and computer-assisted dosing recommendations should not be taken as a fixed approach to therapy in patients with decreased renal function. These are initial attempts to arrive at an effective dose regimen. Physicians using sound clinical judgment in caring for patients with renal disease must evaluate each situation, choose a drug regimen based on all factors, and continually re-evaluate the response to therapy.

Suggested readings

Anderson RJ, Schrier RW. *Clinical use of drugs in patients with kidney and liver disease.* Philadelphia: WB Saunders, 1981.

Aronoff GR, Berns JS, Brier ME, Golper TA, Morrison G, Singer I, Swann SK, Bennett WM. *Drug prescribing in renal failure. Dosing guidelines for adults.* Philadelphia: American College of Physicians, 1999.

Index

Note: Page numbers followed by *f* indicate figures; page numbers followed by *t* indicate tables.